Pain Management: A Clinical Guide

Pain Management: A Clinical Guide

Edited by Lily Hunt

hayle medical

New York

Hayle Medical,
750 Third Avenue, 9th Floor,
New York, NY 10017, USA

Visit us on the World Wide Web at:
www.haylemedical.com

ISBN: 978-1-64647-552-0

Cataloging-in-Publication Data

Pain management : a clinical guide / edited by Lily Hunt.
p. cm.
Includes bibliographical references and index.
ISBN 978-1-64647-552-0
1. Pain. 2. Pain--Treatment. 3. Pain--Physiological aspects. 4. Pain medicine. I. Hunt, Lily.
RB127 .C55 2023
616.047 2--dc23

Table of Contents

Preface IX

Chapter 1 **Comparison of several methods for pain management after video-assisted thoracic surgery for pneumothorax** 1
Pierre-Antoine Allain, Michele Carella, Apostolos C. Agrafiotis, Julien Burey, Jalal Assouad, El-Mahdi Hafiani, Yacine Ynineb, Francis Bonnet, Marc Garnier and Christophe Quesnel

Chapter 2 **A randomized controlled trial on analgesic effect of repeated quadratus lumborum block versus continuous epidural analgesia following laparoscopic nephrectomy** 10
Dita Aditianingsih, Pryambodho, Naufal Anasy, Aida Rosita Tantri and Chaidir Arif Mochtar

Chapter 3 **Analgesic efficacy of ultrasound-guided paravertebral block in percutaneous nephrolithotomy patients** 20
Ferda Yaman and Devrim Tuglu

Chapter 4 **Retrospective study of quadratus lumborum block for postoperative analgesia in patients undergoing percutaneous nephrolithotomy** 28
Luning Chen, Jingjing Ji, Yali Tian, Qing Sun, Xuefeng Qiu, Xiaogong Li and Bingbing Li

Chapter 5 **Comparison of analgesic efficacy between rectus sheath blockade, intrathecal morphine with bupivacaine and intravenous patient-controlled analgesia in patients undergoing robot-assisted laparoscopic prostatectomy** 37
Jung-Woo Shim, Yun Jeong Cho, Minhee Kim, Sang Hyun Hong, Hyong Woo Moon, Sung Hoo Hong and Min Suk Chae

Chapter 6 **Adding dexmedetomidine to morphine-based analgesia reduces early postoperative nausea in patients undergoing gynecological laparoscopic surgery** 48
Huai Jin Li, Shan Liu, Zhi Yu Geng and Xue Ying Li

Chapter 7 **The analgesic efficacy compared ultrasound-guided continuous transverse abdominis plane block with epidural analgesia following abdominal surgery** 55
Chaosheng Qin, Yuanming Liu, Jijun Xiong, Xiaogang Wang, Qinghua Dong, Tingshi Su and Jingchen Liu

Chapter 8 **Antinociceptive effects of magnesium sulfate for monitored anesthesia care during hysteroscopy** 64
Peng-fei Gao, Jing-yan Lin, Shun Wang, Yun-feng Zhang, Guo-qiang Wang, Qi Xu and Xiao Guo

Chapter 9 **Postoperative analgesic efficacy of ear acupuncture in patients undergoing abdominal hysterectomy** 72
Hamdy A. Hendawy and Mohamed E. Abuelnaga

Chapter 10 **Using four different clinical tools as predictors for pain after total hip arthroplasty** 80
Anja Geisler, Josephine Zachodnik, Jens Laigaard, Laura S. Kruuse, Charlotte V. Sørensen, Magnus Sandberg, Eva I. Persson and Ole Mathiesen

Chapter 11 **The effect of transversus abdominis plane block on the chronic pain after colorectal surgery** 88
Zi-Ye Pan, Zhong-Hua Hu, Fan Zhang, Wen-Xiu Xie, Yong-Zhong Tang and Qin Liao

Chapter 12 **Preemptive oxycodone is superior to equal dose of sufentanil to reduce visceral pain and inflammatory markers after surgery** 94
Yi An, Lei Zhao, Tianlong Wang, Jiapeng Huang, Wei Xiao, Ping Wang, Lixia Li, Zhongjia Li and Xiaoxu Chen

Chapter 13 **A preliminary assessment of vital-signs-integrated patient-assisted intravenous opioid analgesia (VPIA) for postsurgical pain** 101
Ban Leong Sng, Daryl Jian'an Tan, Chin Wen Tan, Nian-Lin Reena Han, Rehena Sultana and Alex Tiong Heng Sia

Chapter 14 **Efficacy of different dose of dexmedetomidine combined with remifentanil in colonoscopy** 108
Li Jia, Meng Xie, Jing Zhang, Jingyu Guo, Tong Tong and Yuying Xing

Chapter 15 **Comparative evaluation of epidural bupivacaine alone and bupivacaine combined with magnesium sulfate in providing postoperative analgesia** 115
Li-Qin Li, Mei-Dan Fang, Cong Wang, Hong-Liu Lu, Li-Xue Wang, Hong-Yu Xu and Hou-Zhong Zhang

Chapter 16 **Infraclavicular nerve block reduces postoperative pain after distal radial fracture fixation** 126
Stanley S. Wong, Wing S. Chan, Christian Fang, Chi W. Chan, Tak W. Lau, Frankie Leung and Chi W. Cheung

Chapter 17 **Cerebrospinal fluid of chronic osteoarthritic patients induced interleukin-6 release in human glial cell-line T98G** 137
Weiling Liu, Chunmei Li, Francis Chee Kuan Tan, Hong Jye Neo, Yiong Huak Chan, Chian-Ming Low and Tat Leang Lee

Chapter 18 **Gradual withdrawal of remifentanil delays initial post-operative analgesic demand after thyroid surgery** 144
Sarah Saxena, Kimberly Gonsette, Willy Terram, Isabelle Huybrechts, Daniel A. Nahrwold, Matteo Cappello, Luc Barvais and Edgard Engelman

Chapter 19 **Efficacy and safety of pulsed radiofrequency as a method of dorsal root ganglia stimulation for treatment of non-neuropathic pain** 151
Ivana Vuka, Svjetlana Došenović, Tihana Marciuš, Lejla Ferhatović Hamzić, Katarina Vučić, Damir Sapunar and Livia Puljak

Chapter 20 **Doxapram alleviates low SpO_2 induced by the combination of propofol and fentanyl during painless gastrointestinal endoscopy** 172
Zhengfeng Gu, Lian Xin, Haoxing Wang, Chunxiao Hu, Zhiping Wang, Shunmei Lu, Jingjing Xu, Yiling Qian and Jun Wang

Chapter 21 **Intrathecal morphine is associated with reduction in postoperative opioid requirements and improvement in postoperative analgesia in patients undergoing open liver resection** 178
Jefferson Tang, Leonid Churilov, Chong Oon Tan, Raymond Hu, Brett Pearce, Luka Cosic, Christopher Christophi and Laurence Weinberg

Chapter 22 **Enhanced preoperative education about continuous femoral nerve block with patient-controlled analgesia improves the analgesic effect for patients undergoing total knee arthroplasty and reduces the workload for ward nurses** 189
Xiaona Lin, Yang Zhou, Hongcai Zheng, Jing Zhang, Xiaoxiao Wang, Kaixi Liu, Jun Wang, Xiangyang Guo, Zhengqian Li and Bin Han

Chapter 23 **The effects of different doses of dexmedetomidine on the requirements for propofol for loss of consciousness in patients monitored via the bispectral index** 194
Yang Gu, Fan Yang, Yonghai Zhang, Junwei Zheng, Jie Wang, Bin Li, Tao Ma, Xiang Cui, Kaimei Lu and Hanxiang Ma

Chapter 24 **The analgesic efficacy of ultrasound-guided transversus abdominis plane block for retroperitoneoscopic renal surgery** 201
Xue Li, Zhen-Zhen Xu, Xue-Ying Li, Ting-Ting Jiang, Zeng-Mao Lin and Dong-Xin Wang

Chapter 25 **The erector spinae plane block causes only cutaneous sensory loss on ipsilateral posterior thorax** 210
Jingxiong Zhang, Yuting He, Shi Wang, Zhengjie Chen, Yu Zhang, Yuan Gao, Quanguang Wang, Yun Xia, Thomas J. Papadimos and Riyong Zhou

Chapter 26 **Effects of dexmedetomidine on stress hormones in patients undergoing cardiac valve replacement** 218
Hanhua Wu, Jinqing Tang, Jiamei Pan, Ming Han, Huijun Cai and Hong Zhang

Permissions

List of Contributors

Index

Preface

The purpose of the book is to provide a glimpse into the dynamics and to present opinions and studies of some of the scientists engaged in the development of new ideas in the field from very different standpoints. This book will prove useful to students and researchers owing to its high content quality.

Pain refers to a type of distressing sensation that is frequently triggered by strong or harmful stimuli. It is the primary sign of a variety of illnesses, wounds and infections. It may also be caused from treatments for ailments and disorders. Chronic pain and acute pain are the two primary categories of pain. The techniques for decreasing and regulating the amount of pain a person experiences over a long period of time is referred to as pain management. Various forms of pain can be managed using a variety of methods. Complementary therapies, pain medications and physical therapy are a few pain management strategies. The majority of pain management methods aim to enhance a person's coping strategies or lessen chronic pain. This book elucidates the concepts and innovative models around prospective developments with respect to pain management. It is appropriate for students seeking detailed information in this area of medicine as well as for experts.

At the end, I would like to appreciate all the efforts made by the authors in completing their chapters professionally. I express my deepest gratitude to all of them for contributing to this book by sharing their valuable works. A special thanks to my family and friends for their constant support in this journey.

Editor

1

Comparison of several methods for pain management after video-assisted thoracic surgery for pneumothorax

Pierre-Antoine Allain[1], Michele Carella[1], Apostolos C. Agrafiotis[2], Julien Burey[1,3], Jalal Assouad[2,3], El-Mahdi Hafiani[1], Yacine Ynineb[1], Francis Bonnet[1,3], Marc Garnier[1,3]* and Christophe Quesnel[1,3]

Abstract

Background: There is no defined gold standard for pain management after video-assisted thoracic surgery (VATS) for pneumothorax. In addition to systemic analgesia, various loco-regional analgesic techniques have been proposed but remain poorly evaluated in this context. We aimed to assess the analgesic efficacy of several of these techniques for the management of postoperative pain.

Methods: We conducted a monocentric prospective observational cohort study from February 2017 to April 2018 in patients suffering from spontaneous pneumothorax and scheduled for VATS ($n = 59$). Patients received systemic analgesia (i) alone ($n = 15$); (ii) combined with a continuous paravertebral block ($n = 9$); (iii) combined with a continuous serratus plane block ($n = 19$); or (iv) single-shot serratus plane block ($n = 16$) as decided by the attending physician. Pain scores and analgesic-related side effects were prospectively collected by an independent observer during the first postoperative 72 h. The primary endpoint criterion was the cumulative oral morphine consumption at the end of the third postoperative day. Statistical analysis used univariate and multivariate step-by-step forward logistic regression models to determine risk factors associated with the main criteria.

Results: Mean pain scores and morphine consumption were not significantly different between the 4 groups. In the multivariate analysis, the use of a continuous serratus plane block through a catheter was the only technique associated with a reduced incidence of high-dose oral morphine consumption (OR 0.09–95%CI [0.01–0.79], $p = 0.03$).

Conclusion: This study suggests that serratus plane block combined with continuous infusion through a catheter may have some benefits, although further studies are needed to confirm these results and determine the true place of the serratus plane block in pain management after VATS for pneumothorax.

Keywords: Video-assisted thoracic surgery , Pneumothorax , Postoperative pain , Serratus plane block , Paravertebral block

Background

Spontaneous pneumothorax (SP) has an overall incidence of 24/100,000 in caucasian males [1]. Recurent and/or complete pneumothorax, compromising normal breathing and oxygenation, requires chest drainage and prevention of further recurrences. Thus, surgical treatment of pneumothorax is indicated in cases of SP relapse, bilateral pneumothorax and persistent air leak. Among the surgical procedures performed to avoid pneumothorax recurrence, the most common is pleurodesis by mechanical abrasion of the parietal pleura. The second most common is pleurectomy followed by chemical pleurodesis by intrathoracic instillation of talc [2]. These procedures are performed either through video-assisted thoracic surgery (VATS) or thoracotomy. Although VATS is associated with less intense postoperative pain [3], it remains a painful surgical procedure.

* Correspondence: marcgarnier@gmail.com
[1]Service d'Anesthésie-Réanimation et Médecine Péri-opératoire, AP-HP Hôpital Tenon, 4 rue de la Chine, 75020 Paris, France
[3]Faculté de médecine Sorbonne Université (Paris VI), Paris, France

Indeed, a moderate to intense postoperative pain is reported during the first postoperative 72 h and especially within the first 24 h [4]. The use of loco-regional analgesia is recommended to control postoperative pain after VATS as it allows morphine sparing and facilitates early postoperative rehabilitation [5]. Different loco-regional analgesic techniques could be used to control pain after pneumothorax surgery such as a paravertebral block, an intercostal block, an intrapleural block or more recently a serratus plane block [5]. However, some of them have limitations such as the requirement for multiple injections in the case of an intercostal block. In addition, when a pleurectomy is performed, the loss of the parietal lining of the pleura decreases the efficacy of a paravertebral block [6]. Moreover, the comparative performances of these techniques have been poorly evaluated. Thus, in current practice, there is no gold standard analgesic strategy for pneumothorax surgery.

Every year, more than one hundred patients are referred to the on-call emergency unit for pneumothorax management in our institution, among whom 60% require surgical treatment. Postoperative analgesia is commonly ensured by a loco-regional analgesic technique, but the choice of technique remains at the discretion of the attending anesthesiologist. Consequently, we evaluated the efficacy and the side effects of several techniques in a cohort of patients scheduled for VATS to treat SP.

Methods

This study followed the STROBE statements [7].

Patient selection

This study is a monocentric prospective observational cohort study conducted at Tenon Hospital, Paris, France. Consecutive patients over 18 years old and suffering from pneumothorax requiring VATS treatment between February 2017 and April 2018 were included in the study. The exclusion criteria were: secondary pneumothorax, pregnancy, chronic preoperative analgesic treatment and opioid addiction, associated hemothorax, supra-segmental parenchymal resection and the lack of social health insurance coverage. Intraoperative conversions of VATS into thoracotomy and revision surgery within the first postoperative 72 h were also excluded from the study.

Anesthesia, surgery and analgesia management

Except for the choice of the postoperative loco-regional analgesic technique, the anesthetic management of patients undergoing VATS for pneumothorax is standardized in our institution. All the patients were anesthetized using a targeted concentration infusion of propofol (Fresenius Kabi; Bad Homburg vor der Höhe, Germany) and sufentanil (Mylan; Canonsburg, PA, USA), while the depth of anesthesia was monitored with a bispectral index coupled with standard anesthetic monitoring. Atracurium (Hospira; Lake Forest, IL, USA) was used for muscle relaxation. Dexamethasone 8 mg IV (Mylan) was systematically used to reduce postoperative nausea and vomiting. Intraoperative ketamine administration (0.3 mg/kg – Panpharma; Boulogne-Billancourt, France) was considered as a co-analgesic except in cases of high blood pressure in the operating room, or significant active cannabis intoxication. Oral postoperative multimodal analgesia routinely included acetaminophen (1 g 4 times a day – Sanofi-Aventis, Paris, France), nefopam (20 mg 4 times a day – Biocodex; Gentilly, France) and tramadol (50 mg 4 times a day – Meda Pharma, Solna, Sweden). Intraoperative IV lidocaine (0.3 to 0.5 mg/kg – Aguettant; Lyon, France) and postoperative ketoprofen (50 mg 4 times a day – Sanofi-Aventis) administrations were left to the discretion of the attending anesthesiologist. All patients were immediately extubated at the end of the surgical procedure.

Surgery was conducted under one-lung ventilation after intubation with a double-lumen tube. Single-port VATS was the first choice method; multi-port surgery being reserved for cases when that failed. VATS was standardized as previously described [8], with a 1.5–2 cm single incision performed on the axillary anterior line in the seventh intercostal space. Wound retractors were used to protect intercostal tissues. All the instruments were introduced through this single port. Surgery consisted of resection of apical parenchymal dystrophies using an articulated stapler, followed by a talc effusion pleurodesis. A single 24F chest tube was introduced through the single incision under visual control at the end of the procedure.

The loco-regional analgesic technique was left to the discretion of the physician in charge of the patient and was performed at the end of the surgical procedure. A paravertebral block was performed by the surgeon through a transparietal approach with insertion of a catheter under direct vision until placement of the tip into the paravertebral space [9], and then injected with an initial bolus of 15 mL lidocaine 20 mg/mL + epinephrine 50 μg/mL (Aguettant), followed by a continuous injection of 10 mL/h ropivacaine 2 mg/mL (Fresenius Kabi) through an elastomeric pump. A serratus plane block was performed by the injection of local anesthetics between the serratus anterior and the latissimus dorsi muscles, with ultrasound guidance, as described initially by Blanco et al. [10]. A serratus plane block was performed either by single injection (ropivacaine 2 mg/mL, 20 mL for patients under 175 cm and 30 mL for patients taller than 175 cm) or by injection of an initial bolus (lidocaine 20 mg/mL + epinephrine 50 µg/mL, 15 mL) followed by the placement of a catheter between the two muscles and the continuous injection of 10 mL/h ropivacaine 2 mg/mL through an elastomeric pump. In addition, 10 mg on-demand oral rapid-release morphine (Actiskenan®, Ethypharm, Saint-Cloud, France) was given to patients in case of residual pain (Visual Analog Scale (VAS) value > 3/10). We predefined a threshold of 50 mg of morphine over the first 3 postoperative days as being "high-dose morphine consumption", based on the mean amount of morphine consumption observed in our institution and the limited data available from recent studies reporting postoperative morphine consumptions in patients scheduled for VATS [11, 12].

Data collection

We collected demographic data (age, sex, weight, height, body mass index), as well as information about active smoking status and chronic drugs consumption (especially cannabinoids and opioids) for each patient. The following surgical data were also collected: the number, side and site of surgical incisions and thoracic drains, the duration of surgery, the surgical technique used (pleurodesis or pleural abrasion, with or without resection of dystrophic parenchyma) and the duration of postoperative drainage. We also recorded the anesthetic and analgesic agents administered to patients during anesthesia, such as ketamine, intravenous lidocaine, dexamethasone, paracetamol, nefopam, tramadol, ketoprofen and/or morphine.

The morphine titration cumulative dose and pain intensity score (graded from 0 to 10 on a VAS) at rest and on coughing were collected in the recovery room upon the patient's arrival and after one hour. Finally, pain VAS values were also collected at rest and on coughing in the wards at 2, 12, 24, 48 and 72 h after surgery. Cumulative oral morphine consumption was collected as well as daily and total doses of other analgesics such as acetaminophen, nefopam, tramadol, IV lidocaine and ketoprofen. The occurrence of nausea, vomiting and urinary retention were noted for each patient. The hospital length-of-stay was recorded.

Definition of endpoints and statistical analysis

The primary endpoint was the cumulative oral morphine consumption (expressed in mg) during the first postoperative 72 h. The secondary endpoints were: 1) the intensity of postoperative pain at rest and on coughing, and 2) the incidence of side effects most frequently associated with opioid consumption such as nausea, vomiting and urinary retention. Quantitative data were expressed as median values [25-75th percentiles] and qualitative data were expressed as numbers (percentages). Primary and secondary endpoints for each analgesic technique used were compared using the Kruskall-Wallis test with Dunn's correction. We defined a priori a morphine consumption > 50 mg within the first postoperative 72 h as a reasonable marker of difficult pain control and high-dose morphine consumption. Factors associated with a high-dose morphine consumption were assessed by univariate logistic regression and chi-square for quantitative and qualitative variables, respectively. All variables with p value ≤0.2 were integrated into the multivariate step by step forward logistic regression model. $P < 0.05$ was considered significant. Statistical analysis was performed using SPSS version 23 (SPSS, IBM Corp, Armonk, NY).

Results

Sixty-seven patients underwent VATS for SP during the study period, out of whom 61 were included in the study (Fig. 1). Among the 6 patients who were not included, 2 were under 18 years of age, 2 had pneumothorax secondary to trauma and bullous emphysema, 1 had bilateral pneumothorax and 1 refused to participate. Additionally, 2 more patients were excluded due to intraoperative conversion to thoracotomy and early reoperation for hemorrhage, respectively (Fig. 1). The demographics of the patients and the surgical procedures are described in Table 1. Among the 59 patients analyzed, 10 (17%) had a past history of lung disease and 17 (28%) had recurrent SP. A standardized single port procedure was performed in 92% of the cases. The median operative time was 75 [60–100] minutes.

Sixteen patients (27%) had a serratus plane block with a single injection and 19 (32%) had a serratus plane block with insertion of a catheter for continuous loco-regional analgesic infusion. A paravertebral block with insertion of a catheter was performed in 9 patients (15%). Fifteen (25%) patients received oral multimodal analgesia alone, including rapid-release morphine. Values of pain intensity score corresponding to the analgesic technique used are reported in Table 2.

Morphine consumptions are reported in Fig. 2. Morphine consumption and VAS values were not different for the 4 groups ($p > 0.05$ - Table 3 & Fig. 2). There were no significant differences in the incidence rates of postoperative nausea, vomiting or urinary retention across the groups. The cumulative postoperative oral morphine consumption at 72 h was 30 [10–60] mg. Over the study-period, 19 (32%) patients required > 50 mg of oral morphine to control their pain. In the univariate analysis, parameters with a p value ≤0.2 when comparing patients with low-dose and high-dose morphine consumption were the use of a continuous serratus plane block ($p = 0.06$), the use of systemic analgesia alone ($p = 0.02$), a single-port incision ($p = 0.16$) and the postoperative use of tramadol as a co-analgesic ($p = 0.19$) (Table 3). In the multivariate analysis, the continuous serratus plane block was the only

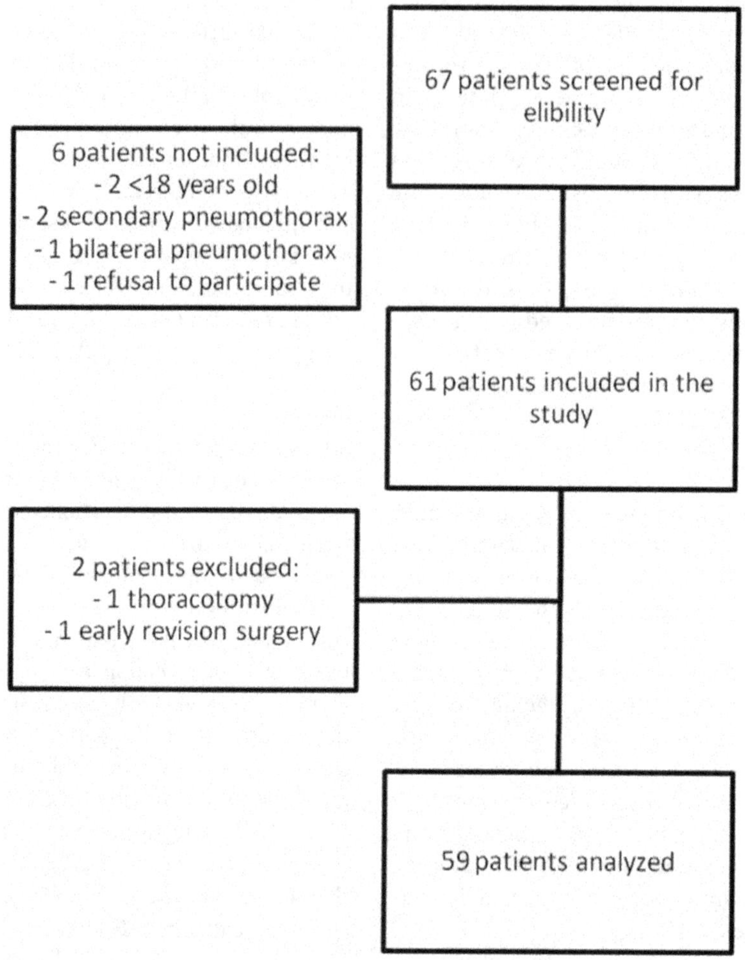

Fig. 1 Flow diagram of the study

variable independently associated with reduced high-dose morphine consumption (OR 0.09, 95%CI [0.01–0.79]; $p = 0.03$) (Table 4). Non-significant association were found between reduced high-dose morphine consumption and the postoperative use of tramadol ($p = 0.057$) and a single-port surgical procedure ($p = 0.052$) (Table 4).

Discussion

This prospective cohort study shows relatively high pain intensity and morphine consumption after VATS for pneumothorax. In this context, the serratus plane block with insertion of a catheter for continuous local anesthetic infusion, in addition to multimodal systemic analgesia, provided satisfactory pain control during the first postoperative 72 h and decreased high-dose morphine consumption.

Pain treatment after thoracic surgery is challenging, thoracotomy being considered as one of the most painful surgical procedures. The gold standard for pain treatment after thoracotomy is epidural analgesia [13]. However, there is evidence to suggest that a paravertebral block could be equally effective with less side effets [13–15]. As thoracic surgery patients take part in enhanced rehabilitation strategies that require capability to deambulate, and aim to achieve rapid recovery, side effects induced by epidural analgesia, such as orthostatic hypotension and urinary retention, are especially deleterious and may preclude the application of such a postoperative rehabilitation program. That said, a paravertebral block could be less efficient after pleurodesis due to pleural inflammation or surgical dilaceration of the parietal lining of the pleura [6]. This may explain the trend towards higher pain scores in patients having undergone a paravertebral block in our study, and could make the use of a paravertebral block unsuitable for ensuring analgesia in this context.

VATS is considered less painful than thoracotomy [3], explaining why anesthesiologists consider epidural analgesia less appropriate [16]. Nevertheless, loco-regional analgesic techniques are still included routinely in postoperative analgesic protocols to provide good quality analgesia in VATS patients [5]. The choice of the appropriate loco-regional analgesic technique is determined by

Table 1 Patients' characteristics

Patient's characteristics ($n = 59$)	n (%) or median [25^e-75^e percentiles]
Preoperative characteristics, *n (%) or median [IQR]*	
Gender (male)	44 (75%)
Age (years)	34 [26–42]
BMI (kg.m^{-2})	20.9 [18.9–23.0]
ASA I class	40 (68%)
Respiratory comorbidity	10 (17%)
Past history of pneumothorax	17 (29%)
Past history or active smoking	40 (68%)
Cannabis consumption	19 (32%)
Hypertension	5 (9%)
Surgical procedure, *n (%) or median [IQR]*	
One-port VATS	54 (92%)
Chemical pleurodesis	46 (78%)
Bullous/wedge resection	36 (61%)
Duration of surgery (min)	75 [60–100]
Single chest tube	54 (92%)
Duration of postoperative thoracic drainage (days)	4 [3.0–5.0]
Recovery room, *n (%) or median [IQR]*	
Extubation immediately after surgery	59 (100)
Dose of morphine titration	10 [5.5–14.0]

the extent and duration of the pain. In the context of pneumothorax surgery, the duration of pain is mainly related to the duration of postoperative chest drainage. In this cohort of patients, despite the fact that all loco-regional analgesic techniques resulted in satisfactory pain control after a couple of hours, the serratus plane block was the only technique that reduced the number of patients requiring high-dose oral morphine as an analgesic rescue treatment. The serratus plane block, as described by Blanco et al. was initially introduced in patients scheduled for breast surgery [10]. In a previous study, Okmen et al. reported that performing a single-bolus serratus

Table 2 Postoperative Visual Analog Scale values and incidence of postoperative nausea and vomiting and urinary retention according to the analgesic protocol

Visual Analog Scale values								PONV	Urinary retention
time	H0	H1	H2	H12	H24	H48	H72		
Systemic analgesia alone *(n = 15)*									
At rest	4.5 [2–7]	4 [4–6]	3 [2–4]	3 [2–6]	3 [2–6]	2 [1.5–4]	2 [0–4]	3 (21%)	1 (7%)
On coughing	6.5 [5–8]	7 [5–8]	5 [4–6]	5 [4–7]	5 [4–7]	5 [4–5]	3 [2.5–5]		
Paravertebral block with continuous infusion through a catheter *(n = 9)*									
At rest	5 [1–6]	6 [1–6]	4 [1–4]	4 [2–5]	3 [2–4]	2 [2–4]	2 [0–4]	2 (22%)	2 (22%)
On coughing	8 [4.5–9]	8 [4.5–9]	4 [3.5–5.5]	6 [4–9.5]	4.5 [3–6]	5 [3–7.5]	4 [2.5–5]		
Single-injection serratus plane block *(n = 16)*									
At rest	4.5 [0.5–7]	5.5 [3–6]	3 [1–3.5]	3 [3–4]	3.0 [3–4]	3 [2–4]	2 [0–3]	2 (13%)	1 (6%)
On coughing	6.5 [1–8]	6 [3–7]	4 [2–5]	5 [4–7.5]	4.5 [3–6]	5 [4–6]	3 [2–4]		
Serratus plane block with continuous infusion through a catheter *(n = 19)*									
At rest	4.5 [0–6]	3 [0–6]	1 [0–3]	3 [2–5.5]	2 [1.5–4.5]	2 [0–4]	1 [0–2]	8 (42%)	0 (0%)
On coughing	6 [1–8]	5 [3–7]	3 [3–5]	4.5 [3–6]	3 [3–6]	4 [1–5]	2 [2–3]		

Values are expressed as median [25^e-75^e percentiles] or n (%)
PONV postoperative nausea and vomiting

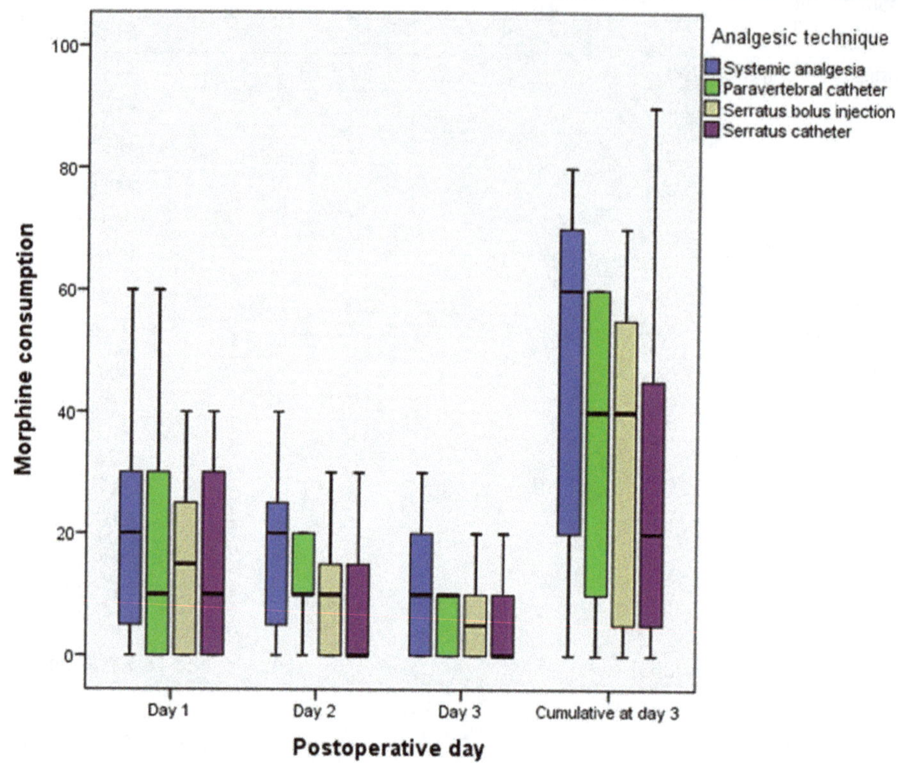

Fig. 2 Daily and cumulative oral morphine consumption during the first postoperative 72 h according to the postoperative analgesic technique used

plane block resulted in lower pain intensity and smaller quantities of tramadol being administered as intravenous patient-controlled analgesia (PCA) after VATS [17]. However, the control group that only received IV tramadol PCA was far from the standard of care for this procedure, and the study was restricted to the first postoperative 24 h while postoperative pain is supposed to last over a longer time period. Park et al. documented that a single-injection serratus plane block performed before surgery decreased both intraoperative remifentanil requirements and postoperative fentanyl consumption compared with a sham block [18]. In another study using a comparable design, Kim et al. documented lower pain scores, reduced morphine consumption and a higher degree of satisfaction in patients treated with a serratus plane block compared to a sham block [19]. Although properly designed and showing the efficacy of the serratus plane block, these two prospective studies, as well as the Okmen et al. study, did not compare the serratus plane block to a standard of care considered appropriate for this kind of surgical procedure. Kalil et al. have compared thoracic epidural anesthesia to serratus plane block with insertion of a catheter and documented no difference in pain scores in a limited number of patients scheduled for VATS [20]. Conversely, in our study, the serratus plane block was associated with an opioid sparing effect that was not found for the other locoregional analgesic techniques. In addition, the fact that continuous infusion through a catheter was associated with reduced high-dose morphine consumption over the first postoperative 3 days, unlike a single-injection serratus plane block, supports the placement of such a catheter to maintain an effective postoperative analgesia over several days. Taken altogether, these data suggest that the serratus plane block may be a technique to ensure good pain relief and morphine sparing after VATS for pneumothorax.

This study has several limitations. First of all, the number of patients included in the study is limited making it only a preliminary assesment of the effect of a serratus plane block. Indeed, although the serratus plane block with continuous infusion through a catheter is associated with reduced high-dose morphine consumption, we did not observe any significant difference in the global morphine consumption between the different groups. Although a serratus plane block is theoretically advantageous in the context of pleurodesis, we did not report any superiority of the serratus plane block over the paravertebral block regarding pain score or global morphine consumption. However, it could be hypothesized that our study lacks power to demonstrate such a superiority, in particular as a trend towards a lower morphine consumption in the continuous serratus plane block group existed. Further larger studies are required to confirm these preliminary results.

Table 3 Univariate analysis of parameters in patients with cumulative oral morphine consumption ≤50 mg and > 50 mg during the first postoperative 72 h

Cumulative morphine at D3	≤ 50 mg (*n* = 40)	> 50 mg (*n* = 19)	P
Age > 40 years old	11 (28%)	7 (36.8)	0.46
Gender (male)	31 (78%)	13 (68.4)	0.45
ASA class > I	14 (35%)	5 (26.3)	0.50
BMI (kg.m^{-2})	21 [19–23]	21 [18–22]	0.88
Preoperative chest tube > 24 h	26 (65%)	15 (79%)	0.27
Hypertension	4 (10%)	1 (5%)	0.54
Diabetes mellitus	1 (3%)	0 (0%)	0.48
Respiratory comorbidity			0.65
Asthma	3 (8%)	1 (5%)	
COPD	3 (8%)	0 (0%)	
Interstitial lung disease	1 (3%)	0 (0%)	
Emphysema	1 (3%)	1 (5%)	
Past history of pneumothorax	11 (28%)	6 (32%)	0.74
Cannabis chronic use	12 (30%)	7 (37%)	0.59
Single-port incision	38 (95%)	16 (84%)	0.16
Chemical pleurodesis	32 (80%)	14 (74%)	0.58
Pulmonary resection	23 (58%)	13 (68%)	0.42
Postoperative chest tube duration > 1 day	4 (10%)	1 (5%)	0.54
Duration of surgery > 60 min	21 (53%)	13 (68%)	0.24
Anesthetic and analgesic agents			
Total dose of sufentanil used (*µg/kg*)	0.89 [0.69–1.11]	0.81 [0.71–1.22]	0.76
Ketamine	31 (78%)	15 (79%)	0.90
Intravenous Lidocaine	26 (65%)	11 (58%)	0.59
Dexamethasone	38 (95%)	17 (90%)	0.43
Acetaminophen	40 (100%)	19 (100%)	–
Nefopam	39 (98%)	18 (95%)	0.58
Ketoprofen	22 (55%)	11 (58%)	0.83
Tramadol	39 (98%)	17 (90%)	0.19
Loco-regional analgesic technique			
Systemic analgesia alone	6 (15%)	9 (47%)	0.02
Paravertebral catheter	6 (15%)	3 (16%)	0.93
Serratus single injection	12 (30%)	4 (21%)	0.47
Serratus catheter	16 (40%)	3 (16%)	0.06

Values are expressed as median [25^{e}-75^{e} percentiles] or n (%)
COPD: chronic obstructive pulmonary disease

Table 4 Multivariate analysis of factors associated with high-dose cumulative oral morphine consumption during the first postoperative 72 h

Variables	Odd ratio [95%CI]	P
Postoperative tramadol use	0.04 [0.002–1.09]	0.057
Serratus catheter	0.09 [0.01–0.79]	0.03
Single-port surgery	0.07 [0.005–1.01]	0.052

Secondly, since it is not a double-blind randomized study, several biases may have been introduced. However, pain scores and morphine administration were not evaluated by the physicians who performed the block in the operating theatre, providing an acceptable assessment of postoperative pain and morphine consumption. However, it can not be ruled out that certain differences in intra-operative features (such as duration of the surgery, actual doses of anesthetics and analgesics delivered, use of a non-steroidal anti-inflammatory drug that was left to the discretion of the attending anesthesiologist, etc.) may have impacted the pain scores and postoperative morphine consumptions, which could only have been avoided with a randomized design. It could also be hypothesized that, in the absence of randomization, surgical features may have impacted both postoperative pain scores and locoregional analgesia efficacy. However, 92% of patients had single-port VATS, which is a standardized procedure in our structure [8], thus limiting the risk of non-balanced effects of the surgery between groups.

Thirdly, the definition of the morphine consumption threshold used in our study could be challenged. We chose a threshold of 50 mg of cumulative oral morphine administration over the first postoperative 72 h to define high-dose consumption and assess the efficacy of the loco-regional analgesic techniques. As there is no agreed definition of what constitutes high-dose morphine consumption after VATS for pneumothorax, we chose the mean value from our institution. It should be noted that the validity of this threshold is reinforced by other recent studies reporting close postoperative morphine consumptions in patients scheduled for VATS [11, 12]. The clinical relevance of the opoid sparing effect of serratus plane block could also be challenged as the multivariate analysis suggests a link between single-port surgery and a reduced need for postoperative high-dose morphine; a finding in line with a previous retrospective study [4]. However, most of the patients of this cohort had single port surgery as it has been reported to be a safe and less invasive technique for SP surgery [8], suggesting that even with an optimized surgical technique a serratus plane block with catheter remains a valid choice for postoperative pain management. Along the same lines, tramadol administration tended to reduce the need for high-dose morphine. Using more tramadol postoperatively resulted in fewer patients using morphine on demand. Tramadol administation also explains why the incidence in postoperative nausea and vomiting was comparable in all the groups independently of morphine consumption.

Conclusions

This study suggests that serratus plane block combined with continuous infusion through placement of a catheter may have some benefits, although further studies are needed to confirm these results and determine the true place of the serratus plane block in pain management after VATS for pneumothorax.

Abbreviations

PCA: Patient-Controlled Analgesia; SP: Spontaneous Pneumothorax; VAS: Visual Analog Scale; VATS: Video-Assisted Thoracic Surgery

Acknowledgments

The authors thank Francesca McVeigh for English proofreading.

Authors' contributions

PAA conceived the protocol, analyzed the collected data, and drafted the manuscript. MC participated in the protocol conception, recorded the data and corrected the manuscript. AA, JB, JA, EM-H and YY contributed to patient care and corrected the manuscript. FB, MG and CQ participated in the protocol conception, analyzed the collected data, and drafted the manuscript. All authors have read and approved the final version of the manuscript.

Author details

[1]Service d'Anesthésie-Réanimation et Médecine Péri-opératoire, AP-HP Hôpital Tenon, 4 rue de la Chine, 75020 Paris, France. [2]Service de chirurgie thoracique, AP-HP Hôpital Tenon, 4 rue de la Chine, 75020 Paris, France. [3]Faculté de médecine Sorbonne Université (Paris VI), Paris, France.

References

1. Bintcliffe O, Maskell N. Spontaneous pneumothorax. BMJ. 2014;348:g2928.
2. Hallifax RJ, Yousuf A, Jones HE, Corcoran JP, Psallidas I, Rahman NM. Effectiveness of chemical pleurodesis in spontaneous pneumothorax recurrence prevention: a systematic review. Thorax. 2017;72:1121–31.
3. Bendixen M, Jørgensen OD, Kronborg C, Andersen C, Licht PB. Postoperative pain and quality of life after lobectomy via video-assisted thoracoscopic surgery or anterolateral thoracotomy for early stage lung cancer: a randomised controlled trial. Lancet Oncol. 2016;17:836–44.
4. Tamura M, Shimizu Y, Hashizume Y. Pain following thoracoscopic surgery: retrospective analysis between single-incision and three-port video-assisted thoracoscopic surgery. J Cardiothorac Surg. 2013;8:153.
5. Steinthorsdottir KJ, Wildgaard L, Hansen HJ, Petersen RH, Wildgaard K. Regional analgesia for video-assisted thoracic surgery: a systematic review. Eur J Cardiothorac Surg. 2014;45:959–66.
6. Komatsu T, Sowa T, Kino A, Fujinaga T. The importance of pleural integrity for effective and safe thoracic paravertebral block: a retrospective comparative study on postoperative pain control by paravertebral block. Interact Cardiovasc Thorac Surg. 2015;20:296–9.
7. von Elm E, Altman DG, Egger M, Pocock SJ, Gøtzsche PC, Vandenbroucke JP, et al. The strengthening the reporting of observational studies in epidemiology (STROBE) statement: guidelines for reporting observational studies. J Clin Epidemiol. 2008;61:344–9.
8. Masmoudi H, Etienne H, Sylvestre R, Evrard D, Ouede R, Le Roux M, et al. Three hundred fifty-one patients with pneumothorax undergoing Uniportal (single port) video-assisted thoracic surgery. Ann Thorac Surg. 2017;104:254–60.
9. Komatsu T, Kino A, Inoue M, Sowa T, Takahashi K, Fujinaga T. Paravertebral block for video-assisted thoracoscopic surgery: analgesic effectiveness and role in fast-track surgery. Int J Surg. 2014;12:936–9.
10. Blanco R, Parras T, McDonnell JG, Prats-Galino A. Serratus plane block: a novel ultrasound-guided thoracic wall nerve block. Anaesthesia. 2013;68: 1107–13.
11. Perna V, Carvajal AF, Torrecilla JA, Gigirey O. Uniportal video-assisted thoracoscopic lobectomy versus other video-assisted thoracoscopic lobectomy techniques: a randomized study. Eur J Cardiothorac Surg. 2016; 50:411–5.
12. Duclos G, Charvet A, Resseguier N, Trousse D, D'Journo X-B, Zieleskiewicz L, et al. Postoperative morphine consumption and anaesthetic management of patients undergoing video-assisted or robotic-assisted lung resection: a prospective, propensity score-matched study. J Thorac Dis. 2018;10:3558–67.
13. Joshi GP, Bonnet F, Shah R, Wilkinson RC, Camu F, Fischer B, et al. A systematic review of randomized trials evaluating regional techniques for postthoracotomy analgesia. Anesth Analg. 2008;107:1026–40.
14. Fibla JJ, Molins L, Mier JM, Sierra A, Carranza D, Vidal G. The efficacy of paravertebral block using a catheter technique for postoperative analgesia in thoracoscopic surgery: a randomized trial. Eur J Cardiothorac Surg. 2011; 40:907–11.
15. Yeung JHY, Gates S, Naidu BV, Wilson MJA, Gao Smith F. Paravertebral block versus thoracic epidural for patients undergoing thoracotomy. Cochrane Database Syst Rev. 2016;2:CD009121.
16. Shanthanna H, Moisuik P, O'Hare T, Srinathan S, Finley C, Paul J, et al. Survey of postoperative regional analgesia for thoracoscopic surgeries in Canada. J Cardiothorac Vasc Anesth. 2018;32:1750–5.
17. Ökmen K, Metin Ökmen B. Evaluation of the effect of serratus anterior plane block for pain treatment after video-assisted thoracoscopic surgery. Anaesth

Crit Care Pain Med. 2018;37:349–53.
18. Park MH, Kim JA, Ahn HJ, Yang MK, Son HJ, Seong BG. A randomised trial of serratus anterior plane block for analgesia after thoracoscopic surgery. Anaesthesia. 2018;73:1260–4.
19. Kim D-H, Oh YJ, Lee JG, Ha D, Chang YJ, Kwak HJ. Efficacy of ultrasound-guided serratus plane block on postoperative quality of recovery and analgesia after video-assisted thoracic surgery: a randomized, triple-blind, placebo-controlled study. Anesth Analg. 2018;126:1353–61.
20. Khalil AE, Abdallah NM, Bashandy GM, TA-H K. Ultrasound-guided serratus anterior plane block versus thoracic epidural analgesia for thoracotomy pain. J Cardiothorac Vasc Anesth. 2017;31:152–8.

2

A randomized controlled trial on analgesic effect of repeated quadratus lumborum block versus continuous epidural analgesia following laparoscopic nephrectomy

Dita Aditianingsih[1*], Pryambodho[1], Naufal Anasy[1], Aida Rosita Tantri[1] and Chaidir Arif Mochtar[2]

Abstract

Background: Epidural analgesia as the effective pain management for abdominal surgery has side effects such as paresthesia, hypotension, hematomas, and impaired motoric of lower limbs. The quadratus lumborum block (QLB) has potential as an abdominal truncal block, however, its analgesic efficacy has never been compared to epidural analgesia on laparoscopic nephrectomy. This prospective randomized controlled study compared the effectiveness of QLB with the epidural analgesia technique in relieving postoperative pain following transperitoneal laparoscopic nephrectomy.

Methods: Sixty-two patients underwent laparoscopic donor nephrectomy and were randomized to receive QLB ($n = 31$) or continuous epidural ($n = 31$). The QLB group received bilateral QLB using 0.25% bupivacaine and the epidural group received 6 ml/h of 0.25% bupivacaine for intraoperative analgesia. As postoperative analgesia, the QLB group received repeated bilateral QLB with the same dose and the epidural group received 6 ml/h of 0.125% bupivacaine for 24 h after surgery completion. The primary outcome was the 24-h cumulative morphine requirement after surgery. The secondary outcome was the postoperative pain scores. Sensory block coverage, hemodynamic changes, Bromage score, postoperative nausea-vomiting (PONV), paresthesia, and duration of urinary catheter usage were recorded and analyzed.

Result: The 24-h cumulative morphine requirement and pain scores after surgery were comparable between the QLB and epidural groups. The coverage of QLB was extended from T9 to L2 and the continuous epidural block was extended from T8 to L3 dermatomes. The mean arterial pressure (MAP) measured at 24 h after surgery was lower in the epidural group ($p = 0.001$). Bromage score, incidence of PONV, and paresthesia were not significantly different between the two groups. Duration of urinary catheter usage was shorter ($p < 0.001$) in the QLB group.

Conclusion: The repeated QLB had a similar 24-h cumulative morphine requirement, comparable postoperative pain scores and sensory blockade, higher postoperative MAP, a similar degree of motoric block, no difference in the incidence of PONV and paresthesia, and shorter urinary catheter usage, compared to the continuous epidural analgesia following transperitoneal laparoscopic nephrectomy.

Keywords: Epidural analgesia, Laparoscopic nephrectomy, Postoperative analgesia, Patient-controlled analgesia, Quadratus lumborum block

* Correspondence: ditaaditiaa@gmail.com
[1]Department of Anesthesiology and Intensive Care, Cipto Mangunkusumo General Hospital, Universitas Indonesia, 6th Salemba Raya, DKI Jakarta 10430, Indonesia

Background

The management of postoperative pain holds an important role in laparoscopic living donor nephrectomy patient's recovery [1, 2]. The postoperative pain after laparoscopic nephrectomy remains a major concern because some patients still demonstrate acute pain that is not different between laparoscopic or open nephrectomy [2, 3]. Epidural analgesia is the gold standard for abdominal surgery including for laparoscopic nephrectomy, however, it has unfavorable side effects such as paresthesia, hypotension, hematomas, impaired motoric of lower limbs and urinary retention that could delay recovery. Administration of intravenous patient-controlled analgesia (PCA) opioid has potential side effects such as sedation, pruritus, nausea, vomiting, and respiratory depression [4].

Blanco and colleagues first introduced the quadratus lumborum block (QLB) by injecting local anesthetic in the interfascial plane at the anterolateral margin of quadratus lumborum muscle (the lateral QLB) under ultrasound guidance and then modified the point of injection into the posterior wall of quadratus lumborum muscle (the posterior QLB) for postoperative analgesia after cesarean delivery [5]. Børglum and colleagues refined the technique, by adopting the posterior approach of QLB and using the 'Shamrock' sign to place the needle tip anterior to the quadratus lumborum muscle, then injecting the local anesthetic agent into the plane between the quadratus lumborum and psoas muscles (the anterior QLB) [6].

Clinical trials of QLB are still limited, but evidence has shown the efficacy of QLB in reducing opioid requirement and postoperative pain to promote recovery after cesarean section, laparoscopic or laparotomy procedure, and hip surgery [5, 7–10]. Transperitoneal laparoscopic donor nephrectomy patients reveal the significant postoperative pain related to the Pfannenstiel incision, port sites wounds, and deep intra-abdominal nociception [2, 3]. For the abdominal surgery, QLB became an alternative to epidural without central neuraxial block side effects [5, 11], however, the efficacy of QLB as perioperative pain management in transperitoneal laparoscopic nephrectomy is unclear. We hypothesized that repeated QLB could be superior to a continuous epidural block in relieving postoperative pain with fewer side effects in living donor patients. Our study compared the effectiveness of QLB to the continuous epidural analgesia in relieving postoperative pain following transperitoneal laparoscopic nephrectomy. The primary outcome was the 24-h cumulative morphine requirement after surgery. The secondary outcome was the 24-h postoperative pain scores. The sensory block coverage, hemodynamic changes, Bromage score, postoperative nausea-vomiting (PONV) occurrence, and duration of urinary catheter usage were recorded during observation.

Methods

Patients and study design

This prospective open-label randomized controlled study adheres to CONSORT guideline. This study was approved by the Ethics and Research Committee of Universitas Indonesia (0211/UN2.F1/ETIK/2018) and was retrospectively registered in ClinicalTrials.gov (NCT03520205) on May 9th, 2018 with predicted subject recruitment time from May 1st – October 30th, 2018. Written informed consents were obtained from all adult patients with American Society of Anesthesiologists (ASA) I–II who underwent laparoscopic living donor nephrectomy in Cipto Mangunkusumo Hospital, DKI Jakarta. The inclusion criteria included age 18–60 years with body mass index (BMI) < 30 kg/m^2. The exclusion criteria included the inability to communicate, history of allergy or contraindication to local anesthetics, contraindication to epidural or QLB (coagulopathy or infections on the injection site).

The research protocol was explained to the patient who met the inclusion criteria. All patients were educated about QLB and continuous epidural procedures, how to describe the degree of pain with the numerical rating scale (NRS), and how to use the PCA morphine pump when the pain level (NRS) ≥ 4 after the surgery. After obtaining written approval, the patients were randomized either into the QLB group (intervention group) or the epidural group (control group). Randomization was conducted in a block size of 4 using a computerized randomization sequence by independent research assistants. The randomization allocation number for each subject was written on paper and put in a closed envelope. The envelope was opened by the anesthesiologist who was appointed to perform epidural or QLB for this study. Primary investigators and statisticians were blinded to data collection throughout the study.

General management

Standard monitoring was placed such as electrocardiogram, oxygen saturation, non-invasive blood pressure monitors and cardiometry ICON™. General anesthesia induction was conducted with the administration of fentanyl 2 μg/kg as co-induction, proceeded with propofol 1–2 mg/kg. Endotracheal tube intubation was facilitated with atracurium 0.5 mg/kg. The ventilator was set to volume control with positive end-expiratory pressure 5 cmH_2O and FiO_2 30–50%, breathing frequency was adjusted with the end-tidal carbon dioxide target of 35–45 mmHg. The anesthesia was maintained using sevoflurane with 0.8–1.3 minimum alveolar concentration, fresh gas flow 1 L/minute with oxygen compressed air ratio of 40:60, atracurium 0.5 mg/kg/h, to achieve bispectral index of 40–60, end-tidal fraction of sevoflurane 1.6–2.2%, and train of four ratios ≤25% during surgery. All subjects received fentanyl 1 μg/kg i.v. if there was an increase of change in systolic blood pressure or pulse rate > 20% from the initial value during surgery and the total intraoperative fentanyl usage was recorded. Ephedrine was given if there is a decrease in mean arterial pressure (MAP) less than 65 mmHg during the study observation.

All patients were planned for the transperitoneal left laparoscopic nephrectomy and kidney extraction through a Pfannenstiel incision, that was performed by the surgeon (CAM, IW, ARH) who had more than 5 years of experience to performed transperitoneal laparoscopic live donor nephrectomy. At the end of surgery, neostigmine 0.04–0.07 μg/kg was given to reverse residual neuromuscular block and the patient was extubated when had reached train of four ratio of 0.9–1.0.

Technique of epidural analgesia

Two experienced anesthetist consultants (P, DA) performed all the thoracic epidural and QLB procedures. Patients in the epidural group had an epidural catheter placement procedure in the left lateral decubitus position after intubation under general anesthesia. After ensuring skin asepsis and draping the area with a sterile cover, an 18G Tuohy epidural needle was inserted in vertebral interspace T10–11 and catheter was advanced 5 cm length within the epidural space [12]. We observed vacuum epidural catheter aspiration and a test dose of 3 ml 0.25% bupivacaine with adrenaline 1:200,000 without any change in pulse rate or blood pressure to confirm the position of catheter within the epidural space. Then a continuous epidural infusion of 6 ml/h 0.25% bupivacaine was maintained for intraoperative analgesia. For 24 h postoperative pain management, after completion of the surgery, the continuous epidural dosage was decreased into 0.125% bupivacaine 6 ml/h at the start and the dose was increased in 2 ml/h increments up to 10 ml/h if the pain is still uncontrolled on PCA morphine setting.

Technique of Quadratus Lumborum block

All patients in the QLB group received the first bilateral ultrasound-guided transmuscular QLB (anterior QLB or QLB3) after induction and intubation under general anesthesia for intraoperative analgesia. Patients were in supine position with the site to be blocked slightly facing upward by pillow underneath it and the tilted operating table. After ensuring skin asepsis of the area, a 2.0–5.5 MHz convex transducer (C5-1E, DC-70, Mindray, Shenzen China) covered with sterile drapes attached in the transverse plane to the inferior lumbar (Petit's) triangle that consisted of iliac crest in the inferior edge, the latissimus dorsi muscle in the posterior side and external abdominal oblique muscle in the anterior region. The transducer was advanced posteriorly until the Shamrock sign (the erector spinae, quadratus lumborum, and psoas muscles being the leaves, and the transverse process of L4 as the stem) appeared on the ultrasound. A 21G 100-mm peripheral block needle (Stimuplex®, BBraun, Mesulngen Germany) was inserted in-plane with ultrasound probe passing in anterior to posterior direction through the QL muscle and reached the border between the QL and psoas major muscle [6, 11]. After confirming negative for blood aspiration, 1 ml normal saline was injected to obtain hydrodissection sign for verifying the needle tip, then a volume of 0.3–0.4 ml/kg 0.25% bupivacaine with a maximum volume of 25 ml was injected on each side (See Additional file 1). For 24 h postoperative analgesia, the second bilateral QLB procedures were repeated one time at the end of surgery using a similar regimen of 0.3–0.4 ml/kg 0.25% bupivacaine with a maximum volume of 25 ml on each side. (See Additional file 1).

Postoperative patient-controlled morphine

In the recovery room, patient-controlled morphine i.v. using a portable programmed pump (Perfusor® Space PCA Infusion Pump System, BBraun, Germany) was connected after the patient was fully awake and able to follow the instruction. All patients were informed first at preoperative anesthesia visit and once again at the recovery room after the surgery, how to press the PCA button if they experienced moderate to severe pain. The PCA setting was 1 mg bolus, lockout time 10 min and maximum dosage 6 mg/h, without basal opioid infusion. Ondansetron 4 mg i.v. and omeprazole 40 mg i.v. were administered every 12 h to prevent PONV.

Study parameters and statistical analysis

This study aimed to compare the analgesic efficacy of QLB to continuous epidural analgesia as postoperative pain management. The primary outcome was the cumulative morphine requirement in 24 h after surgery. Time to first morphine requirement was also recorded. The secondary outcomes were pain scores at rest and movement, and motoric block at time points 2, 6, 12 and 24 h after anesthesia recovery. Pain scores were assessed using NRS (0 = no pain; 1–3 = mild pain, 4–6 = moderate pain, 7–10 = severe pain). Sensory block was assessed after anesthesia recovery using pinprick and cold loss sensation with ice and alcohol. The motoric block was evaluated using Bromage score (grade 1 = free movement of leg and feet; 2 = just able to flex knees with free movement of the feet; 3 = unable to flex knees, free movement of feet; 4 = unable to move the legs or feet). The MAP, pulse rate, and cardiometry cardiac index were recorded at baseline, during surgery, and 24 h after anesthesia recovery. The occurrence of PONV and paresthesia within 24 h postoperatively and urinary catheterization duration were recorded. All of the outcomes were documented by the acute pain service team and ward nurses.

Sample size calculation was based on the primary hypothesis that opioid requirement in 24 h after surgery. Based on the previous study, the mean (standard deviation (SD)) cumulative morphine requirement 24 h after surgery was 4 mg (SD = 4.723) [13]. From a preliminary study, the mean (SD) cumulative morphine requirement 24 h after surgery was 4 mg (SD = 6.09). A sample size of 28 patients in each group was determined with a statistical power of 0.8 and type-1 error of 0.05. This study recruited 62 patients to allow 10% dropouts.

All statistical studies were analyzed using Statistical Package for the Social Sciences version 20 (IBM Corp. 2011, Armonk, NY). Differences between numerical variables were analyzed using the unpaired t-test for normal distribution data and Mann-Whitney test for abnormal distribution data. Differences between categorical variables were analyzed using Chi square test. Numerical data with normal distribution was displayed in a mean (SD), abnormal distribution was displayed in the median (95% confidence interval (CI)) values, and as a percentage for categorical variables. The analysis was statistically significant if the *p*-value was less than 0.05.

Results

We enrolled 62 patients who met the inclusion criteria and signed the informed consent to take part in the study from May 1st – October 30th, 2018. The subjects were randomly assigned into two groups and received their allocated intervention. All patients underwent transperitoneal left laparoscopic nephrectomy and had a Pfannenstiel incision. None of the subjects had subcostal incision or the conversion from laparoscopic to open nephrectomy. None of the subjects were excluded from the study; therefore, all patients were followed-up and included in the final analysis (Fig. 1).

Forty-one (66%) subjects are male. Between the QLB and epidural group, the demographic baseline and perioperative characteristics of the study subjects were similar. The intraoperative fentanyl requirement was not significantly different between the two groups. However, ephedrine requirement was higher in the epidural group compared to QLB group (0 (0–50) vs 10 (0–50) mg, $p = 0.026$) (Table 1). The mean total dosage of bupivacaine used in the QLB group was significantly lower than the epidural group (Table 1).

Figure 2 shows the 24-h cumulative morphine requirement at each time point after surgery were comparable between the QLB and epidural group. Time to first morphine initiation using PCA was not significantly different between the QLB and epidural groups (120 (95% CI: 137.61–354.45) vs 125 (95% CI: 133.56–370.31) minutes, $p = 0.703$) (See Additional file 2). There were 3 subjects in the QLB group and 4 subjects in the epidural group did not need additional morphine at all in 24 h after anesthesia recovery.

Pain scores at rest and in movement at each time point in 24 h after anesthesia recovery were not significantly different between the QLB and epidural groups (Table 2). The lowest pain scores at rest and in

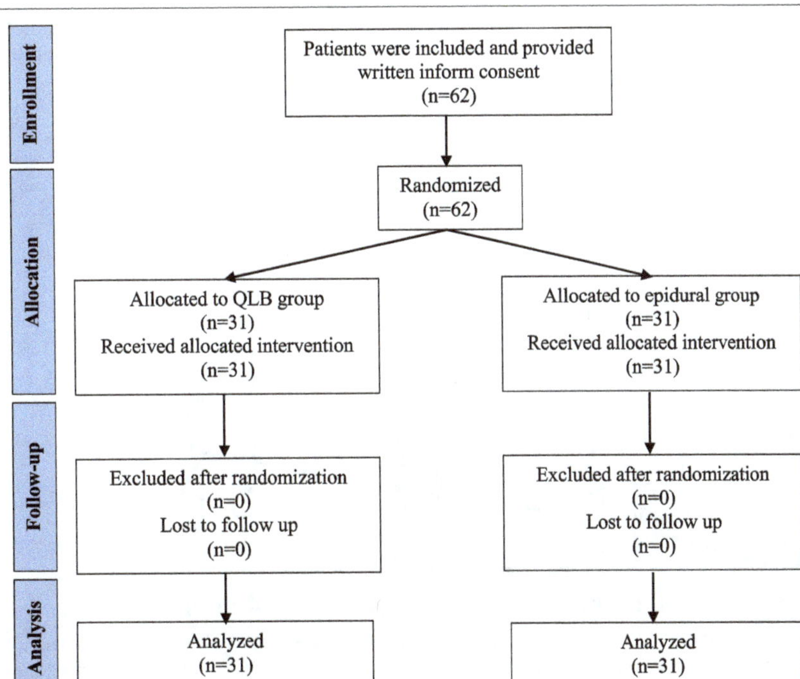

Fig. 1 CONSORT flow diagram

Table 1 Patient baseline and perioperative characteristics

Variables	QLB group (n = 31)	Epidural group (n = 31)	p value
Men (%)	21 (67.74)	20 (64.51)	1.000
Age (years)	38.29 ± 12.97	39.97 ± 11.49	0.447
Body weight (kg)	64.34 ± 10.10	62.72 ± 10.06	0.530
Body height (cm)	164.06 ± 7.62	161.80 ± 8.74	0.277
BMI (kg/m^2)	24.06 ± 3.82	24.13 ± 4.06	0.940
ASA			0.794
ASA 1 (%)	18 (58.06)	20 (64.51)	
ASA 2 (%)	13 (41.94)	11 (35.49)	
Intraoperative fentanyl dosage (µg)	50 (34.66–83.08)	50 (40.73–101.21)	0.442
Intraoperative ephedrine dosage (mg)	0 (1.37–9.59)	10 (5.48–14.39)	0.026
Duration of surgery (minute)	285.6 ± 42.6	292.2 ± 44.4	0.551
Duration of anesthesia (minute)	354.6 ± 36.6	357.6 ± 33.6	0.796
Total bupivacaine dosage (mg)	200.00 ± 0.00	253.19 ± 11.12	< 0.001

QLB Quadratus lumborum block, *BMI* Body mass index, *ASA* American Society of Anesthesiologist. Data are presented in number (percentage), mean ± standard deviation or median (95% confidence interval).

movement were at 2 and 6 h after anesthesia recovery in both groups.

The bar in Fig. 3 shows the variable degree of sensory block spread in both groups. The majority of patients in the QLB group had the loss of cold and pinprick sensations from T10 to L2, compared with the majority of patients the epidural group had the loss of cold and pinprick sensations from T9 to L2. None of patients in the QLB group showed sensory blockade on level T8 and L3.

Intraoperative MAP, pulse rate and cardiac index (Fig. 4) were not significantly different between the QLB and epidural groups, however, postoperative MAP measured at 24 h after surgery was significantly lower in the

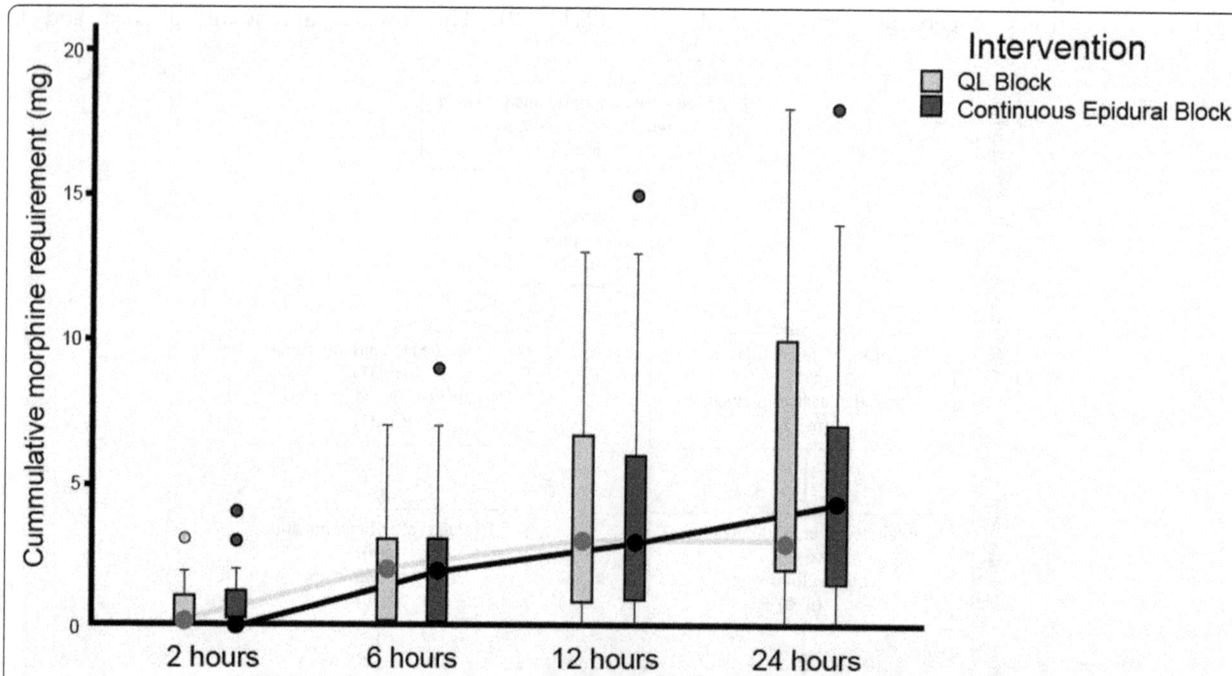

Fig. 2 Cumulative morphine requirement of QLB versus continuous epidural analgesia. Median (95% CI) values of cumulative morphine requirement (mg) after anesthesia recovery at each time point are as follows: 2 h, 0 (0.34–1.05) vs 0 (0.28–1.10) (p = 0.857); 6 h, 2 (0.69–2.08) vs 2 (0.68–1.93) (p = 0.977); 12 h, 3 (1.11–2.74) vs 3 (0.97–2.49) (p = 0.764); 24 h, 3 (0.69–2.62) vs 4 (0.66–1.88) (p = 0.792). The p-values were analyzed using Mann-Whitney test, the horizontal lines indicate medians; boxes indicate interquartile range; whiskers indicate range

Table 2 Postoperative pain scores of QLB versus continuous epidural analgesia

Parameter	QLB group (*n* = 31)	Epidural group (*n* = 31)	*p*-value	Mean difference (95% CI)
NRS at rest after anesthesia recovery				
Immediately	1 (1.37–2.78)	2 (1.74–3.34)	0.377	– 0.46 (– 1.50–0.58)
At 2 h	2 (1.44–2.56)	2 (1.48–2.83)	0.719	−0.15 (– 1.01–0.70)
At 6 h	1 (1.38–2.47)	2 (1.53–2.54)	0.751	−0.12 (– 0.84–0.61)
At 12 h	2 (1.54–2.69)	2 (1.59–2.56)	0.916	0.04 (−0.69–0.77)
At 24 h	2 (1.59–2.56)	2 (1.60–2.71)	0.831	−0.08 (– 0.80–0.64)
NRS in movement after anesthesia recovery				
Immediately	3 (2.48–3.98)	3 (2.58–4.18)	0.774	−0.15 (– 1.23–0.92)
At 2 h	3 (2.62–3.84)	3 (2.48–3.83)	0.862	0.08 (−0.81–0.96)
At 6 h	3 (2.59–3.64)	3 (2.62–3.13)	0.916	−0.04 (– 0.77–0.69)
At 12 h	3 (2.90–4.10)	3 (2.85–3.84)	0.685	0.15 (−0.60–0.91)
At 24 h	3 (2.84–3.78)	3 (2.68–3.78)	0.827	0.08 (−0.63–0.78)

QLB Quadratus lumborum block, *NRS* Numerical rating scale. Data are presented as mean or median (95% confidence interval). Numerical values are compared using unpaired t-test or and Mann-Whitney test. *P*-values of 0.05 or less are considered significant.

epidural group 72.26 (95% CI: 67.69–76.83) mmHg than those in QLB group 83.33 (95% CI: 78.72–87.95) mmHg ($p = 0.001$) (See Additional file 3).

The Bromage scores were not significantly different between the groups. In the epidural group, only 1 subject had postoperative mild paresthesia and improving when the continuous epidural analgesia was discontinued at the end of study. The incidence of PONV in the QLB group was not significantly higher than the epidural group. Subjects in the QLB block group had a significantly shorter duration of urinary catheterization than the epidural group (Table 3). Block-related complications such as local anesthetic systemic toxicity (LAST), bleeding, infection or neurological deficits, and epidural catheter-related problems (dislodge, blocking, or leakage) were not found in this study.

Discussion

Living laparoscopic nephrectomy donors suffer more pain and are associated with more morphine consumption than other laparoscopic nephrectomy patients [14, 15]. Our study was the first randomized controlled trial

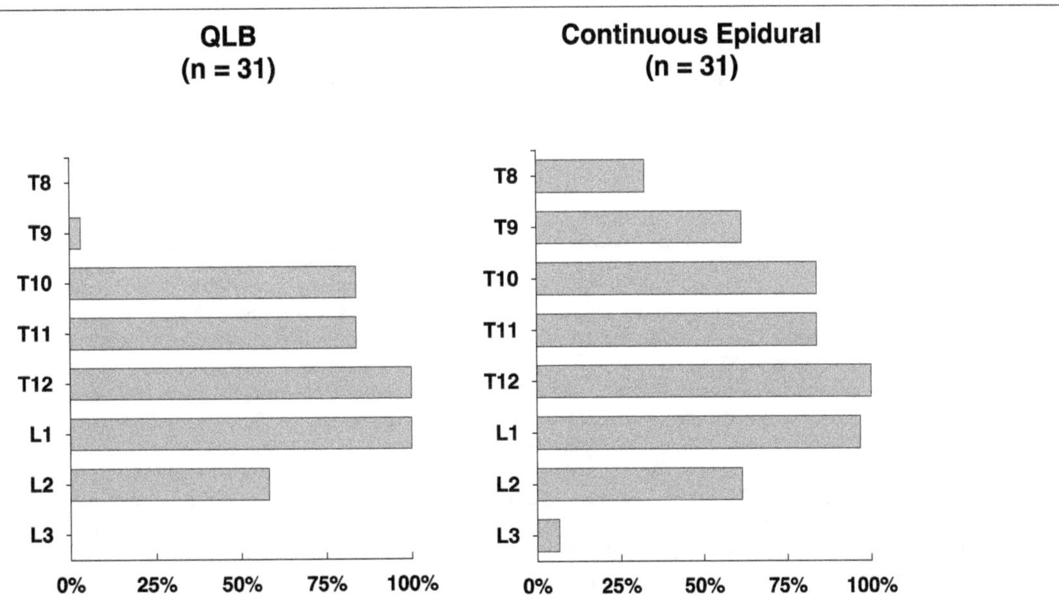

Fig. 3 Dermatomal effects of QLB and continuous epidural analgesia. The QLB and epidural group showed similar percentage of sensory blockade on level T12–L1 (97–100%), T10–T11 (84%), L2 (58–61% of patients). The QLB group showed percentage of sensory blockade on level T9 (3% vs 61.3%), T8 (0% vs 32.3%), L3 (0% vs 6.5%) less than epidural group patients. QLB, quadratus lumborum block

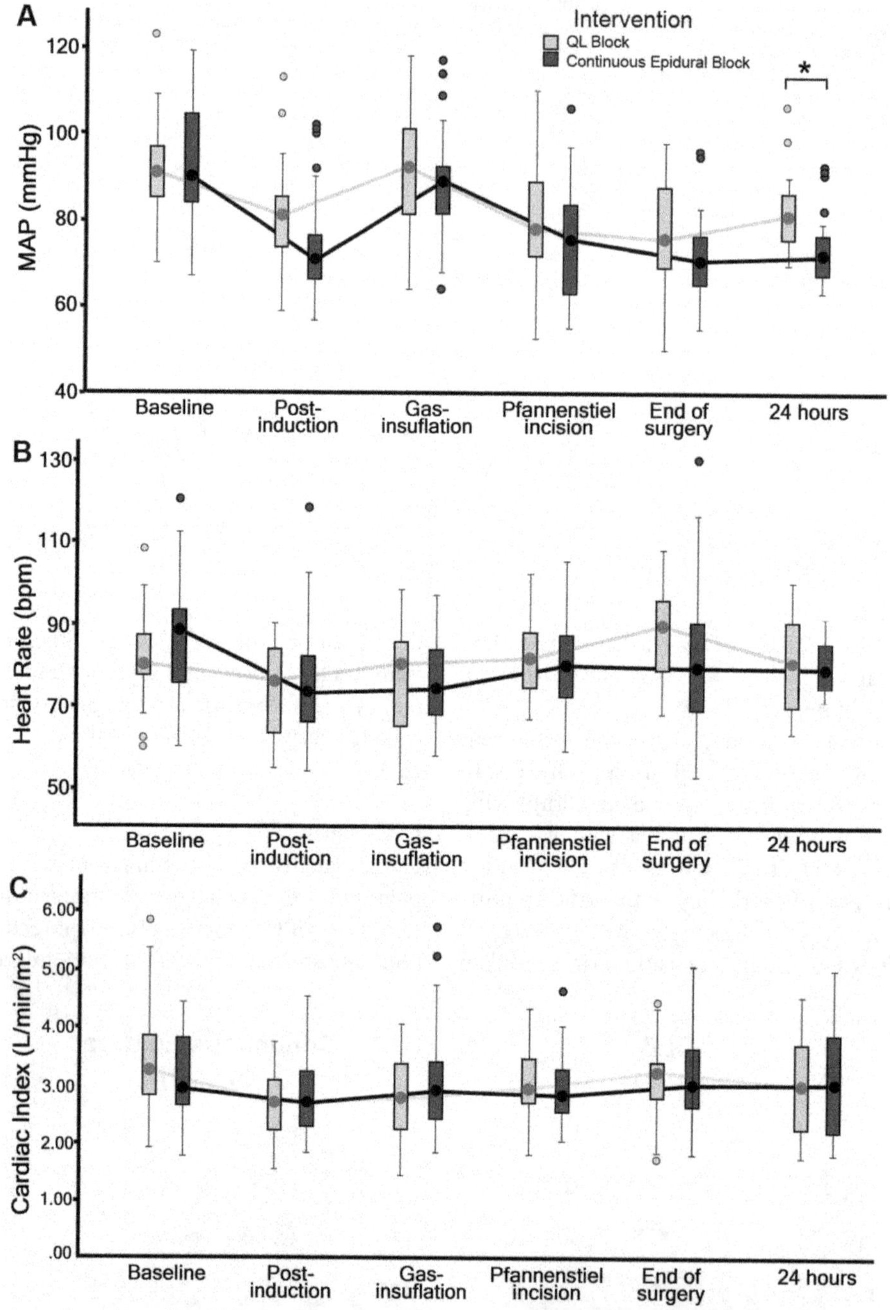

Fig. 4 Intraoperative hemodynamic profile of QLB versus continuous epidural analgesia**.** The horizontal lines indicate medians; boxes indicate interquartile range; whiskers indicate range. Median (95%CI) values of hemodynamic parameters at time points as follows: MAP: baseline 91 (87.34–95.76) to 90 (88.36–98.99) ($p = 0.524$); post-induction, 81 (75.76–85.15) to 71 (70.36–79.06) ($p = 0.072$); gas-insufflation 92 (86.84–97.48) to 88 (82.90–92.52) ($p = 0.210$); pfannenstiel incision 78 (75.60–84.47) to 75 (73.91–82.03) ($p = 0.486$); end of surgery 75 (72.48–81.32) to 71 (68.22–75.17) ($p = 0.063$); 24 h 83.33 (78.72–87.95) to 72.26 (67.69–76.83) ($p = 0.001$); HR: baseline 80 (77.67–85.30) to 88 (80.16–90.93) ($p = 0.215$); post-induction 76 (70.87–78.10) to 73 (70.00–80.45) ($p = 0.816$); gas-insufflation 80 (71.48–81.16) to 74 (72.27–79.80) ($p = 0.855$); pfannenstiel incision 81 (77.95–90.89) to 80 (76.75–84.73) ($p = 0.447$); end of surgery 90 (83.64–92.17) to 80 (75.14–88.02) ($p = 0.049$); 24 h, 82 (64–100) to 82 (72–92) ($p = 0.991$); CI: baseline 3.20 (3.06–3.74) to 2.90 (2.81–3.38) ($p = 0.173$); post-induction 2.70 (2.43–3.01) to 2.70 (2.59–3.11) ($p = 0.499$); gas-insufflation 2.80 (2.44–2.98) to 2.90 (2.73–3.41) ($p = 0.095$); pfannenstiel incision 2.90 (2.78–3.25) to 2.80 (2.70–3.18) ($p = 0.669$); end of surgery 3.20 (2.79–3.33) to 3.00 (2.75–3.37) ($p = 0.987$); 24 h 3.08 (2.67–3.49) to 2.63 (2.34–2.93) ($p = 0.071$). The *p*-values were analyzed using Mann-Whitney test, $*p < 0.05$ is significant. QL, quadratus lumborum; MAP, mean arterial pressure

comparing the analgesic efficacy of bilateral transmuscular anterior QLB with continuous thoracic epidural analgesia following transperitoneal laparoscopic living donor nephrectomy. During surgery, the intraoperative fentanyl consumption was not significantly different between the QLB and continuous epidural group. After surgery, the 24-h cumulative morphine requirement and the pain scores at rest and in movement were not significantly different between the two groups. Our results suggested that the QLB had comparable analgesic effects with continuous epidural analgesia for the first 24 h after laparoscopic nephrectomy. However, we found the pain level assessment was challenging. The PCA morphine after surgery was intended to treat surgical pain but the urinary catheter discomfort also became a trigger for the patient to use the PCA.

In our study, the dermatomal coverage of QLB extended from T10 to L2 that was lower compared to the QLB coverage from T7 to T12 in a study by Murouichi and colleagues [8]. However, the spread of local anesthetic covered the dermatome area of the Pfannenstiel incisions at T12–L1 and the analgesic effect was sufficient for surgical wound pain relief [2, 3, 16]. Although local anesthetic was injected at L4 level, the studies in cadavers and volunteers demonstrated the extensive cephalad distribution of local anesthetic to the thoracic level that may be associated with the anterolateral penetration of quadratus lumborum and anterior thoracolumbar fascia [17]. This spread has not been clearly proven, however, the QLB has the potential to provide both somatic and visceral analgesia due to the spreads of local anesthetics to the thoracolumbar fascia that was extensively innervated by the A- and C-fiber nociceptors and mechanoreceptors. The transmuscular anterior QLB (or QLB3) facilitates the spread of local anesthetic into the thoracic paravertebral space, which produces prolonged block from 6 to 48 h and achieving visceral pain relief similar to epidural block [6, 18].

As a comparison to the bilateral QLB using 0.25% bupivacaine, postoperative epidural analgesia using 6 mL/h of 0.125% bupivacaine without opioid was considered a weak analgesic treatment to achieve mild to moderate analgesia after surgery. The total dose of local anesthetic determines the quality of block and the analgesic effect that could affect our study result. A meta-analysis showed a comparable pain score between the low and high concentrations of local anesthetic, however, a higher dose may have improved and prolonged the analgesic effect [19]. The epidural block remained the effective approach to produce a reliable analgesia for abdominal surgery compared to the QLB because of the spread of local anesthetic was vary depending on the site of injection that was highly associated with the coverage and quality of analgesia [20, 21]. Therefore, the optimal dose of local anesthetic for QLB still needs to be determined.

The epidural group showed lower MAP and required more ephedrine during observation compared to the QLB group. Epidural analgesia especially using high concentration more than 0.1% bupivacaine or equivalent ropivacaine dose has unfavorable side effects such as hypotension, especially in patients at risk of hemodynamic instability [10, 19] Zhu and colleagues found the combination of thoracic epidural and general anesthesia had lower systolic, diastolic and pulse pressure compared with general anesthesia alone in laparoscopic cholecystectomy [22].

We found the QLB using 0.25% bupivacaine relieved the pain in abdominal area as effective as epidural analgesia using 0.125% bupivacaine without limb motor blockade. Both groups showed the absence of lower extremity motor blockade represented by the Bromage score (0–1). A meta-analysis summarized that 0.1% or less bupivacaine and equivalent ropivacaine epidural concentration resulted in less motor blockade, earlier ambulation, and reduced urinary retention although most of the studies analyzed were using opioid additives

Table 3 Postoperative side effects of QLB versus continuous epidural analgesia

Parameter	QLB group ($n = 31$)	Epidural group ($n = 31$)	p-value	Mean difference (95% CI)
Bromage score after anesthesia recovery				
Immediately	1 (0.96–1.12)	1 (0.96–1.12)	1.000	0 (0.11–0.11)
At 2 h	1 (0.96–1.12)	1 (0.96–1.12)	1.000	0 (− 0.11–0.11)
At 6 h	1 (0.96–1.12)	1 (1–1)	0.327	0.04 (− 0.41–0.12)
At 12 h	1 (1–1)	1 (1–1)	1.000	–
At 24 h	1 (1–1)	1 (1–1)	1.000	–
Paresthesia (%)	0 (0.00)	1 (3.22)	0.05	–
Postoperative nausea and vomiting (%)	7 (22.58)	5 (16.12)	0.07	–
Duration of urinary catheter (hours)	37.03 ± 9.14	42.97 ± 5.72	0.004	− 6.73 (− 11.25 – − 2.21)

QLB Quadratus lumborum block. Data are presented as mean ± standard deviation or median (95% confidence interval) or number (percentage). Numerical values are compared using unpaired t-test or and Mann-Whitney test as appropriate. Categorical values are compared using Fisher's Exact Test-Exact sig. (1-sided) or Pearson Chi-square-Asymp. Sig. (2-sided). *P*-values of 0.05 or less are considered significant.

[19]. Paddalwar and colleagues reported the less motor block intensity without affecting the quality of analgesia in epidural analgesia using 0.125% bupivacaine [23]. The incidence of PONV was low and comparable between the QLB and epidural groups since there was no significant difference in the opioid requirement between the two groups.

Patients receiving QLB showed a significantly shorter duration of urinary catheterization than patients with continuous epidural analgesia. Early removal of the urinary catheter when it is no longer needed is recommended regarding postoperative early recovery because longer urinary catheterization can affect mobilization [24]. We noticed that some surgeons decided to remove the urinary catheter after the discontinuation of epidural analgesia due to the concern of urinary retention. From our observation, none of our patients in both groups required urinary re-catheterization, which was different from the study by Niraj and colleagues that found more patients with continuous epidural analgesia required urinary re-catheterization due to urinary retention than patients with continuous transversus abdominis plane block. Epidural analgesia acts on lumbar and sacral nerve fibers and blocks the bladder detrusor function [25]. Hayami and colleagues demonstrated that the urinary catheter removal before discontinuing epidural analgesia had higher incidences of postoperative urinary retention regardless of the amount of opioid use [25].

From the technical aspects and safety perspective, LAST was a concern in our study as the QLB was the bilateral high-volume local anesthetic block. However, the mean total bupivacaine requirement in the QLB group was significantly lower than the epidural group. We did not find any LAST symptoms during study observation given that the total dosage of local anesthetic in both groups were lower than the recommendation for bupivacaine to not exceed 2.5–3 mg/kg or 175 mg per injection with maximum dosage 400 mg in 24 h [26–28]. The thoracic epidural procedure is more challenging especially for the mid to high thoracic level compare to the lower thoracic or lumbar level. The sonoanatomic markers of the lateral (QLB1), posterior (QLB2) and intramuscular QLB are easy to find and safe to be performed in a supine position. The transmuscular anterior approach (QLB3) is considered as an invasive technique which is better performed in the lateral or supine slightly lateral position by the experienced practitioners [29].

Our study had several limitations. We did not include a control group using i.v. morphine PCA alone or the multimodal analgesia (MMA) regimen as the comparator in our study. Given that the results showed the low 24-h morphine consumption and NRS pain score, determining the true analgesic value of QLB and continuous epidural analgesia might be uncertain. However, our pain score results were lower than the pain score from a study by Gorevski and colleagues that compared i.v. PCA without any regional block to those using MMA [14]. Our results also showed the lower 24-h morphine consumptions in comparison to a study by Wang and colleagues on the laparoscopic nephrectomy patients using i.v PCA alone for the 24 h after surgery [14, 15]. Since the postoperative pain score of our study was relatively low, there was still a possibility that MMA without any regional block can achieve the same level of analgesia as the QLB or epidural analgesia alone. However, Capdevila and colleagues had proven the open nephrectomy patients receiving thoracic epidural analgesia experienced significantly less postoperative pain and morphine consumption compared to patients receiving the MMA regimen [30].

There was a lack of blinding because of the epidural block had a catheter inserted and the QLB was the bilateral injections without insertion of the catheter, but those are the common approach of the procedure in our clinical practice. The extent of block was confirmed only once after anesthesia recovery, and the analgesic efficacy was assessed only in 24 h after surgery following the policy in our institution that retains epidural catheter only for 24 h after laparoscopic surgery. Our subjects were representative of the normal BMI population that underwent laparoscopic nephrectomy in our institution. Therefore, generalizability is limited in the different population such as obese patient or other clinical contexts in which continuous QLB is available or epidural block can be maintained longer than 24 h.

Conclusion

The QLB has potential as the alternative pain management following laparoscopic nephrectomy. The QLB had a similar 24-h cumulative morphine requirement, higher postoperative mean arterial pressure, similar postoperative pain intensity, time of first analgesics, PONV, degree of motor and sensory blockade, and shorter duration of urinary catheterization in comparison with continuous epidural analgesia after transperitoneal laparoscopic nephrectomy. Further studies of the QLB regarding the optimal dosage of local anesthetic is needed.

Supplementary information

Additional file 1. Quadratus lumborum block sonography.

Additional file 2. Postoperative analgesic requirement of QLB versus continuous epidural analgesia.

Additional file 3. Perioperative hemodynamic profile of QLB versus continuous epidural analgesia.

Abbreviations

ASA: American Society of Anesthesiologists classification; BMI: Body mass index; L1, L2, L3, L4: First, second, third, fourth lumbar vertebral body; LAST: Local anesthetic systemic toxicity; MAP: Mean arterial pressure; MMA: Multimodal analgesic; NRS: Numerical rating scale; PCA: Patient-controlled analgesia; PONV: Postoperative nausea and vomiting; QLB: Quadratus lumborum block; T7, T8, T9, T10, T11, T12: Seventh, eighth, ninth, tenth, eleventh, twelfth thoracic vertebral body

Acknowledgements

Not applicable.

Authors' contributions

DA designed the study, performed the blocks, interpreted the results and drafted the manuscript. P participated in the design of the study, performed the blocks and interpreted the results. NA drafted the manuscript. AT participated in the interpretation of the results. CAM participated in the interpretation of the results. All authors read and approved the final manuscript.

Author details

[1]Department of Anesthesiology and Intensive Care, Cipto Mangunkusumo General Hospital, Universitas Indonesia, 6th Salemba Raya, DKI Jakarta 10430, Indonesia. [2]Department of Urology, Cipto Mangunkusumo General Hospital, Universitas Indonesia, DKI Jakarta, Indonesia.

References

1. Wisbono E, Wahyudi I, Mochtar CA, Hamid ARA, Sukmono RB. Laparoscopic living donor nephrectomy in cipto mangunkusumo hospital: Postoperativepain and recovery analysis. Adv Sci Lett. 2018;24:6704–8. https://doi.org/10.1166/asl.2018.12816.
2. Alper I, Yuksel E. Comparison of acute and chronic pain after open nephrectomy versus laparoscopic nephrectomy: a prospective clinical trial. Medicine (Baltimore). 2016;95(16):e3433. https://doi.org/10.1097/MD.0000000000003433.
3. Ergün M, Berkers AW, van der Jagt MF, Langenhuijsen JF, van Özdemir-Brunschot D, van der Vliet JA. F. C. D'Ancona, Warlé MC. Components of pain assessment after laparoscopic donor nephrectomy. Acta Anaesthesiol Scand. 2014;58(2):219–22. https://doi.org/10.1111/aas.12236.
4. Sahajananda H. Jyothi, Punithavathy. Renal transplantation with and without epidural analgesia. Indian J Anesth. 2006;50(3):187–92.
5. Blanco R, Ansari T, Riad W, Shetty N. Quadratus lumborum block versus transversus abdominis plane block for postoperative pain after cesarean delivery: a randomized controlled trial. Reg Anesth Pain Med. 2016;41(6):757–62. https://doi.org/10.1097/AAP.0000000000000495.
6. Onwochei DN, Børglum J, Pawa A. Abdominal wall blocks for intra-abdominal surgery. BJA Educ. 2018;18(10):317–22. https://doi.org/10.1016/j.bjae.2018.07.002.
7. Ishio J, Komasawa N, Kido H, Minami T. Evaluation of ultrasound-guided posterior quadratus lumborum block for postoperative analgesia after laparoscopic gynecologic surgery. J Clin Anesth. 2017;41:1–4. https://doi.org/10.1016/j.jclinane.2017.05.015.
8. Murouchi T, Iwasaki S, Yamakage M. Quadratus lumborum block: analgesic effects and chronological ropivacaine concentrations after laparoscopic surgery. Reg Anesth Pain Med. 2016;41(2):146–50. https://doi.org/10.1097/AAP.0000000000000349.
9. McCrum CL, Ben-David B, Shin JJ, Wright VJ. Quadratus lumborum block provides improve immediate postoperative analgesia and decreased opioid use compared with a multimodal pain regimen following hip arthroscopy. J Hip Preserv Surg. 2018;5(3):233–9. https://doi.org/10.1093/jhps/hny024.
10. Corso RM, Pirracini E, Sorbello M, Bellantonio D, Tedesco M. Ultrasound-guided transmuscular quadratus lumborum block for perioperative analgesia in open nephrectomy. Minerva Anestesiol. 2017;83(12):1334–5. https://doi.org/10.23736/S0375-9393.17.12167-X.
11. Ueshima H, Otake H, Lin J. Ultrasound-guided quadratus lumborum block: an updated review of anatomy and techniques. Biomed Res Int. 2017. https://doi.org/10.1155/2017/2752876.
12. Afsham G, Chohan U, Khan A, Chaudry N, Khan ZE, Khan AA. Appropriate length of epidural catheter in the epidural space for postoperative analgesia: evaluation by epidurography. Anaesthesia. 2011;66:913–8. https://doi.org/10.1111/j.1365-2044.2011.06820.x.
13. Abdelsalam K, Mohamdin OW. Ultrasound-guided rectus sheath and transversus abdominis plane blocks for perioperative analgesia in upper abdominal surgery: A randomized controlled study. Saudi J Anaesth. 2016;10(1):25–8. https://doi.org/10.4103/1658-354X.169470.
14. Gorevski E, Wead S, Tevar A, Succop P, Volek P, Martin-Boone J. Retrospective evaluation of donor pain and pain management after laprascopic nephrectomy. Transplant Proc. 2011;43(7):2487–91. https://doi.org/10.1016/j.transproceed.2011.06.038.
15. Wang J, Mab H, Fua Y, Wang N. Comparison of postoperative morphine requirements in renal donors and patients with renal carcinoma undergoing laparoscopic nephrectomy. Transplant Proc. 2016;48:31–4. https://doi.org/10.1016/j.transproceed.2015.12.032.
16. Lavoie A, Toledo P. Multimodal postcesarean delivery analgesia. Clin Perinatol. 2013;40(3):443–55. https://doi.org/10.1016/j.clp.2013.05.008.
17. Dam M, Moriggl B, Hansen CK, Hoerman R, Bendtsen TF, Borglum J. The pathway of injectate spread with the transmuscular quadratus lumborum block: a cadaver study. Anesth Analg. 2017;125(1):303–12. https://doi.org/10.1213/ANE.0000000000001922.
18. Elsharkawy H, El-Boghdadly K, Barrington M. Quadratus lumborum block: anatomical concepts, mechanism, and techniques. Anesthesiology. 2019;130(2):322–35. https://doi.org/10.1097/ALN.0000000000002524.
19. Sultan P, Murphy C, Halpern S, Carvalho B. The effect of low concentrations versus high concentrations of local anesthetics for labour analgesia on obstetric and anesthetic outcomes: a meta-analysis. Can J Anesth. 2013;60(9):840–54. https://doi.org/10.1007/s12630-013-9981-z.
20. Ng SC, Habib AS, Sodha S, Carvalho B, Sultan P. High-dose versus low-dose local anaesthetic for transversus abdominis plane block post-caesarean delivery analgesia: a meta-analysis. Br J Anaesth. 2018;120(2):252–63. https://doi.org/10.1016/j.bja.2017.11.084.
21. Kang W, Lu D, Yang X, Zhou Z, Chen X, Chen K, Zhou X, Feng X. Postoperative analgesic effects of various quadratus lumborum block approaches following cesarean section: a randomized controlled trial. J Pain Res. 2019;12:2305–12. https://doi.org/10.2147/JPR.S202772.
22. Zhu J, Zhang X, Yang H. Effects of combined epidural and general anesthesia on intraoperative hemodynamic responses, postoperative cellular immunity, and prognosis in patients with gallbladder cancer: a randomized controlled trial. Medicine (Baltimore). 2017;96(10):e6137. https://doi.org/10.1097/MD.0000000000006137.
23. Paddalwar S, Nagrale M, Chandak A, Shrivastava D, Papalkar J. A randomized, double-blind, controlled study comparing bupivacaine 0.125% and ropivacaine 0.125%, both with fentanyl 2 μg/ml, for labor epidural analgesia. Indian J Pain. 2013;27(3):147–53. https://doi.org/10.4103/0970-5333.124599.
24. Akerman M, Nada P, Ivan V. A review of the quadratus lumborum block and ERAS. Front Med (Lausanne). 2018;5:44. https://doi.org/10.3389/fmed.2018.00044.
25. Hayami S, Ueno M, Kawai M, Kuriyama T, Kawamata T, Yamaue H. Optimal timing of removal of epidural and urethral catheters to avoid postoperative urinary retention undergoing abdominal surgery. Dig Surg. 2018;36(3):261–5. https://doi.org/10.1159/000490199.
26. University of Iowa Health Care. Maximum recommended doses and duration of local anesthetics. https://medicine.uiowa.edu/iowaprotocols/maximum-recommended-doses-and-duration-local-anesthetics (2018). Accessed: 1 Apr 2018.
27. McGee DL. Local and topical anesthesia. In: Roberts JR, Custalow CB, Thomsen TW, editors. Roberts and hedges' clinical procedures in emergency medicine and acute care. Amsterdam: Elsevier Academic Press; 2019. p. 519–40.
28. Nolan JP. Anaesthesia and neuromuscular block. In: Brown MJ, Sharma P, Mir FA, Bennett PN, editors. Clinical pharmacology. Amsterdam: Elsevier Academic Press; 2019. p. 308–23.
29. Manion SC, Brennan TJ. Thoracic epidural analgesia and acute pain management. Anesthesiology. 2011;115(1):181–8. https://doi.org/10.1097/ALN.0b013e318220847c.
30. Capdevila X, Moulard S, Plasse C, Peshaud JL, Molinari N, Dadure C, Bringuier S. Effectiveness of epidural analgesia, continuous surgical site analgesia, and patient-controlled analgesic morphine for postoperative pain management and hyperalgesia, rehabilitation, and health-related quality of life after open nephrectomy: a prospective, randomized, controlled study. Anesth Analg. 2017;124(1):336–45. https://doi.org/10.1213/ANE.0000000000001688.

3

Analgesic efficacy of ultrasound-guided paravertebral block in percutaneous nephrolithotomy patients

Ferda Yaman[1*] and Devrim Tuglu[2]

Abstract

Background: Paravertabral blocks (PVB) are in use to adequately manage pain arising from a variety of operations on the thorax, abdomen or pelvis. PVB is straightforward, efficacious in operations performed. This study was undertaken to evaluate how efficacious ultrasound-guided thoracic paravertebral block is when used in patients undergoing percutaneous nephrolithotomy (PCN).

Methods: A total of 44 patients, falling in categories I to III of the American Society of Anesthesiologists, and aged between 18 and 65 years, who were scheduled for PCN, were randomly distributed into two groups. The anaesthetic intervention group (PVB) contained 22 individuals, who were injected at level T8-T9 with 20 mL 0.25% bupivacaine as a single administration. In the control group C, also containing 22 individuals, the intervention was not carried out. The groups were compared after PCN in terms of opioid use, pain score, opioid adverse effects profile and the need for supplemental analgesia.

Results: Visual analogue scale pain scores whilst at rest or moving were lower at the level of statistical significance in the PVB group compared to controls at 2 and 4 h post-surgery. At 6 and 8 h post-surgery, the control group had a lower VAS score when moving, and this result reached statistical significance ($p < 0.05$). The controls used more opioid relief than the PVB group and had lower scores for satisfaction ($p < 0.05$).

Conclusion: Ultrasound-guided PVB using bupivacaine and an in-plane technique provides effective analgesia in PNL. It is associated with high scores on patient satisfaction and minimal complications.

Keywords: Ultrasound, Paravertebral block, Percutaneous nephrolithotomy

Background

PCN (percutaneous nephrolithotomy) is a frequently employed, minimally invasive operative technique technique used to remove renal calculi [1]. The technique remains associated with significant demand for analgesic interventions post-surgically. The application of regional anaesthesia is known to possess the highest efficacy in managing pain following surgery of this sort [2]. There are a number of methods available which may potentially reduce postoperative pain associated with nephrostomy tube placement in PCN, namely intercostal nervous blockade, epidural analgesia, peritubal infiltration of local anaesthetic and paravertebral blockade [3–5]. Paravertabral blocks (PVB) are in use to adequately

* Correspondence: ferdayaman@gmail.com; fyaman@ogu.edu.tr
[1]Department of Anesthesiology and Reanimation, Faculty of Medicine, University of Eskişehir Osmangazi, 26040 Eskişehir, Turkey

manage pain arising from a variety of operations on the thorax, abdomen or pelvis. PVB is straightforward, low risk and is efficacious in operations performed unilaterally. It rarely creates hypotension, urinary retention or nausea and vomiting following surgery [6]. PVB performed under ultrasonic guidance (PVB-US) targets the region of emergence of the spinal nerves through the foramina of the vertebrae. It blocks somatic and sympathetic fibres supplying several adjacent dermatomal segments both superior and inferior to where the injection is given [7].

The study's main aim was evaluating analgesic efficacy in PVB-US to the thorax, whilst the secondary aim was assessment of how satisfied patients were with the procedure and how much rescue analgesia was needed in such cases.

Methods

Ethical approval was obtained from the Local Ethics Committee of Kırıkkale University, Kırıkkale, Turkey (No.04/03) and registered retrospectively on the ClinicalTrials.gov database under registration number NCT04406012. The inclusion criteria of this study were an age of 18–65 years and an American Society of Anesthesiologists classification of I or III scheduled for PCN from February 2016 to july 2016. Patients participating the study is shown in the CONSORT diagram (Fig. 1). (No.04/03) and registered retrospectively on the ClinicalTrials.gov database under registration number NCT04406012. Of the 53 individuals with eligibility to join the trial, 5 refused to join and 4 had significant haemorrhage during PCN, so that open surgery was then needed. Thus 44 individuals, ranging from category I to III in the classification scheme of the American Society of Anesthesiologists, were actually enrolled. All trial participants provided written, informed consent. The exclusion criteria were: age below 18 years; current pregnancy; allergy to local anaesthetic drugs; bleeding disorder; depressive illness or anxiety disorder; being obese (i.e. BMI above 35); previous pneumothorax; phrenic nerve paralysis; stenotic aorta of severe degree. The participants in the trial were allocated into one of two groups – those receiving the anaesthetic intervention (thoracic paravertebral block: PVB) and control subjects – using the closed envelope randomisation technique 1 h prior to surgery before admission to the operating room by the nurse of urology yard. Monitoring electrocardiogram (ECG), peripheral pulse oximetry and external blood pressure measurement) was set up at 5 min intervals.

Postoperative analgesia requirements were evaluated using the visual analogue scale (VAS), which ranges in value from 0, indicating an absence of pain, to 10, indicating pain of high severity. The evaluations were performed at 1, 2, 4, 6, 8, 10, 12 and 24 h post-surgery. The score was checked when the patient was resting and when moving (such as when deeply inspiring or coughing). A VAS score above 4 was taken to indicate a need for extra pain relief. The control group were given a standard post-surgical analgesia regime, i.e. dexketoprofen 50 mg i.v. Where administering dexketoprofen did not result in a VAS score below 4, tramadol was co-administered at a dosage of 1 mg per kg body weight.

The individuals in the PVB group all received paravertebral blocks. This group all underwent monitoring via ECG, external BP measurement and pulse oximetry within theatre before PVB was undertaken. Anaesthetic induction occurred after PVB placement. The patient assumed a seated position and a linear 10–18 MHz ultrasound probe (EsaoteMyLab 30, Geneva, Italy) was positioned paramedially over the space between two transverse processes. The transverse processes of the T9 and T10 vertebrae and the superior pleura and costotransverse ligament were visualised. An 80 mm long needle of 22 gauge (Pajunk, Geisingen, Germany) was inserted under ultrasonic guidance and 10 mL bupivacaine hydrochloride (Marcaine 0.5%, Astra Zeneca) dissolved in 20 ml solution was infiltrated into the paravertebral space. The needle is advanced to the point where the superior costotransverse ligament crosses the space. The dispersal of the local anaesthetic agent over the pleura was observed, along with its displacement. All PVBs were undertaken by the same, experienced anaesthetist.

After the paravertebral block was performed, all patients received standardized general anesthetic technique with 2–2.5 mg kg^{-1} propofol, 0.6 mg kg^{-1} rocuronium, 1–2 mcg kg^{-1} fentanyl and anesthesia was maintained with sevoflurane and oxygen-air mixture. Intraoperative dose of additional opioid was different and noted in anesthesia follow-up form.

The pain scores using VAS were noted in both groups post-procedure. The degree of patient comfort was also noted. The occurrence of nausea and vomiting and any need for further pain relief was noted. At 24 h post surgery patient satisfaction was noted. A scale of 1 to 5 was employed for this, ranging from 1 (very unsatisfied) to 5 (very satisfied). The same urologist performed the surgery in all cases.

A power calculation was performed with the G * Power 3.1.9.4 statistical package application using the following parameters: n1 = 22, n2 = 22, $\alpha = 0.05$, (effect size) d = 0.9; (power $(1-\beta)) = 0.83$. The data obtained were evaluated using the IBM SPSS 25.0 statistical application. The Chi-Square statistic was used in comparisons. Descriptive statistics were obtained for the data (frequency, percentage, mean, standard deviation, median, min-max), both continuous and categorical. The

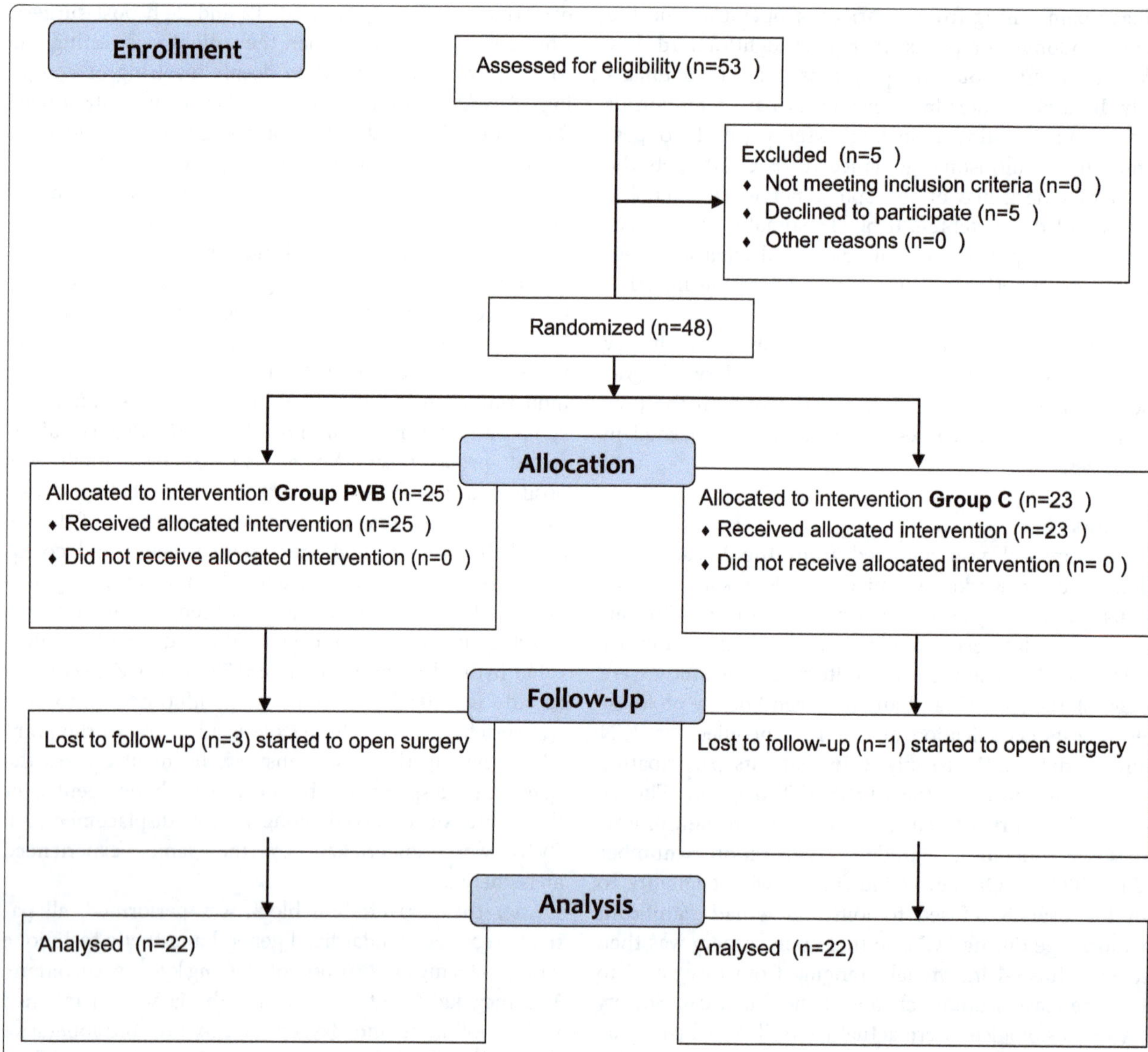

Fig. 1 CONSORT flow diagram. Consolidated Standards of Reporting Trials (CONSORT) flow diagram showing patients' recruitment and allocation

data were tested for normal distribution using the Shapiro-Wilk test. The independent samples t Test was employed for comparisons involving normally distributed quantitative data in the groups, and the Mann–Whitney U test was used in the analysis of non-normally distributed data. The paired samples t test (t test in dependent groups) was employed for within-group comparisons. A p value below 0.05 was taken to indicate statistical significance.

Results

The groups did not differ at the level of statistical significance in terms of sex, age, weight, BMI or classification under the ASA rubric ($p > 0.05$). Both groups were the same from a statistical point of view in terms of opioid use during the surgery and in post-surgical satisfaction score ($p > 0.05$). In the post-surgical period, group C used a greater amount of opioid for pain relief than group PVB, and they were less satisfied with the procedure overall ($p < 0.05$). See Table 1.

The length of time for the operation was between 115 and 127 min. Figure 2 provides the variation in mean arterial pressure and Fig. 3 the cardiac rate during surgery.

At 1 h post-operatively, the VAS score was higher during movement (deep breath, "dynamic") than at rest and this differnce attained statistical significance. In group C, VAS was higher during movement than at rest ($p < 0.05$).

At 2 and 4 h post-operatively, the VAS score was higher in group C, both at rest and while moving. These results were statistically significant.

Table 1 Demographic data of patients, intraoperatively opioid consumption and patient satisfaction scores between groups

		Block (*n* = 22)	Control (*n* = 22)	P
Gender	female	6 (%27,3)	12 (%54,5)	0,125 [a]
	male	16 (%72,7)	10 (%45,5)	
Age (year-old)		50,3 ± 10,5	48,7 ± 14,1	0,673 [b]
Body Mass Index (kg/m^2)		28,0 ± 4,1	30,7 ± 5,2	0,059 [b]
ASA	I	5 (%22,7)	2 (%9,1)	0,447 [a]
	II	15 (%68,2)	17 (%77,3)	
	III	2 (%9,1)	3 (%13,6)	
Intraoperative opioid consumption		98,0 ± 27,5	132,3 ± 39,8	**0,002** [b]
Patient Satisfaction Score		4,0 ± 0,7	3,0 ± 0,7	**0,000** [b]

[a]Chi Square Test
[b]Independent Samples t Test

At 6 and 8 h post-operatively, the VAS "at rest" score did not differ significantly between groups ($p > 0.05$) but the VAS score "moving" was significantly higher in group C ($p < 0.05$). Additionally, the VAS scores differed significantly within the C group when "at rest" and "moving" scores were compared ($p < 0.05$), with the latter being higher, i.e. indicating more discomfort.

At 10 and 12 h post-operatively, the VAS "moving" scores were significantly higher in group C ($p < 0.05$).

At 24 h post-operatively, both dynamic and resting VAS scores did not differ at the level of statistical significance, neither resting nor moving ($p > 0.05$). See Table 2: Evaluation of VAS scores at rest and while moving (mean ± SD)).

There was a statistical difference found in the rate of requiring extra pain relief at 1, 2, 4, 8 10, 12 and 24 h post-surgically. In all cases, group C had greater need for analgesia ($p < 0.05$). See Table 3.

The two groups did not differ at the level of statistical significance for nausea and vomiting at any point ($p > 0.05$).

No complications, e.g. local anaesthetic toxicity, vascular puncture, pneumothorax, inadvertent epidural injection or spinal anesthesia were noted.

Discussion

The satisfaction score following percutaneous nephrolithotomy was high in the group PVB, indicating that PVB is sufficient to provide post-surgical analgesia after such a procedure. Up to 6 h after surgery, the individuals who underwent PVB scored significantly better on VAS than those in whom this anaesthetic procedure was not undertaken. This superiority did not persist after the 6 h post-surgical interval.

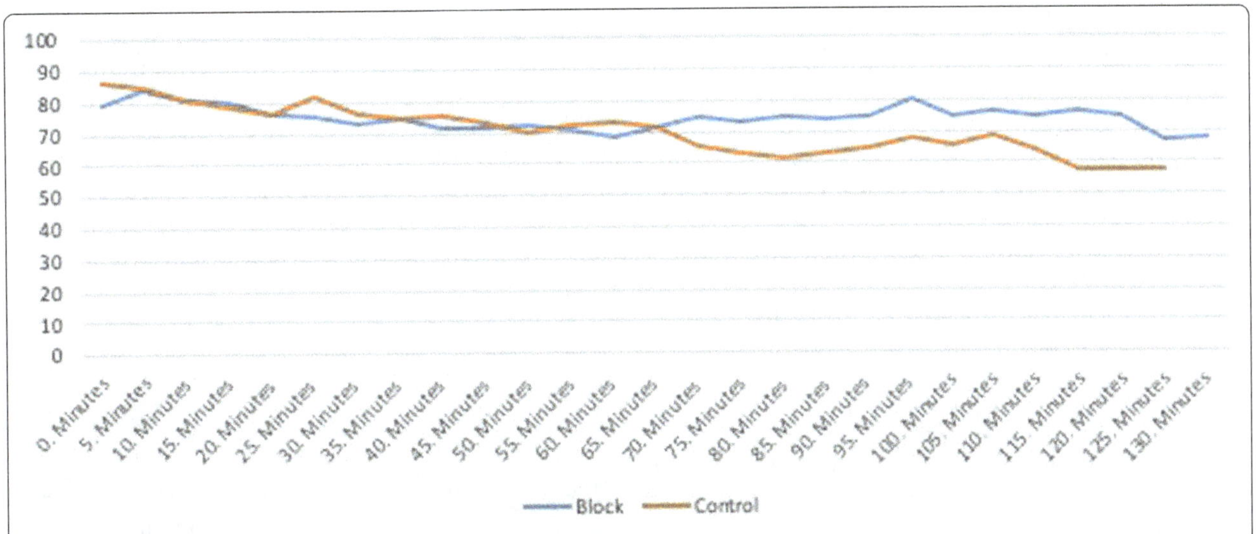

Fig. 2 Changes in Mean Arterial Pressure between the groups intraoperatively

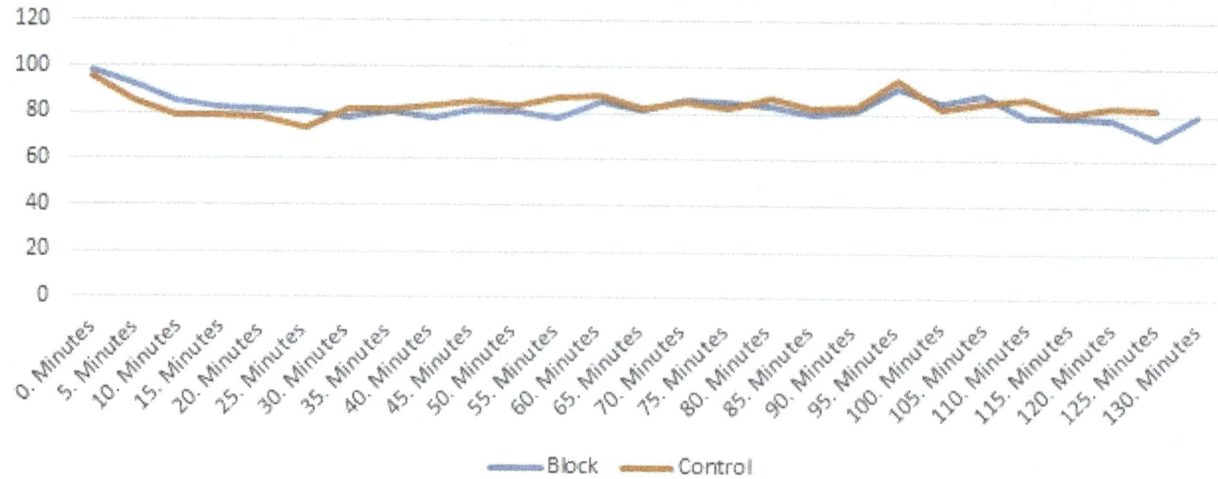

Fig. 3 Changes in Heart Rate between the groups intraoperatively

Table 2 Evaluation of the visual analog score at rest (Mean ± SD)

VAS		Block (*n* = 22)	Control (*n* = 22)	P*
1. hour	rest	0,5 ± 1,2	2,5 ± 3,2	**0,016**
	dynamic	0,7 ± 1,5	2,8 ± 3,5	**0,014**
	P**	0,083	**0,017**	
2. hour	rest	2,4 ± 2,1	4,6 ± 3,5	**0,014**
	dynamic	2,8 ± 2,2	5,0 ± 3,9	**0,022**
	P**	**0,001**	**0,025**	
4. hour	rest	1,5 ± 1,2	3,2 ± 3,2	**0,029**
	dynamic	1,9 ± 1,5	4,0 ± 3,5	**0,011**
	P**	**0,002**	**0,000**	
6. hour	rest	1,3 ± 1,1	3,0 ± 2,6	**0,010**
	dynamic	1,5 ± 1,4	4,0 ± 2,9	**0,001**
	P**	0,104	**0**	
8. hour	rest	1,2 ± 1,2	2,2 ± 2,2	0,071
	dynamic	1,4 ± 1,3	3,0 ± 2,6	**0,016**
	P**	0,057	**0,000**	
10. hour	rest	1,0 ± 1,0	1,8 ± 2,0	0,079
	dynamic	1,3 ± 1,2	2,1 ± 2,5	0,172
	P**	**0,005**	0,056	
12. hour	rest	0,6 ± 0,8	1,0 ± 1,6	0,354
	dynamic	0,9 ± 1,2	1,3 ± 2,0	0,462
	P**	**0,011**	0,056	
24. hour	rest	0,2 ± 0,7	0,4 ± 0,8	0,413
	dynamic	0,0 ± 0,2	0,5 ± 1,3	0,080
	P**	0,186	0,162	

* Independent Samples t Test
** Paired Samples t Test

The results from this study are in line with other published research on using PVB in PCN. However, there are disparities in the other studies in terms of timing, optimal concentration of local anaesthetic and the level at which to inject. It is also unclear whether one or more infiltrations of local anaesthetic are needed [5, 8–11].

Different techniques have been employed previously for PVB. A technique relying on loss of resistance has been described, which was in use before ultrasound guidance became available within operating theatres. Ak, K. et al. described injecting 0.5% levobupivacaine at the level of the tenth, eleventh and twelfth thoracic

Table 3 Additional analgesic consumption between the groups

Additional tramadol		Block (*n* = 22)	Control (*n* = 22)	P[a]
1. hour	no	22 (%100,0)	20 (%90,9)	0,488
	yes	0 (%0,0)	2 (%9,1)	
2. hour	no	13 (%59,1)	9 (%40,9)	0,366
	yes	9 (%40,9)	13 (%59,1)	
4. hour	no	21 (%95,5)	18 (%81,8)	0,345
	yes	1 (%4,5)	4 (%18,2)	
6. hour	no	21 (%95,5)	14 (%63,6)	**0,021**
	yes	1 (%4,5)	8 (%36,4)	
8. hour	no	22 (%100,0)	20 (%90,9)	0,488
	yes	0 (%0,0)	2 (%9,1)	
10. hour	no	22 (%100,0)	19 (%86,4)	0,233
	yes	0 (%0,0)	3 (%13,6)	
12. hour	no	22 (%100,0)	22 (%100,0)	1000
	yes	0 (%0,0)	0 (%0,0)	
24. hour	no	22 (%100,0)	22 (%100,0)	1000
	yes	0 (%0,0)	0 (%0,0)	

[a]Chi Square Test

vertebrae. 4 mL were infiltrated at each level as the surgery, conducted under general anaesthesia, ended. These researchers noted that pain at rest as assessed by VAS was significantly improved following PVB, for 2 h post-surgery [10]. The present study differed in how PVB was used. In the present study, the patient was conscious and sitting upright as 20 mL bupivacaine 0.25% was infiltrated. We found pain relief lasted for 6 h post-surgically. The difference in observed outcome compared to other studies may relate to the difference in injection volume and the prolonged action duration of bupivacaine compared to levobupivacaine.

Hatipoğlu et al. reported on performing PVB at levels T11, T12, L1 prior to surgery but with the patient under general anaesthesia and placed in a prone position. They employed 0.5% bupivacaine, injecting 5 ml per level under ultrasound guidance. Thus the total volume of local anaesthetic was 15 mL. These authors state that analgesia was mantained up to 24 h post-surgery [9]. Our findings reveal that the VAS-rated discomfort was significantly lower in group PVB than in group C until 12 h post-surgery when the patient was moving, but not while at rest. We performed the procedure without patient sedation, with the patient sitting upright before the operation.

Patient positioning may affect the distribution of local anaesthetic from a single injection when the concentration is low. This may be the explanation for the difference of duration of analgesia.

Yayık et al. investigated analgesia procured through PVB vs peritubal infiltration. VAS dynamic and resting scores were significantly lower in the PVB group than the peritubal infiltration group or a control group at all time points following surgery up to 24 h post-surgery. They performed the PVB procedure with the patient in the prone position. They employed 0.25% bupivacaine injected at levels T8–9, at the end of surgery [11]. Our study used the same concentration and volume of bupivacaine, however PVB was undertaken prior to surgery.

A different study also employed PVB in percutaneous nephrolithotomy. A catheter was inserted into the paravertebral space at level T10 prior to commencing surgery. Catheter insertion was in awake patients, sitting upright. Ultrasonic guidance was not used. Twenty mL bupivacaine 0.5% was injected prior to surgery. Rescue analgesia was noted to be required first at 275 min post-surgery [8]. The duration of analgesia achieved with this volume and concentration indicates that PVB involving a single injection is insufficient for complete analgesia postoperatively over the first 24 h post-surgery. However, it does lead to a decreased need for systemic analgesic drugs. In our study, we used a lower concentration but the same volume of bupivacaine. For the first 4 h post-surgery, VAS scores, both dynamic and resting, were significantly lower in group PVB than in the control group. Our results indicate that the duration of PVB is 6 h using bupivacaine 0.25% in 20 mL total volume.

Baldea et al. report on a study in which PVB block was performed at the level of T10 by means of a single injection of 20 mL 0.5% bupivacaine. The block was performed prior to surgery with the patient seated and under ultrasound guidance. The first dose of opioids for relief analgesia was given at 119.7 min post-surgically in the PVB group [12].

It is clear that PVB is efficacious in providing analgesia for percutaneous nephrolithotomy. Indeed, PVB, together with epidural anaesthesia, are considered Gold Standard procedures. Newer studies have focused on lengthening the duration of analgesia through the addition of adjuvant therapy, notably clonidine and dexmedetomidine [13, 14].

Kamble et al. compared PVB for PCNL using either 0.5% Bupivacaine alone or 0.5% Bupivacaine plus 1 µg/kg of clonidine: PVB was performed prior to surgery in awake patients in the sitting position. Clonidine was shown to have an adjunctive role with bupivacaine, providing a higher quality paravertebral block and prolonging analgesia to a significant extent post-surgically. The dosage employed took account of patient weight: 15 ml in patients with a weight below 60 kg and 18 ml in patients with a weight exceeding 60 kg [13]. Our study, did not address whether adjuvant pharmacological agents affect the duration of analgesia, although it did establish that a single injection of 0.25% bupivacaine in 20 mL volume produced an analgesic effect lasting 8 h after surgery ended.

Another study examined the use of PVB in video-assisted thoracic surgery (VATS). In that study, two treatments were compared: ropivacaine 0.5% in a volume of 30 mL with adjuvant dexmedetomidine 50 microgram or ropivacaine 0.5% in 30 mL alone. The level of injection was between T3 and T5. Two injections were given in the lateral decubitus position. The treatment was post-surgical but before the patient recovered consciousness. Adjuvant dexmedetomidine lengthened the duration of analgesia obtainable with bupivacaine alone. The pain score at rest (assessed using VAS) did not differ significantly at any point postoperatively, with the exception of 4 h post-surgery. In the adjuvant therapy group, the maximum VAS pain scores for the 24 h post-operative period while resting or when coughing were lower than those seen in the group receiving ropivacaine alone. This result attained statistical significance [14]. It seems that further research is needed to determine the optimal dose of local anaesthetics with or without adjuvant and to clarify the ideal timing to perform PVB, i.e. before surgery or post-surgically.

Our study showed that patient satisfaction was higher in the PVB group than group C. If PVB is performed in awake patients, a single injection may be preferable to multiple injections. Research on cadavers demonstrated that the spread of infiltrated anaesthetic was no different, whether injection occurred singly or at two levels. This study also employed ultrasonic guidance [15]. Additionally, some research has evaluated single injection vs multiple injection in PVB to the thorax. The trial participants underwent VATS, after which they had PVB using nerve stimulators to guide the injection. In terms of efficacy, the single puncture technique was potentially superior to multiple puncture, since the patients were more satisfied, the procedure took less time and there was a lower risk of developing complications [16].

Whilst PVB has become the de facto Gold Standard in chest surgery, this has yet to be acknowledged in the literature on the subject [17]. A number of studies have demonstrated the safety and efficacy of PVB to provide analgesia perioperatively in procedures affecting the kidney [18, 19].

The reports published so far about the occurrence of complications mention a risk of inadvertent epidural or intrathecal injection in approaching 1% of cases. Ultrasound was not used for guidance where this occurred. Total spinal anaesthesia has occurred on some occasions [20]. Total spinal anaesthesia has even occurred once when ultrasonic guidance was in use, but this case was approached with an out-of-plane technique [21]. This study followed a retrospective design to assess the degree of complications associated with single-puncture, transverse, in-plane PVB with ultrasonic guidance. All participants underwent mastectomy. Some 1427 PVBs were performed on the thorax, with no more than 6 complications occurring. Amongst other complications, bradycardia leading to symptoms with hypotension (n = 3), one vasovagal attack (n = 1), and a potentially toxic reaction to the local anaesthetic (n = 2). Neither inadvertent rupture of the pleura nor a pneumothorax leading to symptoms occurred [22].

Both in this study and in the authors' routine practice, the authors have a preference for the in-plane anaesthetic technique. Complications of the technique, including bleeding or technical issues, did not occur.

This study suffers from certain limitations. For example, we were unable to assess precisely the tramadol dosage needed, since patient-controlled analgesia, which would give a clear picture, was not used. In addition, the area of block achieved was not precisely delineated by performing a sensory neurological examination.

Conclusion

Ultrasound-guided PVB using bupivacaine and an in-plane technique provides effective analgesia in PNL. It is associated with high scores on patient satisfaction and minimal complications.

Abbreviations

PVB: Paravertebral block; BP: blood pressure; VAS: Visual analogue score; PCN: Percutaneous nephrolithotomy; PVB-US: PVB performed under ultrasonic guidance; ASA: Classification of American Society of Anesthesiologists; ECG: Electrocardiogram; BMI: Body Mass Index

Acknowledgements

N/A

Authors' contributions

FY conceived the idea, designed the study, interpreted the data, collected and analyzed the data and wrote the manuscript draft. DT helped to collect data and interpretation of the data. All authors read and approved the final manuscript.

Author details

[1]Department of Anesthesiology and Reanimation, Faculty of Medicine, University of Eskişehir Osmangazi, 26040 Eskişehir, Turkey. [2]Department of Urology, Faculty of Medicine, University of Kırıkkale, Kırıkkale, Turkey.

References

1. Preminger GM. Percutaneous nephrolithotomy: an extreme technical makeover for an old technique. Arch Ital Urol Androl. 2010;82(1):23–5.
2. Rawal N. Current issues in postoperative pain management. Eur J Anaesthesiol. 2016;33(3):160–71. https://doi.org/10.1097/EJA.0000000000000366.
3. Singh I, Yadav OK, Gupta S. Efficacy of intercostal nerve block with 0.25% bupivacaine in percutaneous nephrolithotomy: a prospective randomized clinical trial. Urol Ann. 2019;11(4):363–8. https://doi.org/10.4103/UA.UA_141_18.
4. Wang J, Zhang C, Tan D, et al. The effect of local anesthetic infiltration around nephrostomy tract on postoperative pain control after percutaneous nephrolithotomy: a systematic review and meta-analysis. Urol Int. 2016;97(2): 125–33. https://doi.org/10.1159/000447306.
5. Li C, Song C, Wang W, Song C, Kong X. Thoracic paravertebral block versus epidural anesthesia combined with moderate sedation for percutaneous nephrolithotomy. Med Princ Pract. 2016;25(5):417–22. https://doi.org/10.1159/000447401.
6. Davies RG, Myles PS, Graham JM. A comparison of the analgesic efficacy and side-effects of paravertebral vs epidural blockade for thoracotomy--a systematic review and meta-analysis of randomized trials [published correction appears in Br J Anaesth. 2007 Nov;99(5):768]. Br J Anaesth. 2006; 96(4):418–26. https://doi.org/10.1093/bja/ael020.
7. Richardson J, Lönnqvist PA, Naja Z. Bilateral thoracic paravertebral block: potential and practice. Br J Anaesth. 2011;106(2):164–71. https://doi.org/10.1093/bja/aeq378.
8. Borle AP, Chhabra A, Subramaniam R, et al. Analgesic efficacy of paravertebral bupivacaine during percutaneous nephrolithotomy: an observer blinded, randomized controlled trial. J Endourol. 2014;28(9):1085–90. https://doi.org/10.1089/end.2014.0179.
9. Hatipoglu Z, Gulec E, Turktan M, et al. Comparative study of ultrasound-guided paravertebral block versus intravenous tramadol for postoperative pain control in percutaneous nephrolithotomy. BMC Anesthesiol. 2018;18(1): 24. Published 2018 Feb 17. https://doi.org/10.1186/s12871-018-0479-7.
10. Ak K, Gursoy S, Duger C, et al. Thoracic paravertebral block for postoperative pain management in percutaneous nephrolithotomy patients: a randomized controlled clinical trial. Med Princ Pract. 2013;22(3):229–33. https://doi.org/10.1159/000345381.
11. Yayik AM, Ahiskalioglu A, Demirdogen SO, Ahiskalioglu EO, Alici HA, Kursad H. Ultrasound-guided low thoracic paravertebral block versus peritubal infiltration for percutaneous nephrolithotomy: a prospective randomized study. Urolithiasis. 2020;48(3):235–44. https://doi.org/10.1007/s00240-018-01106-w.
12. Baldea KG, Patel PM, Delos Santos G, et al. Paravertebral block for percutaneous nephrolithotomy: a prospective, randomized, double-blind placebo-controlled study [published online ahead of print, 2020 Jan 25]. World J Urol. 2020. https://doi.org/10.1007/s00345-020-03093-3.
13. Kamble TS, Deshpande CM. Evaluation of the efficacy of bupivacaine (0.5%)

alone or with clonidine (1 µg/kg) versus control in a single level paravertebral blockin patients undergoing PCNL procedure. J Clin Diagn Res. 2016;10(12):UC13–7. https://doi.org/10.7860/JCDR/2016/20890.9033.
14. Hong B, Lim C, Kang H, et al. Thoracic paravertebral block with adjuvant dexmedetomidine in video-assisted thoracoscopic surgery: a randomized, double-blind study. J Clin Med. 2019;8(3):352. Published 2019 Mar 12. https://doi.org/10.3390/jcm8030352.
15. Cowie B, McGlade D, Ivanusic J, Barrington MJ. Ultrasound-guided thoracic paravertebral blockade: a cadaveric study. Anesth Analg. 2010;110(6):1735–9. https://doi.org/10.1213/ANE.0b013e3181dd58b0.
16. Kaya FN, Turker G, Mogol EB, Bayraktar S. Thoracic paravertebral block for video-assisted thoracoscopic surgery: single injection versus multiple injections. J Cardiothorac Vasc Anesth. 2012;26(1):90–4. https://doi.org/10.1053/j.jvca.2011.09.008.
17. D'Ercole F, Arora H, Kumar PA. Paravertebral block for thoracic surgery. J Cardiothorac Vasc Anesth. 2018;32(2):915–27. https://doi.org/10.1053/j.jvca.2017.10.003.
18. Baik JS, Oh AY, Cho CW, Shin HJ, Han SH, Ryu JH. Thoracic paravertebral block for nephrectomy: a randomized, controlled, observer-blinded study. Pain Med. 2014;15(5):850–6. https://doi.org/10.1111/pme.12320.
19. Tan X, Fu D, Feng W, Zheng X. The analgesic efficacy of paravertebral block for percutaneous nephrolithotomy: a meta-analysis of randomized controlled studies. Medicine (Baltimore). 2019;98(48):e17967. https://doi.org/10.1097/MD.0000000000017967.
20. Beyaz SG, Özocak H, Ergönenç T, Erdem AF, Palabıyık O. Total spinal block after thoracic paravertebral block. Turk J Anaesthesiol Reanim. 2014;42(1):43–5. https://doi.org/10.5152/TJAR.2013.60.
21. Albi-Feldzer A, Duceau B, Nguessom W, Jayr C. A severe complication after ultrasound-guided thoracic paravertebral block for breast cancer surgery: total spinal anaesthesia: a case report. Eur J Anaesthesiol. 2016;33(12):949–51. https://doi.org/10.1097/EJA.0000000000000536.
22. Pace MM, Sharma B, Anderson-Dam J, Fleischmann K, Warren L, Stefanovich P. Ultrasound-guided thoracic paravertebral blockade: a retrospective study of the incidence of complications. Anesth Analg. 2016;122(4):1186–91.

4

Retrospective study of quadratus lumborum block for postoperative analgesia in patients undergoing percutaneous nephrolithotomy

Luning Chen[1†], Jingjing Ji[1†], Yali Tian[1], Qing Sun[1], Xuefeng Qiu[2], Xiaogong Li[2] and Bingbing Li[1*]

Abstract

Background: The postoperative analgesic effect of transmuscular quadratus lumborum block (QLB-TM) in patients following lower abdominal surgeries has been identified; however, the efficacy of QLB using the lateral approach (QLB-L) is still in debate. Therefore, this retrospective study was conducted to investigate the effect of a single-shot block with QLB-L on postoperative analgesia for patients undergoing percutaneous nephrolithotomy (PCNL).

Methods: The medical information of the patients undergoing PCNL was retrieved from the electronic charter system (Medisystem, Suzhou, China) in our Nanjing Drum Tower Hospital during the period of Jan/2019 to Jun/2019. Among the total of 57 patients, there are 17, 18, and 22 patients subjected to QLB-L, QLB-TM, or routine treatment, respectively. The primary observational parameter was to assess postoperative pain with visual analog scales (VAS) at rest 30 min after extubation, 24 h, and 48 h after surgery, respectively. The secondary observatory endpoints, including the consumption of intraoperative opioids, the cumulative dose of non-steroid anti-inflammatory drugs (NSAIDs) and the incidence of adverse events related to postoperative analgesia, were evaluated as well.

Results: The static VAS score at 24 h after surgery and the intraoperative consumption of sufentanil were significantly lower in patients receiving either intervention of QLB-L or QLB-TM as compared with those receiving routine treatment. However, one shot of QLB had no impact on VAS scores at 30 min post-extubation, 48 h after PCNL procedure compared with the patients receiving routine treatment. The percentage of non-ambulatory patients within 24 h post-PCNL was significantly higher in the QLB-TM group compared with the routine treatment group ($P = 0.04$). There were no significant differences in the incidence of postoperative nausea and vomit (PONV), itches, respiratory depression, the time for the first defecation, and the length of hospital stay (LOS) among the three groups.

Conclusions: QLB-L procedure may exert as equivalent as QLB-TM in terms of abrogating postoperative pain within 24 h post-surgery and decreasing intraoperative sufentanil consumption in patients undergoing PCNL procedure as well. The caution should be taken to avoid lower extremities weakness in the patients after QLB-TM within the first 24 h post-PCNL procedure.

Keywords: Quadratus lumborum block, Percutaneous nephrolithotomy, Analgesia, Postoperative, Ultrasound-guided block

* Correspondence: icecolor@163.com
[†]Luning Chen and Jingjing Ji contributed equally to this work.
[1]Department of Anesthesiology, Drum Tower Hospital Affiliated Nanjing University Medical School, Road 321#, Nanjing, Zhongshan 210008, China

Background

Percutaneous nephrolithotomy (PCNL) is the treatment of choice for patients with multiple or complex kidney or upper urinary tract stones, which necessitates the meticulous multi-modality analgesia due to mild to moderate pain originated from renal capsule dilation or nephrostomy-tube-related stress during the first 24 h after operation [1]. Hence, alternative options such as thoracic paravertebral block (TPVB) or quadratus lumborum block (QLB) technique are strongly recommended as an appropriate adjunctive to systemic intravenous analgesia for pain control [2–4]. In 2015, Børglum et al. defined transmuscular quadratus lumborum block (QLB-TM) using the Shamrock sign [5]. The injectate trajectory is aiming at the interfascial plane between the anterior border of quadratus lumborum (QL) muscle and psoas major muscle. Relative to the lateral approach of QLB (QLB-L) which was initially introduced by Blanco in 2007 and is only applied in limited clinical practices nowadays [6], the transmuscular approach has gained broader acceptance in a variety of abdominal surgeries comprising of cesarean section, renal, hernioplasty as well as laparoscopic procedures for its strong narcotic sparing effect [7–9]. The efficacy of QLB-L, as a variant of transverse abdominis plane (TAP) block, in postoperative pain control after PCNL was questioned for its incapability of providing the adequate analgesic plane from T9–12 [10]. The studies from Blanco and Kadam et al., however, suggested that QLB-L provided adequate postoperative analgesia in lower abdominal surgeries as well, given the local anesthetics were administered beneath the middle layer of the thoracolumbar fascia lateral to the QL muscle to acquire adequate cephalad-distribution with the blockade of T9–12 spinal nerves [11, 12].

In this study, we investigated the effect of ultrasound-guided QLB, targeting anterior-laterally or transmuscularly to the QL muscle, on pain relief after PCNL. Our hypothesis in this study is that the patients who receive QLB-L procedure record as low visual analog scales (VAS) value at rest as QLB-TM.

Methods

Ethical approval

This study was approved by the ethics committee of Drum Tower Hospital Affiliated with the Nanjing University Medical School (reference number: 2019–304-01).

Methods

The medical information of the patients undergoing PCNL was retrieved from the electronic charter system (Medisystem, Suzhou, China) in our Nanjing Drum Tower Hospital from Jan/2019 to Jun/2019. Query used the following criteria: (a) anesthesia start time within the specified date/time parameters (Jan/2019-Jun/2019); (b) surgical procedure equal to PCNL;(C) patient has a completed pain assessment procedure form indicating the performance of QLB-L or QLB-TM. This is a retrospectively comparative study comparing the analgesic effect of ultrasound-guided QLB with two different approaches (QLB-L group, QLB-TM group) versus routine practice (control group) on postoperative pain following PCNL.

Participants

Those eligible patients with age > 18 years old, American Society of Anesthesiologists (ASA) physical status classification I-III scheduled to undertake the selective PCNL procedure were included in this retrospective study. The patients with the history of severe hypertension (systolic blood pressure > 180 mmHg), diabetes mellitus with neuropathic pain, hepatic cirrhosis, renal function insufficiency, depressant condition, alcohol addiction, chronic intake of oral non-steroid anti-inflammatory drugs (NSAIDs) or analgesics, or with incomplete/loss of clinical data were excluded in this study.

Anesthesia and perioperative management

The decision on which type of QLB approach performed before general anesthesia or intravenous medication alone without the requirement of truncal nerve block for pain control after PCNL was made by practitioners their own according to their daily routine of anesthetic management for those PCNL patients.

QLB-L technique (schematic illustration in Fig 1a and b): The patient was placed securely in the lateral decubitus position. A low-frequency curvilinear probe (SonoSite Edge, transducer C60x/5 2 MHz, Fujifilm Sonosite Inc., US) was attached above the iliac crest. Under the guidance of ultrasound, the 18 gauge 10-cm needle (Stimuplex® D, B. Braun Medical Inc., Germany) was applied to puncture from dorsal to ventral direction aiming at the anterolateral margin of the junction of QL and transversalis fascia, and 5 ml saline solution was injected to confirm the correct position by hydro-dissection phenomenon [13]. The block was completed with the 0.375% ropivacaine at a volume of 0.5 ml/kg thereafter. The range of sensory block was tested 30 min after the procedure. Patients whose block plane of abdominal wall between T10-L1 level 30 min after the block were the eligible candidates receiving truncal nerve block technique for postoperative analgesia.

QLB-TM technique (Fig 1c and d): The patient was placed in the same position as the QLB-L technique. The ultrasound probe was vertically attached above the iliac crest. The transverse process of second lumbar vertebra (L2) and typical shamrock image were identified, and the needle was inserted from the edge of the probe and proceeded further into the fascia between the QLM and psoas major muscle. The local anesthetics were

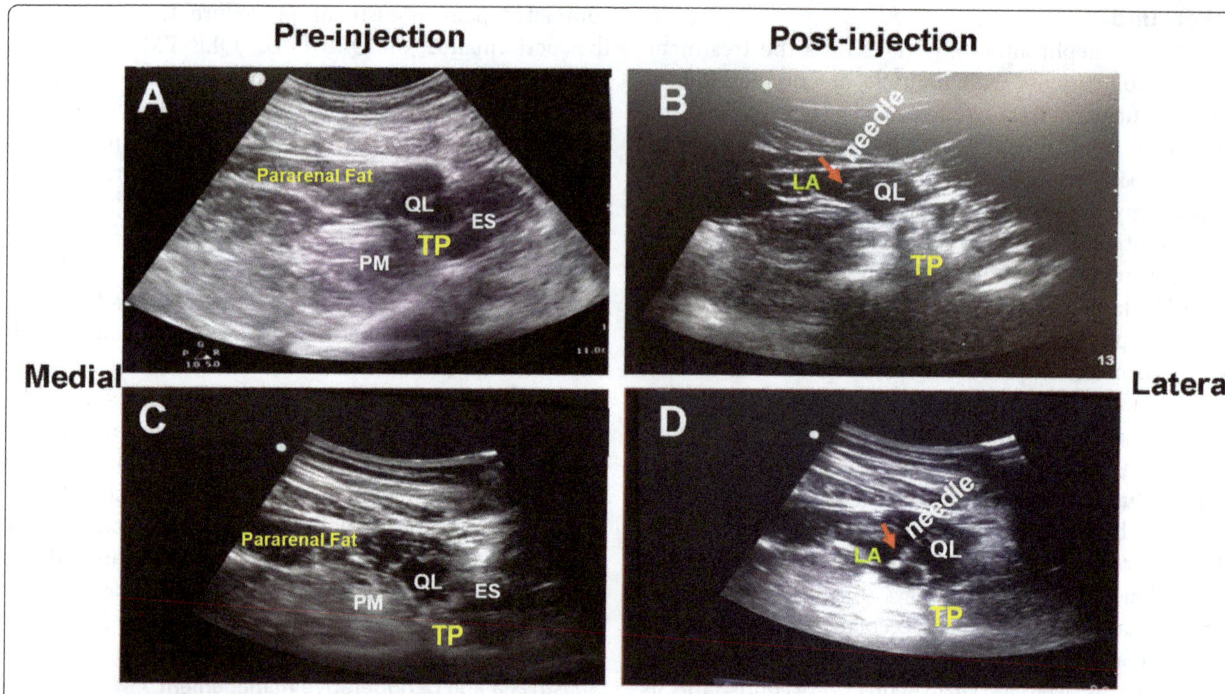

Fig. 1 Schematic illustration of the procedure of QLB-L (**a**: Pre-injection; **b**: Post-injection of local anesthetics) and QLB-TM (**c**: Pre-injection; **d**: Post-injection of local anesthetics). QL: Quadratus lumborum; PM: Psoas major muscle; ES:Erector spinae muscle; TP: Transverse process; LA: local anesthetics; Red arrow: tip of the stimuplex needle®

injected into the accurate interfascial plane between these two muscles.

All patients received standard general anesthesia monitoring, and intravenous infusion commenced with Lactate Ringer's solution at the rate of 400 ml/h to replace the fluid loss owing to 8 h fasting and no drinking. Anesthesia was induced with intermittent bolus injection of (midazolam 0.01 mg/kg), propofol (2 mg/kg), sufentanil (0.2 microgram/kg), and cisatracurium (0.2 mg/kg) facilitated in tracheal intubation. The mechanical ventilation was commenced to maintain the end-tidal PCO_2 at 40 mmHg. General anesthesia was obtained by total intravenous anesthesia with continuous infusion of propofol (4–6 mg/kg/min), cisatracurium (2 microgram/kg/min) to ensure appropriate sedation (BIS at the range of 40–60), substantial analgesia and muscle relaxation, respectively. The invasive arterial pressure monitor was established via left radial artery cannulation with a transducer connected to Philips (IntelliVue MP60, Bothell, Washington, United States) before surgery. Intermittent sufentanil (0.1 microgram/kg) was given if the heart rate (HR), blood pressure, or both increased more than 20% of the baseline. At 10 min before the beginning of the surgical procedure, 50 mg of flurbiprofen dissolved in 100 ml saline were intravenously administered. The hemodynamic parameters and oropharyngeal temperature were recorded automatically by Medisystem electronic charter database (Suzhou, China) in our department.

At the end of the operation, the patient was transferred to the post-anesthesia care unit (PACU), and the tracheal tube was removed after full emergence from anesthesia. The patient was discharged from the PACU to the ward once Steward Scale score (a, Awake degree: fully awake: 2 points; response to stimulation: 1 point; no response to stimulation: 0 point. b, Airway patency: can cough according to the doctor's order: 2 points; can maintain airway patency without support: 1 point; respiratory tract need support: 0 point. c, Limb mobility: limbs can do conscious activities: 2 points; limbs can make unconscious activities: 1 point; no movement of limbs: 0 point.) was higher than five assessed by an experienced physician in PACU. The VAS method was used for postoperative pain intensity quantification with the scale ranges from 0 to10 (0/10: pain-free, 10/10: severe pain that participants could not tolerate). VAS scores were assessed by a well-trained doctor at 30 min immediately after extubation, every other 4 h thereafter till 48 h post-surgery in the ward. When the VAS score of patients was over 3, 50 mg flurbiprofen was titrated to free of pain. Given the VAS score over 5, dizocine (0.1 mg/kg) was administrated for pain control as a rescue dose. The maximal dose of flurbiprofen or dizocine is 200 mg, 0.2 mg/kg daily, respectively.

Data collection

Preoperative demographic variables included the following: age (years); gender; BMI (body mass index: kg/m^2); ASA classification; underlying diseases (Diabetes, Coronary artery disease, Hypertension). Intraoperative variables included the following: duration of operation (minutes); anesthesia time (defined as the time spent in the operating room in minutes); categories of drugs used for general anesthesia; intraoperative mean arterial pressure (MAP) and HR; dosage of intraoperatively administered narcotics. Postoperative variables included the following: additional analgesic requirement (NSAIDs, Dizocine); pain intensity assessed on VAS; the incidence of postoperative nausea and vomiting (PONV), itching, respiratory depression, the time for the first defecation, and the length of hospital stay (LOS).

Outcome measurements

The primary outcome was VAS scores of patients at rest at 30 min post-extubation, 24 and 48 h after surgery, respectively. Secondary outcomes comprised of blood pressure and HR of patients recorded at the following time-points: arrival at the operating room (T0), beginning of surgery (T1), the end of surgery (T2), immediate post-extubation (T3), and leaving PACU (T4); the duration of operation, intraoperative opioid (sufentanil) consumption; LOS; postoperative additional analgesic requirement within 48 h after PCNL as well as the adverse effects (such as PONV, itching, respiratory depression, the time for the first defecation) were recorded for further analysis.

Statistical analysis

Power analysis was based on results of the preliminary estimation of the difference in VAS at 24 h after PCNL procedure among various treatment groups from our electronic charter database; specifically, power was set at 0.8, significance criterion was set at 0.05, sigma was at 0.74. This yielded a sample size of 17 for each group. A Shapiro-Wilk test was used to evaluate whether or not the data are normally distributed; The distribution of each continuous variable was presented with s mean ± standard deviation or median with range (R)/ interquartile range (IQR). The distribution of each categorical variable was summarized in terms of its frequency and percentage. One-way analysis of variance using LSD correction for multiple comparisons of parametric variables and the Kruskal-Wallis test was used for the non-parametric variables followed by Dunn's test for multiple comparisons. Repeated measurement analysis of variance was used to analyze repeated measurements. The test of chi-square or Fisher's exact test was applied for the categorized data. A P value of < 0.05 was accepted as statistically significant. The analysis of the data was carried out using the IBM SPSS 21.0 statistical package software.

Results

As is shown in Table 1, the demographic characteristics including gender, age, BMI, ASA physical status, comorbidities, and duration of surgical procedure of patients were recorded among three groups. There were no differences observed in preoperative or perioperative features among the three groups.

The postoperative pain scores assessed using VAS were collected at 30 min after removal of the endotracheal tube in a PACU, 24, 48 h after surgery in the ward, respectively. The patients receiving either type of QLB had lower VAS values at rest 24 h after surgery compared with the patients under routine analgesic treatment (QLB-TM vs Con: 1(0–2) vs 2(1.9–3.1), $P < 0.01$; QLB-L vs Con: 0(0–1) vs 2(1.9–3.1), $P < 0.01$). As shown in Fig. 2, however, at the time-point of 30 min post-extubation or 48 h after surgery, there is no significant difference in VAS values among three groups. The pain intensity for each group at different timepoints were shown in the supplementary material (Supplementary Table 1) .

As shown in Fig. 3, the intraoperative cumulative consumption (Fig 3a) or the consumption dosage/per hour of sufentanil (Fig 3b) was 40.0 (30.0–48.8) microgram, 20.0 (19.0–26.0) microgram /h in control group respectively, which was higher compared with either of QLB group

Table 1 Demographic characteristics, surgical data of the patients undergoing PCNL

Varibles	Con (**n** = 22)	QLB-TM (**n** = 18)	QLB-L (**n** = 17)	F,Z or χ2	P
Age (years)	48.7 ± 10.0	55.1 ± 8.1	51.1 ± 11.2	2.16	0.12
Gender (M/F)	16/6	9/9	13/4	3.35	0.19
BMI (kg/m2)	26.9 ± 3.3	25.2 ± 3.3	25.6 ± 3.9	1.25	0.30
ASA (II/III)	15/7	12/6	11/6	0.05	0.97
Hypertension n(%)	5 (23%)	5 (28%)	5 (29%)	0.25	0.89
Diabetes n(%)	3 (14%)	3 (17%)	1 (6%)	1.00	0.60
Coronary disease n(%)	0 (0%)	0 (0%)	1 (6%)	2.40	0.30
Duration of Operation (min)	117.6 ± 40.2	114.4 ± 40.4	116.6 ± 44.8	0.03	0.96

Data are presented as mean ± standard deviation, case (%)
BMI Body mass index, *M* Male, *F* Female, *ASA* American Society of Anesthesiologists
Con Control, *QLB-L* QLB-Lateral, *QLB-TM* QLB-transmuscular

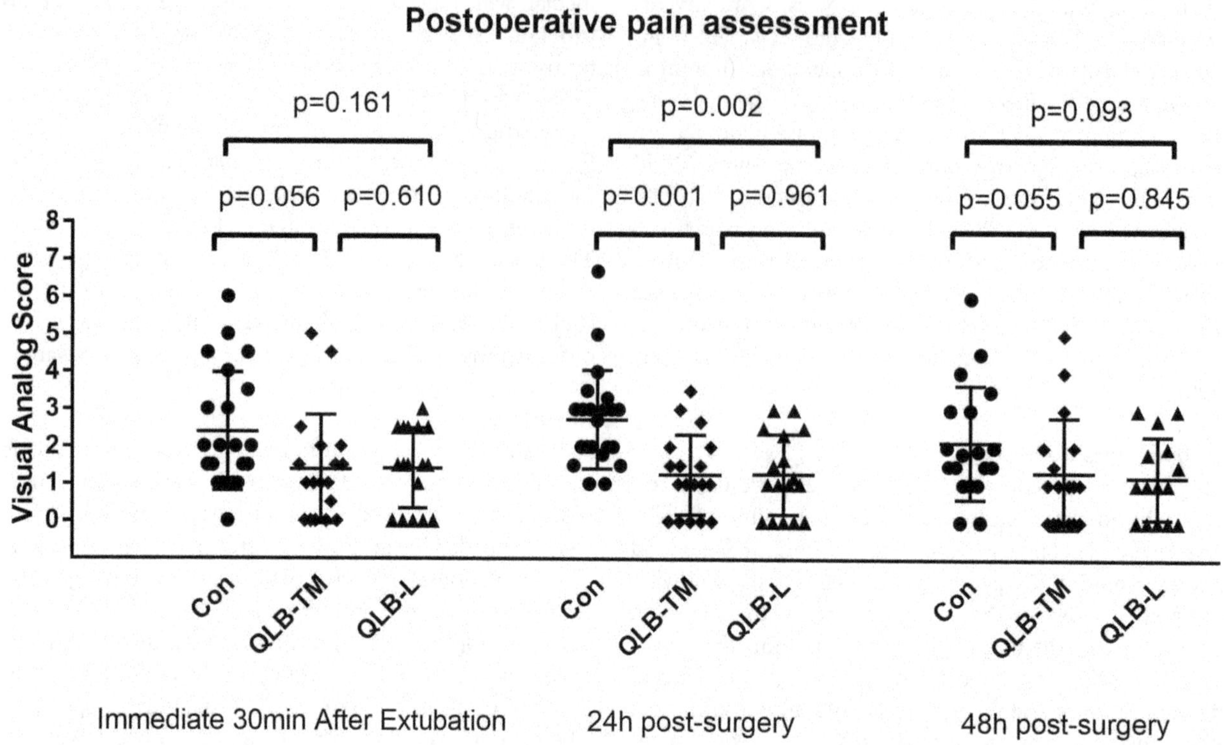

Fig. 2 Effect of either type of QLB on the VAS scores in patients undergoing PCNL. The VAS scores were assessed at 30 min immediately after extubation (**a**), 24 h (**b**), and 48 h after surgery (**c**). The data was presented with mean ± standard deviation if it conformed to normal distribution or median with the range/ interquartile of range if not normally distributed. Con: control; QLB-L: quadratus lumborum –lateral; QLB-TM: quadratus lumborum- transmuscular

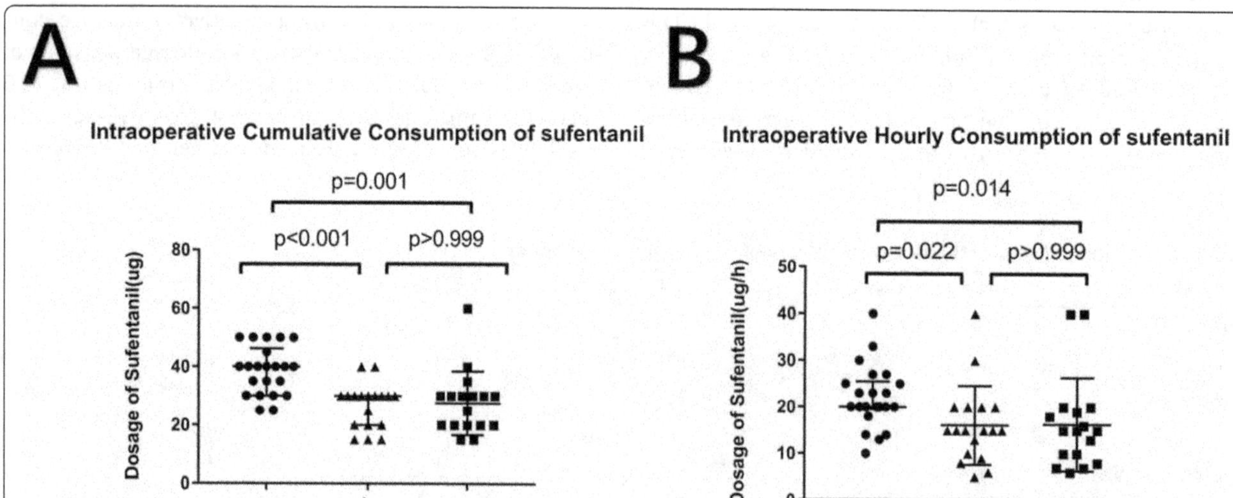

Fig. 3 Effect of either type of QLB on the intraoperative sufentanil consumption (**a**: cumulative dosage; **b**: the dosage of sufentanil consumed per hour in patients undergoing PCNL). The data was presented with the median with an interquartile of range. Con: control; QLB-L: quadratus lumborum –lateral trajectory; QLB-TM: quadratus lumborum- transmuscular trajectory

respectively ($P < 0.05$). The results of each group were shown in the supplementary material (Supplementary Table 2). As shown in Table 2, the median value of the cumulative dose of NSAIDs during the first 24 h after surgery was (75 (0–150) mg) in QLB-TM group and (50 (0–100) mg) in QLB-L respectively, which was equivalent to that consumed in the control group. Furthermore, there is also no significant difference in the rescue dose of dizocine among three groups within 48 h after PCNL. As shown in Table 3, either the first time of flatus or LOS was not shortened in patients receiving QLB treatment. As shown in Fig. 4, the application of either type of QLB had a negligible impact on the perioperative MAP and HR. The results of each group were shown in the supplementary material (Supplementary Table 3).

Consistent with the previous results, the incidence of PONV, itching, respiratory depression were not significantly different among the three groups (Table 3). In this study, we found that there were 8 out of 18 patients in the QLB-TM group who could not get out of bed and ambulated voluntarily without the assistance of an instrument during the first 24 h after surgery, the percentage of which was statistically higher compared with the Con group ($P = 0.04$, Fig. 5a). The lower extremity muscle strength score (Muscle strength grade: grade 0: in a state of complete paralysis, while the muscles cannot contract; grade 1: the muscles can contract, but cannot complete the action; grade 2: the limbs can move in parallel on the bed, but cannot lift off the bed surface; grade 3: the limbs can be raised to leave the bed surface, but cannot resist resistance; level 4: the limbs can resist part of the resistance; grade 5: the muscle strength is normal.) in the ipsilateral side of the block was lower in the QLB-TM group compared with the Con group on postoperative day 1 (POD 1) ($P = 0.003$, Fig. 5c). However, the ratio of the ambulatory patients to all subjects and muscle strength scores in the ipsilateral side of the block in QLB-L group 24 h post-PCNL was not significantly different from Con group ($P = 0.677$, Fig. 5a and c). The lower extremity score in the contralateral side of the block was not significantly different among the three groups on POD 1 (Fig. 5d). Furthermore, the percentage of ambulatory patients on POD 2 was not significantly different among the three groups (Fig. 5b).

Discussion

Our results in the present retrospective study suggest that QLB-L is as effective as QLB-TM in attenuating postoperative pain within 24 h after PCNL. Additionally, either type of QLB procedure similarly decreases the intraoperative consumption of sufentanil without causing hemodynamic instability, albeit it could not lead to further decrease in the incidence of adverse events associated with narcotics use and shortening of LOS.

There are at least four types of QLB approaches performed in the clinic at present. Except for the intramuscular technique reported by Murouchi [14], the other 3 QLB techniques are used by the majority of physicians for pain control following diverse types of surgeries [15]. Actually, QLB-TM has been accepted as one of the most popular approaches in abdominal surgeries as an adjunctive to systemic analgesia, bearing better and reliable pain control advantage [16]. Albeit these distinct approaches of QLB (posterior, lateral, and transmuscular) may have different analgesic efficacy, the quantitative analysis of the analgesic potency of these approaches yet lacks due to the heterogeneity in surgical types [17]. The first prospective study was conducted by Ahmed et al. in the year of 2019 to compare the analgesic efficacy in patients receiving either posterior or transmuscular approach of QLB in unilateral inguinal hernia repair [18]. Their results implicated that QLB-TM is superior to the posterior approach in decreasing the postoperative pain intensity. In the recent two prospective clinical studies conducted by Dam and KılıçE et al. respectively [10, 19], the potency of transmuscular approach of QLB in postoperative pain relief after PCNL procedure was assessed. As a result, QLB-TM rendered the beneficial effect in alleviating the pain of patients during activity after surgery, shortened the time to ambulation, LOS, and promoting the recovery of patients. In line with the previous studies, QLB-TM elicited significant pain relief at rest 24 h-post PCNL in the present study. Furthermore, all patients had an analgesic plane from T9 - L1 30 min after QLB-TM prior to general anesthesia induction and played a role in decreasing the intraoperative sufentanil consumption owing to the blockade of noxious afferent signal from the surgical site.

Nevertheless, there is still no comparison between the transmuscular and lateral approach of QLB after PCNL surgery in a randomized prospective study until now.

Table 2 Postoperative Consumption of flurbiprofen (mg)

Varibles	Con (**n** = 22)	QLB-TM (**n** = 18)	QLB-L (**n** = 17)	F,Z or χ2	P
24 h NSAIDS	50 (0–150)	75 (0–150)	50 (0–100)	0.75	0.69
48 h NSAIDS	0 (0–100)	0 (0–100)	0 (0–100)	0.04	0.98
Dizocine rescue n(%)	1 (5%)	1 (6%)	1 (6%)	0.04	0.98

Data are presented as median (interquartile range)

Table 3 Recovery of patients following PCNL and adverse events

Varibles	Con (**n** = 22)	QLB-TM (**n** = 18)	QLB-L (**n** = 17)	F,Z or χ2	p
LOS (days)	7 (6–10)	8 (7–9)	7 (5–8)	4.0	0.14
First time to Defecation (hours)	48 (48–60)	48 (36–60)	48 (36–48)	3.9	0.14
PONV n(%)	1 (5%)	1 (6%)	1 (6%)	0.4	0.98
Itches n(%)	0 (0%)	0 (0%)	0 (0%)		1
Respiratory depression n(%)	0 (0%)	0 (0%)	0 (0%)		1

Data are presented as median (interquartile range), case (%)
LOS Length of hospital stay (days) *POD* Postoperative day
PONV Postoperative nausea and vomiting

Our results in this retrospective study showed that the loss of cold sensation or pinprick dermatome plane 30 min after QLB-L was not distinct from the QLB-TM group at the extent from T9 to L1, which provided satisfactory intraoperative analgesia and was facilitated to decreasing the sufentanil consumption. Besides, the analgesic effect of QLB-L was equivalent to that of QLB-TM within 24 h post- PCNL surgery in the present study. In the study by Dam et al., they reiterated the importance of the accurate position of needle at the plane between the anterior border of quadratus lumborum muscle and psoas muscle to ensure the cranial spread of local anesthetics beyond arcuate ligament into the thoracic paravertebral region [11]. The trajectory in the lateral approach of QLB, they thought, was directed the fascial plane between the pararenal fat layer and middle thoracolumbar fascia, which prevented local anesthetics entering thoracic paravertebral spaces and barely had the value of clinical significance in pain control for PCNL patients. However, consistent with several other studies [20], our results demonstrate that the lateral type of QLB exerts a favorable effect in controlling postoperative pain after PCNL with the duration of analgesia lasting as long as 24 h. The mechanism underlying the analgesic effect of QLB-L for PCNL patients in the present study is still elusive. The plausive explanations can be attributed as follows: first, the lateral QLB is inclined to spread cephalad beneath the middle layer of thoracolumbar fascia and transversalis fascia in anatomy to interfere the afferent pain signal of T9–12 spinal nerves, which had been identified by several clinical or cadaver studies [15]. Additionally, the injection of 0.5 ml/kg (0.375% ropivacaine) was a relatively larger volume than that used in the previous studies and might be facilitated in the cranial spread of the drug.

We observed that the number of non-ambulatory patients in the QLB-TM group on POD 1 approximated 2-fold of that in the conventional treatment group. The weakness of lower extremities was identified in patients receiving QLB-TM. Previous studies indicated that the QLB-TM reduced postoperative 24 h pain scores and opiates consumption in patients after total hip arthroplasty [21]. The lower extremities weakness was accidentally reported in patients receiving QLB-TM [22]. Recent cadaver study conducted by Carline to assess the dimension of stained nerves using the following three different QLB groups [15]. They observed that a higher rate of lumbar plexus stain (L1–3) occurred in the QLB-TM group. The injection site in the vicinity of lumbar plexus and local anesthetics infiltration accounted for the faintness in lower extremities and better pain control after hip arthroplasty. The LOS was not significantly shortened in QLB groups compared with the routine control group in the present study. One shot of injection has only 24 h duration of pain relief after PCNL; therefore, the advantage of QLB on controlling pain is not evident

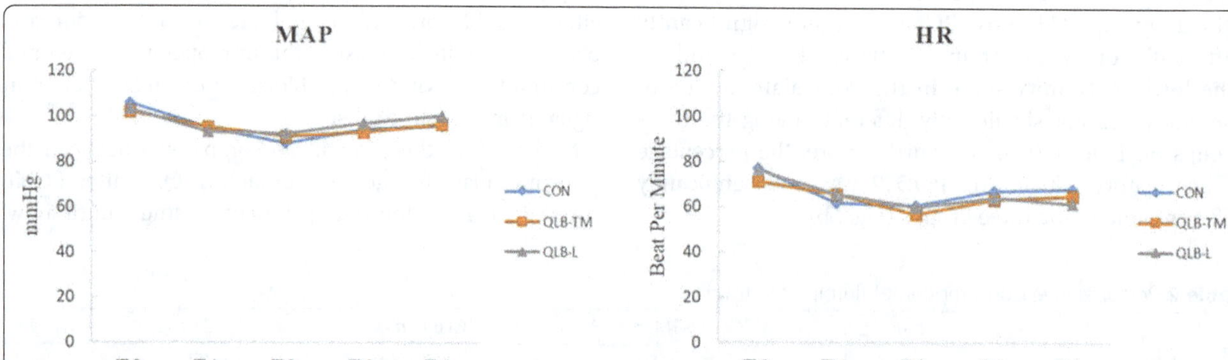

Fig. 4 Effect of either type of QLB on the perioperative mean arterial pressure (MAP) and heart rate (HR). The MAP and HR were recorded at arrival at the operating room(T0), the beginning of operation(T1), the end of the operation(T2), extubation(T3), and transfer from PACU(T4). The data are presented as mean ± standard deviation. Con: control; QLB-L: quadratus lumborum –lateral; QLB-TM: quadratus lumborum- transmuscular

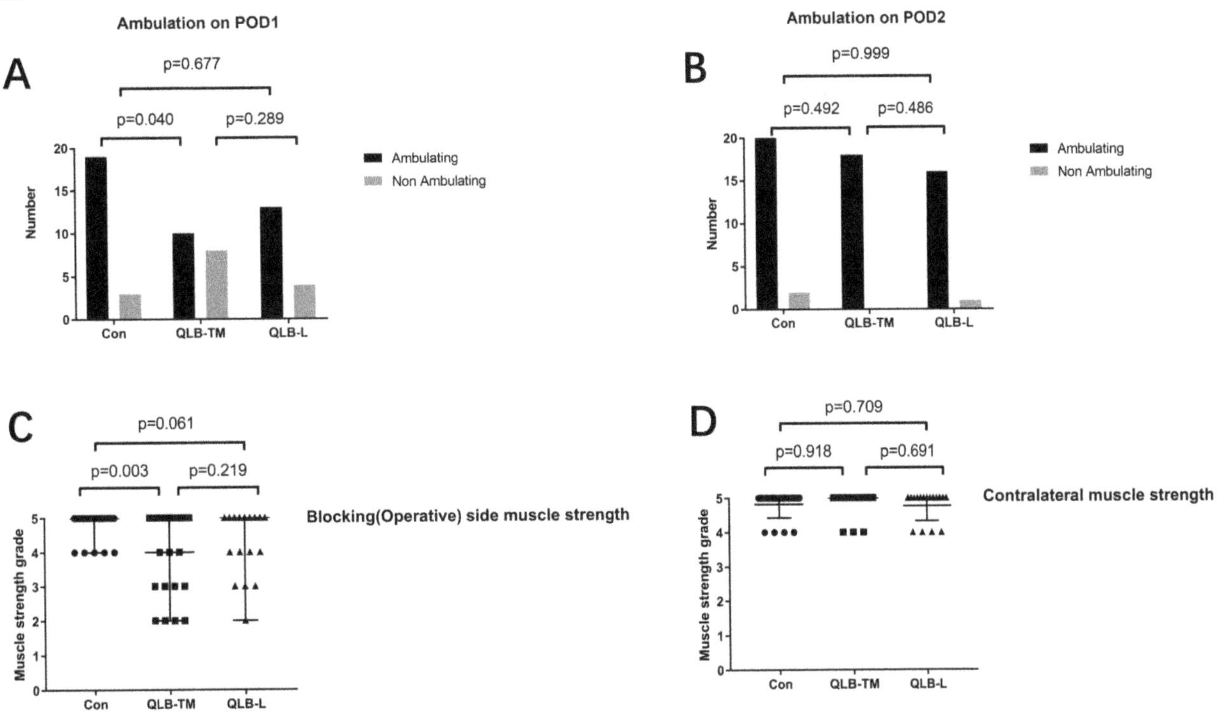

Fig. 5 Effect of either type of QLB on the postoperative motor function of lower extremities and ambulation. The number of ambulatory and non- ambulatory patients on POD 1 (**a**), POD 2(**b**). Muscle strength score in blocking (Operative) side (**c**) or the contralateral side of the block (**d**). The ordinal data was presented median with the range/ interquartile of range. The test of chi-square or Fisher's test was applied for the categorized data. Con: control; QLB-L: quadratus lumborum –lateral; QLB-TM: quadratus lumborum- transmuscular; POD: postoperative day

contrary to the continuous QLB strategy in pain control after liver surgery [23].

There are still several limitations in this study: Given this small size preliminary retrospective cohort study, hence a prospective randomized study is warranted to assess the beneficial pain control effect of QLB-L with ropivacaine compared with placebo in PCNL patients. The larger sample size is needed to detect the difference in lower extremity weakness 24 h after PCNL among QLB groups and the difference in LOS between QLB and routine intervention. Lastly, the optimal concentration and volume for ropivacaine for unilateral QLB are still unknown, and our study cannot give information regarding the adequate dose or volume of QLB in postoperative analgesia.

Conclusions

Collectively, ultrasound-guided QLB-L technique may provide as similar satisfactory pain-control as QLB-TM after PCNL. Cautions should be taken in patients for the latent risk of the weakness of low extremities during the first 24 h after QLB with the transmuscular approach, which can be avoided by being substituted with the lateral approach. Nevertheless, in view of this small-sample retrospective study, high-grade evidence is needed to confirm with confidence the analgesic effect of QLB-L for PCNL patients.

Abbreviations

ASA: American Society of Anesthesiologists; BMI: Body-mass index; HR: Heart rate; LOS: Length of hospital stay; MAP: Mean arterial pressure; NSAIDs: Non-steroid anti-inflammatory drugs; PACU: Post-anesthesia care unit; PCNL: Percutaneous nephrolithotomy; POD: Postoperative day; PONV: Postoperative nausea and vomit; QL: Transmuscular quadratus lumborum block; QLB: Quadratus lumborum block; QLB-L: Lateral approach quadratus lumborum block; QLB-TM: Transmuscular quadratus lumborum block; TAP: Transverse abdominis plane block; VAS: Visual analog scale

Acknowledgments

The authors would like to thank the Department of Anesthesiology, Urology Surgery, Drum Tower Hospital Affiliated Nanjing University Medical School. We also thank Dr. Biyun Xu for her cordial and unselfish assistance in study design and statistical analysis.

Authors' contributions

BBL, LNC, and JJJ designed the research; LNC, JJJ, YLT, QS, XFQ, and XGL performed the research; LNC, JJJ, and YLT analyzed the data; LNC,JJJ, and BBL wrote the paper. All authors have read and approved the manuscript.
Jiangsu Province, No. WSN-147; the Nanjing Health Commission of Nanjing Municipal Government, No. YKK17084.

Author details

[1]Department of Anesthesiology, Drum Tower Hospital Affiliated Nanjing University Medical School, Road 321#, Nanjing, Zhongshan 210008, China.
[2]Department of Surgery, Urology Surgery, Drum Tower Hospital Affiliated Nanjing University Medical School, Road 321#, Nanjing, Zhongshan 210008, China.

References

1. Wang J, Zhang C, Tan D, Tan G, Yang B, Chen W, Tang G. The effect of local anesthetic infiltration around nephrostomy tract on postoperative pain control after percutaneous Nephrolithotomy: a systematic review and meta-analysis. Urol Int. 2016;97(2):125–33.
2. Li C, Song C, Wang W, Song C, Kong X. Thoracic paravertebral block versus epidural anesthesia combined with moderate sedation for percutaneous Nephrolithotomy. Med Princ Pract. 2016;25(5):417–22.
3. Ozkan D, Akkaya T, Karakoyunlu N, Arık E, Ergil J, Koc Z, Gumus H, Ersoy H. Effect of ultrasound-guided intercostal nerve block on postoperative pain after percutaneous nephrolithotomy : prospective randomized controlled study. Anaesthesist. 2013;62(12):988–94.
4. Yayik AM, Ahiskalioglu A, Demirdogen SO, Ahiskalioglu EO, Alici HA, Kursad H. Ultrasound-guided low thoracic paravertebral block versus peritubal infiltration for percutaneous nephrolithotomy: a prospective randomized study. Urolithiasis. 2020;48(3):235–44.
5. Sauter AR, Ullensvang K, Niemi G, Lorentzen HT, Bendtsen TF, Børglum J, Pripp AH, Romundstad L. The shamrock lumbar plexus block: a dose-finding study. Eur J Anaesthesiol. 2015;32(11):764–70.
6. Blanco. Tap block under ultrasound guidance: the description of a "no pops" technique: 271. Reg Anesth Pain Med. 2007;32(5):130.
7. Blanco R, Ansari T, Girgis E. Quadratus lumborum block for postoperative pain after caesarean section: a randomised controlled trial. Eur J Anaesthesiol. 2015;32(11):812–8.
8. Öksüz G, Bilal B, Gürkan Y, Urfalioğlu A, Arslan M, Gişi G, Öksüz H. Quadratus Lumborum block versus Transversus Abdominis plane block in children undergoing low abdominal surgery: a randomized controlled trial. Reg Anesth Pain Med. 2017;42(5):674–9.
9. Zhu M, Qi Y, He H, Lou J, Pei Q, Mei Y. Analgesic effect of the ultrasound-guided subcostal approach to transmuscular quadratus lumborum block in patients undergoing laparoscopic nephrectomy: a randomized controlled trial. BMC Anesthesiol. 2019;19(1):154.
10. Dam M, Hansen CK, Poulsen TD, Azawi NH, Wolmarans M, Chan V, Laier GH, Bendtsen TF, Børglum J. Transmuscular quadratus lumborum block for percutaneous nephrolithotomy reduces opioid consumption and speeds ambulation and discharge from hospital: a single Centre randomised controlled trial. Br J Anaesth. 2019;123(2):e350–8.
11. Dam M, Moriggl B, Hansen CK, Hoermann R, Bendtsen TF, Børglum J. The pathway of Injectate spread with the Transmuscular Quadratus Lumborum block: a cadaver study. Anesth Analg. 2017;125(1):303–12.
12. Kadam VR. Ultrasound-guided quadratus lumborum block as a postoperative analgesic technique for laparotomy. J Anaesthesiol Clin Pharmacol. 2013;29(4):550–2.
13. Ueshima H, Otake H, Lin JA. Ultrasound-guided Quadratus Lumborum block: an updated review of anatomy and techniques. Biomed Res Int. 2017;2017: 2752876.
14. Murouchi T. Quadratus lumborum block intramuscular approach for pediatric surgery. Acta Anaesthesiol Taiwanica : Off J Taiwan Soc Anesthesiol. 2016;54(4):135–6.
15. Carline L, McLeod GA, Lamb C. A cadaver study comparing spread of dye and nerve involvement after three different quadratus lumborum blocks. Br J Anaesth. 2016;117(3):387–94.
16. Hansen CK, Dam M, Steingrimsdottir GE, Laier GH, Lebech M, Poulsen TD, Chan VWS, Wolmarans M, Bendtsen TF, Børglum J. Ultrasound-guided transmuscular quadratus lumborum block for elective cesarean section significantly reduces postoperative opioid consumption and prolongs time to first opioid request: a double-blind randomized trial. Reg Anesth Pain Med. 2019. https://doi.org/10.1136/rapm-2019-100540.
17. Elsharkawy H. Quadratus Lumborum Blocks. Adv Anesth. 2017;35(1):145–57.
18. Ahmed A, Fawzy M, Nasr MAR, Hussam AM, Fouad E, Aboeldahb H, Saad D, Osman S, Fahmy RS, Farid M, et al. Ultrasound-guided quadratus lumborum block for postoperative pain control in patients undergoing unilateral inguinal hernia repair, a comparative study between two approaches. BMC Anesthesiol. 2019;19(1):184.
19. Kılıç E, Bulut E. Quadratus Lumborum block III for postoperative pain after percutaneous Nephrolithotomy. Turkish J Anaesthesiol Reanim. 2018;46(4):272–5.
20. Murouchi T, Iwasaki S, Yamakage M. Quadratus Lumborum block: analgesic effects and chronological Ropivacaine concentrations after laparoscopic surgery. Reg Anesth Pain Med. 2016;41(2):146–50.
21. He J, Zhang L, He WY, Li DL, Zheng XQ, Liu QX, Wang HB. Ultrasound-guided Transmuscular Quadratus Lumborum block reduces postoperative pain intensity in patients undergoing Total hip Arthroplasty: a randomized, double-blind, Placebo-controlled trial. Pain Res Manag. 2020;2020:1035182.
22. Ueshima H, Hiroshi O. Incidence of lower-extremity muscle weakness after quadratus lumborum block. J Clin Anesth. 2018;44:104.
23. Zhu Q, Li L, Yang Z, Shen J, Zhu R, Wen Y, Cai W, Liu L. Ultrasound guided continuous Quadratus Lumborum block hastened recovery in patients undergoing open liver resection: a randomized controlled, open-label trial. BMC Anesthesiol. 2019;19(1):23.

5

Comparison of analgesic efficacy between rectus sheath blockade, intrathecal morphine with bupivacaine and intravenous patient-controlled analgesia in patients undergoing robot-assisted laparoscopic prostatectomy

Jung-Woo Shim[1], Yun Jeong Cho[1], Minhee Kim[2], Sang Hyun Hong[1], Hyong Woo Moon[3], Sung Hoo Hong[3] and Min Suk Chae[1*]

Abstract

Background: We explored the analgesic outcomes on postoperative day (POD) 1 in patients undergoing robot-assisted laparoscopic prostatectomy (RALP) who received intravenous patient-controlled analgesia (IV-PCA), rectus sheath bupivacaine block (RSB), or intrathecal morphine with bupivacaine block (ITMB).

Methods: This was a prospective, observational clinical trial. Patients were divided into three groups: IV-PCA ($n = 30$), RSB ($n = 30$), and ITMB ($n = 30$). Peak pain scores at rest and with coughing, cumulative IV-PCA drug consumption, the need for IV rescue opioids, and Quality of Recovery-15 (QoR-15) questionnaire scores collected on POD 1 were compared among the groups.

(Continued on next page)

* Correspondence: shscms@gmail.com
[1]Department of Anesthesiology and Pain medicine, Seoul St. Mary's Hospital, College of Medicine, The Catholic University of Korea, 222, Banpo-daero, Seocho-gu, Seoul 06591, Republic of Korea

(Continued from previous page)

Results: The preoperative and intraoperative findings were comparable among the groups; the ITMB group required the least remifentanil of all groups. During POD 1, the ITMB group reported lower levels of pain at rest and with coughing, compared with the other two groups. During POD 1, incidences of severe pain at rest (10.0% vs. 23.3% vs. 40.0%) and with coughing (16.7% vs. 36.7% vs. 66.7%) were the lowest in the ITMB group compared with the RSB and IV-PCA groups, respectively. After adjustment for age, body mass index, diabetes mellitus, hypertension, and intraoperative remifentanil infusion, severe pain at rest was 0.167-fold less common in the ITMB group than in the IV-PCA group, while pain with coughing was 0.1-fold lower in the ITMB group and 0.306-fold lower in the RSB group, compared with the IV-PCA group. The ITMB group required lower cumulative IV-PCA drug infusions and less IV rescue opioids, while exhibiting a better QoR-15 global score, compared with the other two groups. Complications (nausea and pruritus) were significantly more common in the ITMB group than in the other two groups; however, we noted no ITMB- or RSB-related anesthetic complications (respiratory depression, post-dural headache, nerve injury, or puncture site hematoma or infection), and all patients were assessed as Clavien-Dindo grade I or II during the hospital stay.

Conclusion: Although ITMB induced complications of nausea and pruritus, this analgesic technique provided appropriate pain relief that enhanced patient perception related to early postoperative recovery.

Keywords: Rectus sheath bupivacaine, Intrathecal morphine with bupivacaine, Robot-assisted laparoscopic prostatectomy

Background

Robot-assisted laparoscopic prostatectomy (RALP) is a technically advanced, minimally invasive surgical method that affords much better surgical view and greater maneuverability than open or laparoscopic prostatectomy [1]. Previous studies have found that RALP is associated with better oncological and functional outcomes, compared with open or laparoscopic radical prostatectomy [2, 3]. However, RALP patients frequently experience unbearable pain that persists over several days after surgery and requires pain-relief medications, such as opioids. This pain arises from skin-port incisions, multiple dissections of prostate-involved and surrounding tissues, bladder spasm, and transurethral catheter irritation [4]. Various central and/or peripheral pain-relief methods have been used to attenuate the severe pain that develops immediately after RALP [5, 6]. A rectus sheath block (RSB) regimen affords peri-umbilical incision site analgesia superior to that achieved via local anesthetic infiltration; this site is the principal source of pain immediately after laparoscopy-based surgery [7]. Compared with transversus abdominis plane (TAP) block, RSB may afford better analgesia when a midline incision is created and more prolonged blockade of noxious input from that site [8]. An intrathecal morphine and bupivacaine block (ITMB) regimen affords pain relief for 20–48 h postoperatively and reduces bladder spasm-related discomfort (a common complication associated with urinary catheter insertion after prostate surgery) [9]. However, no ideal analgesic regimen has been described that affords maximal benefits with minimal side effects; this would improve the quality of early postoperative recovery after RALP.

The aim of this study was to evaluate the analgesic outcomes on postoperative day (POD) 1 in patients undergoing RALP who received RSB or ITMB, compared with patients who received intravenous patient-controlled analgesia (IV-PCA) alone. We also compared postoperative complications and patient satisfaction. We hypothesized that, due to a reduction in surgical pain and bladder spasm-related discomfort, the ITMB regimen would lead to improved pain relief and satisfaction with recovery on the first day after surgery, compared with the other analgesic regimens.

Methods

Ethical considerations

This was a prospective, observational parallel-cohort trial. The protocol was approved by the Institutional Review Board of Seoul St. Mary's Hospital Ethics Committee (approval no. KC20OISI0124) on April 29, 2020. The study was performed in accordance with all relevant principles of the Declaration of Helsinki. The study protocol was prospectively registered on a publicly accessible clinical registration site recognized by the International Committee of Medical Journal Editors (Clinical Research Information Service, Republic of Korea; approval no. KCT0005040) on May 20, 2020. Written informed consent was obtained from all patients enrolled between May 2020 and July 2020. The study adhered to Strengthening the Reporting of Observational Studies in Epidemiology guidelines (Additional file 1); a study flow chart is shown in Fig. 1.

Study population

The inclusion criteria for our study were: age 19–74 years, prostate cancer stage I or II [10], patients

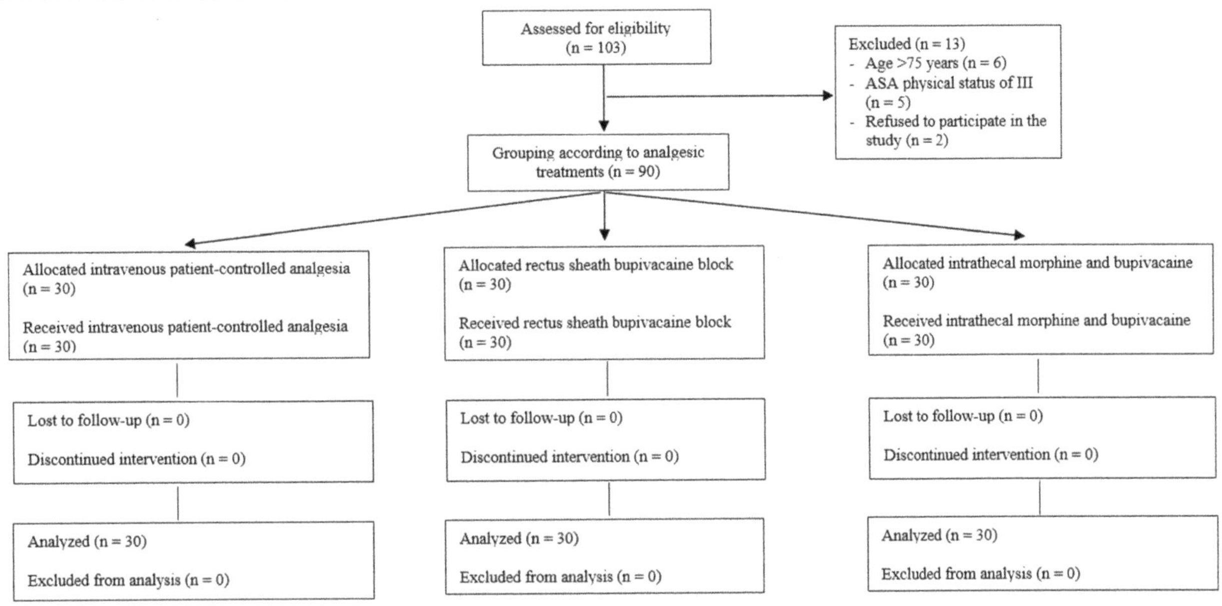

Fig. 1 Flow chart of the study

scheduled for elective RALP, and American Society of Anesthesiologists (ASA) physical status I or II. The exclusion criteria were: a history of allergy to a local anesthetic or opioid drug, coagulopathy (international normalized ratio [INR] > 1.5 for ITMB or INR > 2.0 for a single injection of ultrasound-guided RSB; and platelet count < 100.0×10^9/L) [11, 12], hemodynamic instability that required strong vasopressors (i.e., epinephrine or norepinephrine), hetastarch colloid infusion, or blood product transfusion (i.e., packed red blood cells ≥1 unit due to hemoglobin < 7.0 g/dL) [13], and refusal to participate.

The patients were divided into three groups based on their analgesia preference: IV-PCA alone (reference group), RSB and IV-PCA (RSB group), and ITMB and IV-PCA (ITMB group).

Patient management in the operating room

The RALP surgical technique and balanced anesthetic management were as described previously [14]; patient care was standardized apart from the analgesic treatments. Briefly, balanced anesthesia was performed by attending expert anesthesiologists. Induction of anesthesia was achieved using 1–2 mg/kg of propofol and 0.6 mg/kg of rocuronium; anesthesia was then maintained using 2.0–6.0% desflurane under medical air in oxygen. Remifentanil was continuously infused at a rate of 0.1–0.5 μg/kg/min, as appropriate. The Bispectral Index™ instrument was set between 40 and 50 to ensure appropriate hypnotic depth. Rocuronium was repeatedly infused under train-of-four monitoring (> 1 twitch). End-tidal CO_2 was set between 30 and 40 mmHg with adjustment of the ventilator mode. For fluid therapy, a baseline isotonic crystalloid was prepared based on the estimated fluid maintenance requirements, which were established in accordance with the patient's weight and anticipated tissue trauma. Additional fluid boluses were infused according to blood loss; however, the total amount of fluid was restricted to a maximum of 1 L before vesicourethral anastomosis.

The attending anesthesiologists (whose subspecialty involved regional blocks) and nurses were aware of the group allocations, but were not involved in later patient care or data collection (other than the completion of medical records). RSB was established immediately after the induction of general anesthesia. An ultrasound probe was positioned transversely on the rectus abdominis muscle, above the umbilicus (Fig. 2). Guided by real-time ultrasound, a sterile 22-G Tuohy-type epidural needle was cautiously advanced in-plane (to prevent injury to nearby vessels) from medially to laterally until the tip attained the plane between the lateral side of the rectus abdominis muscle and the posterior rectus sheath. After negative pressure aspiration, 20 mL of 0.25% (w/v) bupivacaine was administered and the block was repeated on the opposite side. ITMB was placed before the induction of general anesthesia. Each patient received 0.2 mg of intrathecal morphine sulfate and 7.5 mg of bupivacaine by means of a sterile 25-G Quincke-type spinal needle inserted between lumbar vertebrae 3 and 4. The drugs were administered through a single injection after collection of cerebrospinal fluid. All patients were allowed access to IV-PCA (1000 μg of fentanyl, 90 mg of ketorolac, and 0.3 mg of ramosetron). The IV-PCA regimen featured

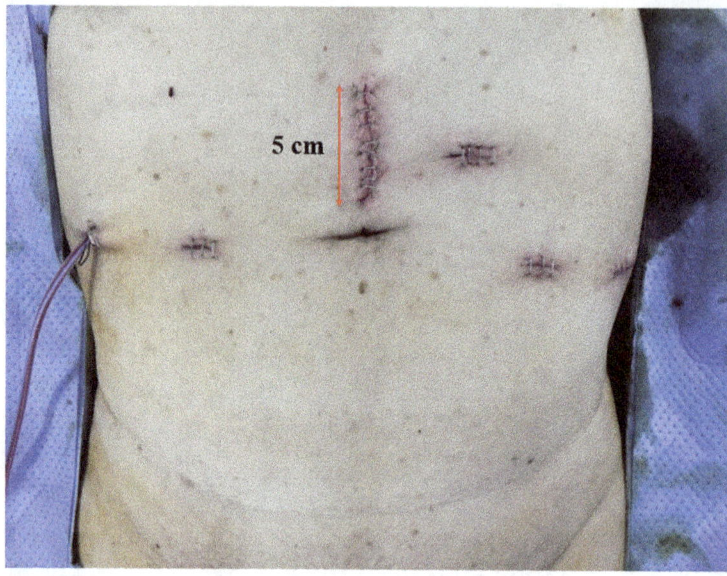

Fig. 2 Peri-umbilical wound site (arrow) that is the principal analgesic target of RSB

a 2-mL bolus injection and 0.5 mL/h basal infusion with a lockout time of 10 min. If a patient experienced acute postoperative breakthrough pain (visual analog scale [VAS] score ≥ 7), 25 mg of pethidine (an IV rescue opioid) was administered based on the discretion of the attending physicians (in the postoperative acute care unit or ward), who were blinded to group assignment.

Pain outcomes

Cumulative IV-PCA drug consumption and the need for IV rescue opioids were primarily assessed during the first 24 h postoperatively. Peak pain scores at rest and with coughing were assessed using a VAS that ranged from 0 to 10, where "0" represented no pain and "10" represented the worst possible pain. Pain severity was classified as mild (VAS scores 0–3), moderate (4–6), or severe (7–10) [15]. Pain was assessed using the VAS three times (i.e., at 1 h postoperatively in the post-anesthesia care unit [PACU], as well as at 6 and 24 h postoperatively in the ward). If a patient experienced acute postoperative breakthrough pain (VAS score ≥ 7), 25 mg of pethidine (an IV rescue opioid) was administered by attending physicians (anesthesiologists in the PACU and urologists in the ward) or nurses, none of whom were aware of the group allocations.

Clinical variables

Preoperative demographic and laboratory parameters were recorded on the day before surgery by attending urologic physicians or nurses in the ward, who were not aware of the group allocations and were not involved in further data collection other than filling in medical record forms. Intraoperative findings, such as surgical duration, hypotension status (systolic blood pressure < 90 mmHg for more than 10 min), total rescue ephedrine infusion, total remifentanil infusion, crystalloid fluid infusion, urine output, and hemorrhage status, were recorded by the attending anesthesiologists or nurses in the operating room, who were not involved in further patient care or data collection (other than filling in anesthetic record forms) and were not aware of the group allocations. Postoperative findings, such as the global quality-of-recovery score on a 15-item questionnaire (the QoR-15) [16]; the incidences of nausea, vomiting, and pruritus; the Clavien-Dindo grade [17]; and laboratory variables, were measured in the ward on the first day after surgery (between 6 and 8 pm). These findings were measured by anesthesiology residents (Y.J.C. and M.K.) who were not aware of the group allocations and were not involved in further patient care or data collection. Additionally, nausea and vomiting were assessed on a binary scale (yes/no). Patients were considered to have nausea, if they responded positively to the question, "are you or have you felt nauseated after surgery?". Using similar questions, vomiting episodes were assessed [18]. Pruritus was assessed using the following scale: 0 = no itch; 1 = itch with no need to scratch, just rubbing (mild); 2 = itch with need to scratch (moderate); 3 = itch with need to scratch and requiring treatment (severe) [19]. We defined overt pruritus as a score ≥ 2. Therefore, nausea, vomiting, and pruritus were considered binary variables in our analysis.

Statistical analyses

The minimum sample size was based on the difference in cumulative IV-PCA drug consumption on POD 1 between patients who received RSB and those who received ITMB, calculated using electronic medical records. Mean cumulative IV-PCA drug consumption on POD 1 by patients who received RSB ($n = 10$) and those who received ITMB ($n = 10$) were 47.1 and 29.1 mL, respectively. The standard deviation (SD) among the 20 patients was 23.6 mL. Therefore, a minimum sample size of 27 patients/group was required to afford an α value of 0.05 and a power of 0.8. We recruited 30 patients for each group; we assumed a dropout rate of 10%.

Data are expressed as means ± standard deviations (SDs), medians with interquartile ranges (IQRs), or numbers with proportions (%), as appropriate. The normality of continuous data distributions was evaluated using the Shapiro–Wilk test. Continuous perioperative variables of the three groups were compared via one-way analysis of variance or the Kruskal–Wallis test; post hoc testing employed the unpaired *t*-test or the Mann–Whitney U test. Perioperative categorical variables were compared among the groups using the Pearson χ^2 test or Fisher's exact test, as appropriate. Trend testing employed a linear-by-linear association method. To determine the clinical analgesic efficacy of the treatments, logistic regression analysis was used to derive odds ratios with 95% confidence intervals of the risks (postoperative peak VAS score ≥ 7 at rest and with coughing) associated with IV-PCA alone (reference), and the RSB and ITMB, after adjusting for age, body mass index, and diabetes mellitus and hypertension statuses (these comorbidities may change in accordance with pain level) [20, 21], and intraoperative remifentanil consumption. Tests for linear trends among patients in terms of cumulative IV-PCA drug consumption on POD 1 were based on stepwise linear regression. All tests were two-sided and a *p*-value < 0.017 was considered statistically significant (multiple comparisons were made). All statistical analyses were performed with the aid of SPSS for Windows (ver. 24.0; IBM Corp., Armonk, NY, USA) and MedCalc for Windows (ver. 11.0; MedCalc Software, Ostend, Belgium).

Results

Study population

In total, 103 patients were assessed for eligibility. Thirteen patients were excluded: six were aged > 74 years, five had ASA physical status III, and two refused to participate. Thus, 90 patients were enrolled and divided into the IV-PCA, RSB, and ITMB groups ($n = 30$ patients per group).

Preoperative and intraoperative findings

Of all patients ($n = 90$), the median age was 65 (62–71) years and the median body mass index was 24.0 (22.5–26.5) kg/m^2. In total, 15 patients (16.7%) had diabetes mellitus and 35 (38.9%) hypertension. None of the patients showed coagulopathic findings preoperatively; the minimum and maximum INRs were 0.8 and 1.0, while the minimum and maximum platelet counts were 120.0×10^9/L and 355.0×10^9/L. Table 1 shows that the preoperative and intraoperative findings were comparable among the three groups. However, during surgery, the ITMB group exhibited the lowest remifentanil consumption, whereas the RSB group required less remifentanil than the IV-PCA group.

Postoperative pain

During POD 1, the ITMB group reported lower pain levels at rest and with coughing than did the RSB and IV-PCA groups (Fig. 3). After adjustment for age, body mass index, comorbidity status, and intraoperative remifentanil infusion, severe pain at rest was 0.167-fold less common in the ITMB group than in the IV-PCA group, while pain with coughing was 0.1-fold lower in the ITMB and 0.306-fold lower in the RSB group, compared with the IV-PCA group (Table 2). Table 3 shows that cumulative IV-PCA drug consumption decreased according to analgesic treatment in the following order: IV-PCA alone > RSB > ITMB (linear regression, $p < 0.001$). The ITMB group required less IV-PCA drug infusion and IV rescue opioids than did the RSB and IV-PCA groups. The ITMB group had the lowest peak VAS scores at rest and with coughing, compared with the other two groups, while the RSB group had a lower peak VAS score with coughing, compared with the IV-PCA group (Table 4).

Postoperative clinical findings

The global QoR-15 questionnaire score was higher in the ITMB group than in the RSB and IV-PCA groups (Table 4). Complications (nausea and pruritus) were significantly more common in the ITMB group than in the other two groups; however, we noted no ITMB- or RSB-related anesthetic complications (respiratory depression, post-dural headache, nerve injury, or puncture site hematoma or infection), and all patients were assessed as Clavien-Dindo grade I or II during the hospital stay.

Discussion

Our principal findings were that ITMB may afford superior analgesia and better patient perception of outcome in terms of early postoperative recovery, compared with RSB or IV-PCA alone, in patients undergoing RALP. The analgesic efficacy of ITMB was approximately three-fold and 10-fold better in terms of reducing severe pain during the early postoperative period, compared with RSB and IV-PCA alone, respectively. Although ITMB was associated with more nausea and

Table 1 Comparisons of preoperative and intraoperative findings between the three groups

Group	IV-PCA	RSB	ITMB	
n	30	30	30	*p*
Preoperative findings				
Age (years)	65 (61–69)	67 (64–72)	65 (62–71)	0.286
Body mass index (kg/m^2)	24.4 (22.7–27.7)	23.6 (22.2–25.2)	24.2 (22.3–26.4)	0.276
Comorbidity				
Hypertension	9 (30.0%)	10 (33.3%)	16 (53.3%)	0.134
Diabetes mellitus	7 (23.3%)	3 (10.0%)	5 (16.7%)	0.383
History of abdominal surgery	7 (23.3%)	4 (13.3%)	6 (20.0%)	0.602
Laboratory variables				
White blood cell count (× 10^9/L)	5.4 (4.6–7.4)	7.1 (5.9–7.6)	6.2 (5.2–7.5)	0.133
Neutrophil (%)	54.3 (47.9–57.2)	55.1 (51.6–59.6)	52.9 (51.1–54.5)	0.118
Lymphocyte (%)	33.8 (31.3–38.3)	32.6 (31.1–40.4)	36.5 (34.6–39.0)	0.089
Hemoglobin (g/dL)	14.3 (13.8–14.8)	13.9 (13.1–15.4)	14.7 (13.7–15.6)	0.375
Platelet count (× 10^9/L)	187.0 (160.5–221.0)	193.0 (169.8–242.0)	207.0 (172.3–232.3)	0.52
International normalized ratio	0.9 (0.8–0.9)	0.9 (0.9–0.9)	0.9 (0.8–0.9)	0.148
Intraoperative findings				
Surgical duration (min)	123 (109–145)	123 (100–141)	123 (114–138)	0.713
Hypotension event[a]	10 (33.3%)	15 (50.0%)	17 (56.7%)	0.175
Total rescue ephedrine infusion (mg)	0 (0–4)	2 (0–8)	4 (0–8)	0.139
Total remifentanil infusion (mg)	0.5 (0.4–0.6)	0.4 (0.3–0.4)[*]	0.2 (0.1–0.3)[*,†]	< 0.001
Crystalloid fluid infusion (mL)	500 (400–600)	575 (400–663)	525 (388–800)	0.782
Urine output (mL)	100 (50–100)	50 (50–100)	100 (50–100)	0.496
Hemorrhage (mL)	100 (50–100)	100 (50–100)	100 (50–163)	0.405

Abbreviations: *IV-PCA* Intravenous patient-controlled analgesia, *VAS* Visual analog scale, *PACU* Post-anesthesia care unit
[*]$p < 0.017$ as statistical significance based on the level in the IV-PCA group
[†]$p < 0.017$ as statistical significance based on the level in the RSB group
[a]Hypotension event defined as systolic blood pressure < 90 mmHg over 10 min
NOTE: Values are expressed as the median (interquartile) and number (proportion)

pruritus than RSB and IV-PCA alone, we noted no ITMB-related, postoperative adverse event, such as respiratory depression, lower leg numbness, or post-dural puncture headache.

Our ITMB data are similar to those of previous laparoscopic and open surgery reports [5, 22–24]; thus, ITMB is a feasible and practicable form of pain relief (yielding a lower pain score and lower opioid requirement). Moreover, it was not associated with serious complications (such as nerve injury) during or after surgery, and was better than RSB or IV-PCA alone. The differences between intrathecal and peripheral blocks include the sites affected by the analgesic drugs and subsequent drug actions. Intrathecally injected morphine and bupivacaine become widely dispersed in cerebrospinal fluid, thus more reliably (compared with RSB) preventing nociceptive inputs from multiple somatic dermatome levels in patients undergoing RALP [24, 25]. The principal skin wound created during laparoscopy-based surgery lies in the peri-umbilical area; the orifice is used for camera insertion and specimen (prostate mass) removal. In the past, RSB effectively countered pain caused by injury to the peri-umbilical dermatomes [26, 27]. However, as surgery advanced from open surgery to human-executed laparoscopic surgery to RALP (reducing the operation time and numbers of painful stimuli delivered by surgical wounds in sites such as the umbilicus) [28], the analgesic effect of RSB seems to have gradually decreased along with improvements in surgical wound care techniques. Furthermore, ITMB may deliver visceral analgesia by interacting with spinal μ- and κ-opioid receptors and voltage-gated sodium channels that contain binding sites for local anesthetics. It is now possible to totally (and simultaneously) avoid the surgical stress and pain imparted by intra-abdominal wounds (created when prostate-adjacent tissues are dissected and retracted) and skin wounds (created when the skin is incised, punctured, and retracted) [29, 30].

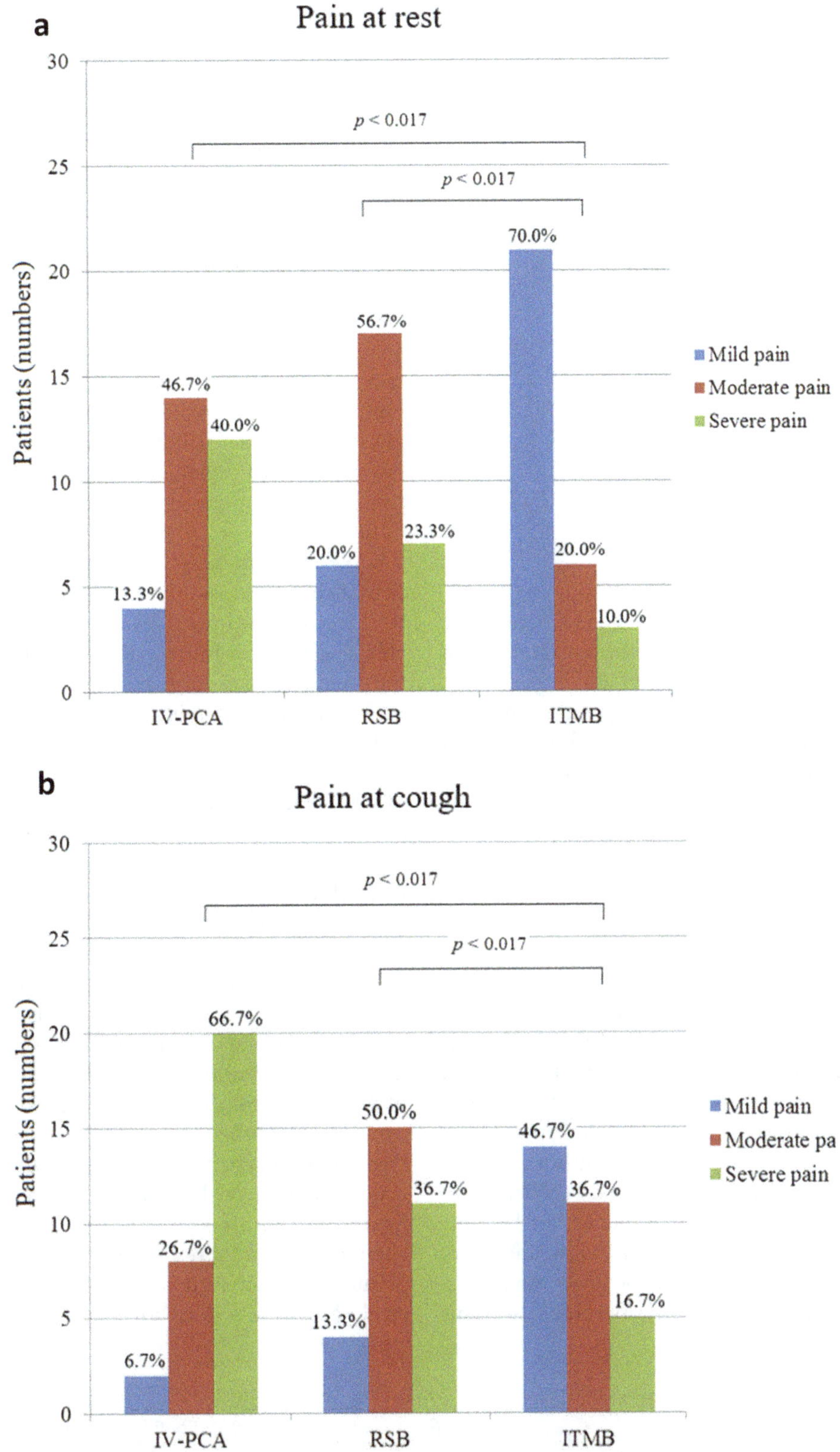

Fig. 3 Pain scores (**a**) at rest and (**b**) with coughing in the three groups ($n = 30$ per group) in the first 24 h postoperatively. Mild pain was defined as a peak VAS score of 0–3, moderate pain as a peak score of 4–6, and severe pain as a peak score of 7–10. $p < 0.017$ indicates statistical significance (adjusted for multiple comparisons). Values are expressed as numbers with proportions (% values)

Table 2 Analgesic efficacy of IV-PCA, the RSB, and ITMB block with severe pain (peak VAS ≥7) at rest and cough during 24 h postoperatively

	ß	Odds ratio	95% Confidence interval	p
Severe pain at rest				
Analgesia adjusted for age, BMI, DM, hypertension, and intraoperative remifentanil consumption				
IV-PCA	Reference			
RSB	−0.74	0.477	0.156–1.464	0.196
ITMB	−1.792	0.167	0.041–0.675	0.012
Severe pain at cough				
Analgesia adjusted for age, BMI, DM, hypertension, and intraoperative remifentanil consumption				
IV-PCA	Reference			
RSB	−1.186	0.306	0.105–0.888	0.029
ITMB	−2.303	0.1	0.029–0.34	< 0.001

Abbreviation: *VAS* Visual analog scale, *IV-PCA* Intravenous patient-controlled analgesia, *RSB* Rectus sheath block, *ITMB* Intrathecal morphine with bupivacaine, *BMI* Body mass index, *DM* Diabetes mellitus

However, RSB inhibits only somatic, afferent nerve pain. Thus, it cannot deliver comprehensive analgesia; pain from the visceral origins is not dulled [26].

In terms of complications, postoperative nausea/vomiting and pruritus compromise the quality of patient recovery [31]. Previous studies suggested that the incidences of such complications were higher in patients who received intrathecal morphine than in those receiving local anesthetic-based analgesia [32–34]. Intrathecal block with low doses of combined morphine (75 or 100 μg) and bupivacaine (5 mg) provided more effective postoperative analgesia than did sham subcutaneous block with normal saline. However, the side effects (e.g., nausea and vomiting) were of comparable incidence and severity between the two groups [35]. Our ITMB regimen included bupivacaine (7.5 mg), which allowed us to reduce the morphine dose to 0.2 mg, thus reducing nausea/vomiting and pruritus while maintaining appropriate analgesia. However, we found higher incidences of nausea and pruritus in patients who received ITMB than in those who received RSB or IV-PCA alone. Notably, our incidences of nausea (30.0%), vomiting (6.7%), and pruritus (16.7%) in the ITMB group may be lower than those of patients who receive intrathecal morphine (without additive bupivacaine). Specifically, the reported incidences of nausea/vomiting and pruritus after surgery were approximately 60–80% and 30–100%, respectively [36–38]. Nguyen et al. [39] suggested that the addition of bupivacaine (15 mg) to intrathecal morphine (0.4 mg) improved pain relief and reduced the incidence of adverse events (such as hypotension) in patients undergoing laparoscopic liver resection. Girgin et al. [40] found that the incidence of pruritus increased as the dose of intrathecal morphine rose from 0.1 to 0.4 mg; however, when morphine was combined with low-dose bupivacaine (7.5 mg), the complication rate was reduced while analgesia remained stable in women undergoing cesarean sections. The good analgesia (i.e., reduced requirement for IV opioid infusion) without adverse complications (Clavien-Dindo grade ≥ III), afforded by our low-dose ITMB regimen, may enhance early postoperative recovery compared with patients treated via RSB or IV-PCA alone.

In our study, there were comparable clinical characteristics, such as surgical duration, hypotension events, and total rescue ephedrine infusion, between the groups. Notably, analgesic treatments (RSB vs. ITMB) may not affect the prolongation of surgical time that possibly results from management by attending anesthesiologists who have excellent technique and sufficient experience with regional blocks, although there were differences in the RSB and ITMB regimens, such as target sites (rectus muscle vs. spine), needle manipulation (ultrasound-based vs. palpation-based), and patient position (supine vs. lateral) [41, 42]. Furthermore, intrathecal injection of bupivacaine may produce a high level of sensory and motor block, as well as arterial hypotension. However, these effects were dose-dependent, such that the lowest dose of bupivacaine (7 mg) provided equally rapid onset and effective anesthesia for cesarean surgery while reducing the incidence of hypotension, compared with bupivacaine doses of 8 and 9 mg, in patients who received combined administration of intrathecal morphine (100 μg) [43]. These findings were consistent with ours in that a low dose of additive intrathecal bupivacaine (7.5 mg) may have minimal impact on the occurrence of persistent hypotension and requirement for rescue inotrope.

Our work had certain limitations. First, we delivered single bupivacaine injections to the rectus sheath when

Table 3 Linear trend for cumulative IV-PCA drug consumption during POD 1 among the IV-PCA vs. RSB vs. ITMB groups

	ß	95% Confidence interval	p
Cumulative IV-PCA drug consumption during POD 1 (mL)			
Adjusted for age, BMI, DM, hypertension, and intraoperative remifentanil consumption			
Linear trend among the IV-PCA vs. RSB vs. ITMB groups	−10.715	– 16.403 - -5.026	< 0.001

Abbreviation: *IV-PCA* Intravenous patient-controlled analgesia, *POD* Postoperative day, *RSB* Rectus sheath block, *ITMB* Intrathecal morphine with bupivacaine, *BMI* Body mass index, *DM* Diabetes mellitus

Table 4 Comparisons of patient outcomes during the first 24 h postoperatively between the three groups

Group	IV-PCA	RSB	ITMB	
n	30	30	30	*p*
Requirement of opioid infusion				
Cumulative IV-PCA infusion (mL)	37.6 (25.9–57.3)	42.8 (29.9–60.8)	18.7 (14.7–26.2)*, †	< 0.001
IV rescue opioid infusion	19 (63.3%)	21 (70.0%)	6 (20.0%)*, †, ‡	< 0.001
Peak visual analog scale				
at rest	6 (4–7)	5 (4–6)	3 (2–4)*, †	< 0.001
at cough	8 (6–9)	6 (5–7)*	4 (3–5)*, †	< 0.001
Quality of early recovery				
Global score of QoR-15 questionnaire on POD 1	124 (122–129)	124 (117–133)	130 (126–141)*,†	0.002
Complications				
Nausea	2 (6.7%)	2 (6.7%)	9 (30.0%)‡	0.012
Vomiting	0 (0.0%)	1 (3.3%)	2 (6.7%)	0.355
Pruritus	0 (0.0%)	0 (0.0%)	5 (16.7%)‡	0.005
Laboratory variables on POD 1				
White blood cell count (× 10^9/L)	13.5 (8.7–16.5)	15.4 (8.2–20.7)	14.3 (11.2–19.3)	0.478
Neutrophil (%)	172.0 (141.0–203.3)	175.5 (154.0–211.8)	168.0 (151.3–201.0)	0.873
Lymphocyte (%)	73.5 (69.1–76.5)	73.1 (68.0–78.7)	71.4 (65.1–78.9)	0.807
Hemoglobin (g/dL)	8.8 (7.4–11.0)	7.8 (7.1–9.1)	8.7 (6.6–10.3)	0.476
Platelet count (× 10^9/L)	12.6 (11.7–13.4)	12.2 (11.0–13.5)	12.3 (11.7–12.9)	0.419
International normalized ratio	1.0 (0.8–1.0)	0.9 (0.9–1.0)	0.9 (0.8–1.0)	0.072

Abbreviations: *QoR-15* Quality of Recovery-15 questionnaire, *POD* Postoperative day
*$p < 0.017$ as statistical significance based on the level in the IV-PCA group
†$p < 0.017$ as statistical significance based on the level in the RSB group
‡$p < 0.05$ using the linear-by-linear method
NOTE: Values are expressed as the median (interquartile) and number (proportion)

comparing the outcomes of the three pain-relief regimens. However, no ideal regional analgesic technique for RALP has yet been established; other regional analgesic models, including catheter-delivered continuous blockade, may be superior to ITMB [44]. Second, because of the absence of robust evidence related to an acceptable range of INRs for single-injection ultrasound-guided subfascial block (i.e., RSB), we presumed that an INR > 2.0 was the highest acceptable level for inclusion in our study. However, because of the risk of hematoma, skillful and meticulous ultrasound-based RSB is required for patient safety and analgesic results. Further RSB analyses are needed to determine the acceptable ranges of coagulopathic parameters, such as the INR. Third, our study was limited in that patients were not randomly allocated, despite the presence of comparable groups. A randomized setting was considered but rejected due to ethical concerns that IV-PCA alone may provide insufficient pain relief, compared with the other two analgesic regimens. Therefore, it was not possible to determine whether the analgesic results were solely related to pain-relief regimens.

Conclusions

ITMB may usefully reduce postoperative pain and aid recovery in patients undergoing RALP. Although robot-assisted surgery is more advanced and less invasive than open or laparoscopic surgery, analgesic care must counter both parietal and visceral pain associated with multi-level skin wounds and intra-abdominal tissue injuries. Our ITMB regimen (a low dose of morphine [0.2 mg] combined with bupivacaine [7.5 mg]) may contribute superior analgesia and better patient perception in terms of early postoperative recovery.

Abbreviations

RALP: Robot-assisted laparoscopic prostatectomy; RSB: Rectus sheath block; TAP: Trasnversus abdominis plane block; ITMB: Intrathecal morphine and bupivacaine block; POD: Postoperative day; IV-PCA: Intravenous patient-controlled analgesia; ASA: American Society of Anesthesiologists; INR: Interntaional normalized ratio; VAS: Visual analogue scale; QoR-15: Quality-of-recovery score on a 15-item questionnaire

Acknowledgements

The authors would like to thank our anesthetic nursing team (Eunju Choi and Hyeji An; Seoul St. Mary's Hospital, The Catholic University of Korea, Seoul, Republic of Korea) for their dedication.

Authors' contributions
J.W.S. and M.S.C. designed the study, wrote the manuscript, and analyzed and interpreted the data. J.W.S., Y.J.C., M.K., S.H.H., H.W.M., S.H.H. and M.S.C. collected the data and provided critical comments. All authors revised the manuscript critically for important intellectual content. All authors read and approved the final manuscript.

Author details
[1]Department of Anesthesiology and Pain medicine, Seoul St. Mary's Hospital, College of Medicine, The Catholic University of Korea, 222, Banpo-daero, Seocho-gu, Seoul 06591, Republic of Korea. [2]Department of Anesthesiology and Pain medicine, Bucheon St. Mary's Hospital, College of Medicine, The Catholic University of Korea, Seoul, Republic of Korea. [3]Department of Urology, Seoul St. Mary's Hospital, College of Medicine, The Catholic University of Korea, Seoul, Republic of Korea.

References

1. Nossiter J, Sujenthiran A, Charman SC, Cathcart PJ, Aggarwal A, Payne H, et al. Robot-assisted radical prostatectomy vs laparoscopic and open retropubic radical prostatectomy: functional outcomes 18 months after diagnosis from a national cohort study in England. Br J Cancer. 2018;118: 489–94.
2. Pearce SM, Pariser JJ, Karrison T, Patel SG, Eggener SE. Comparison of perioperative and early oncologic outcomes between open and robotic assisted laparoscopic prostatectomy in a contemporary population based cohort. J Urol. 2016;196:76–81.
3. Porpiglia F, Fiori C, Bertolo R, Manfredi M, Mele F, Checcucci E, et al. Five-year outcomes for a prospective randomised controlled trial comparing laparoscopic and robot-assisted radical prostatectomy. Eur Urol Focus. 2018; 4:80–6.
4. Woldu SL, Weinberg AC, Bergman A, Shapiro EY, Korets R, Motamedinia P, et al. Pain and analgesic use after robot-assisted radical prostatectomy. J Endourol. 2014;28:544–8.
5. Koning MV, de Vlieger R, Teunissen AJW, Gan M, Ruijgrok EJ, de Graaff JC, et al. The effect of intrathecal bupivacaine/morphine on quality of recovery in robot-assisted radical prostatectomy: a randomised controlled trial. Anaesthesia. 2019;75:599–608.
6. Dal Moro F, Aiello L, Pavarin P, Zattoni F. Ultrasound-guided transversus abdominis plane block (US-TAPb) for robot-assisted radical prostatectomy: a novel '4-point' technique-results of a prospective, randomized study. J Robot Surg. 2019;13:147–51.
7. Gupta M, Naithani U, Singariya G, Gupta S. Comparison of 0.25% Ropivacaine for Intraperitoneal instillation v/s rectus sheath block for postoperative pain relief following laparoscopic cholecystectomy: a prospective study. J Clin Diagn Res. 2016;10:Uc10.
8. Yasumura R, Kobayashi Y, Ochiai R. A comparison of plasma levobupivacaine concentrations following transversus abdominis plane block and rectus sheath block. Anaesthesia. 2016;71:544–9.
9. Bae J, Kim HC, Hong DM. Intrathecal morphine for postoperative pain control following robot-assisted prostatectomy: a prospective randomized trial. J Anesth. 2017;31:565–71.
10. Buyyounouski MK, Choyke PL, McKenney JK, Sartor O, Sandler HM, Amin MB, et al. Prostate cancer - major changes in the American joint committee on cancer eighth edition cancer staging manual. CA Cancer J Clin. 2017;67: 245–53.
11. Horlocker TT, Vandermeuelen E, Kopp SL, Gogarten W, Leffert LR, Benzon HT. Regional anesthesia in the patient receiving antithrombotic or thrombolytic therapy: American Society of Regional Anesthesia and Pain Medicine evidence-based guidelines (fourth edition). Reg Anesth Pain Med. 2018;43:263–309.
12. Sites BD, Chan VW, Neal JM, Weller R, Grau T, Koscielniak-Nielsen ZJ, et al. The American Society of Regional Anesthesia and Pain Medicine and the European Society of Regional Anaesthesia and Pain Therapy joint committee recommendations for education and training in ultrasound-guided regional anesthesia. Reg Anesth Pain Med. 2010;35:S74–80.
13. American Society of Anesthesiologists Task Force on Perioperative Blood Management. Practice guidelines for perioperative blood management: an updated report by the American Society of Anesthesiologists Task Force on perioperative blood management*. Anesthesiology. 2015;122:241–75.
14. Shim JW, Moon HK, Park YH, Park M, Park J, Lee HM, et al. Intraoperative changes in whole-blood viscosity in patients undergoing robot-assisted laparoscopic prostatectomy in the steep Trendelenburg position with pneumoperitoneum: a prospective nonrandomized observational cohort study. BMC Anesthesiol. 2020;20:7.
15. Hawker GA, Mian S, Kendzerska T, French M. Measures of adult pain: visual analog scale for pain (VAS pain), numeric rating scale for pain (NRS pain), McGill pain questionnaire (MPQ), short-form McGill pain questionnaire (SF-MPQ), chronic pain grade scale (CPGS), short Form-36 bodily pain scale (SF-36 BPS), and measure of intermittent and constant osteoarthritis pain (ICOAP). Arthritis Care Res. 2011;63(Suppl 11):S240–52.
16. Stark PA, Myles PS, Burke JA. Development and psychometric evaluation of a postoperative quality of recovery score: the QoR-15. Anesthesiology. 2013; 118:1332–40.
17. Clavien PA, Barkun J, de Oliveira ML, Vauthey JN, Dindo D, Schulick RD, et al. The Clavien-Dindo classification of surgical complications: five-year experience. Ann Surg. 2009;250:187–96.
18. de Souza DS, Costa AF, Chaves GV. Predisposing factors for postoperative nausea and vomiting in gynecologic tumor patients. Support Care Cancer. 2016;24:4661–7.
19. Lockington PF, Fa'aea P. Subcutaneous naloxone for the prevention of intrathecal morphine induced pruritus in elective caesarean delivery. Anaesthesia. 2007;62:672–6.
20. Feldman EL, Nave KA, Jensen TS, Bennett DLH. New horizons in diabetic neuropathy: mechanisms, bioenergetics, and pain. Neuron. 2017;93:1296–313.
21. Bruehl S, Chung OY, Diedrich L, Diedrich A, Robertson D. The relationship between resting blood pressure and acute pain sensitivity: effects of chronic pain and alpha-2 adrenergic blockade. J Behav Med. 2008;31:71–80.
22. Boisen ML, McQuaid AJ, Esper SA, Holder-Murray J, Zureikat AH, Hogg ME, et al. Intrathecal morphine versus nerve blocks in an enhanced recovery pathway for pancreatic surgery. J Surg Res. 2019;244:15–22.
23. Tang Y, Tang X, Wei Q, Zhang H. Intrathecal morphine versus femoral nerve block for pain control after total knee arthroplasty: a meta-analysis. J Orthop Surg Res. 2017;12:125.
24. Lui MW, Li TKT, Lui F, Ong CYT. A randomised, controlled trial of rectus sheath bupivacaine and intrathecal bupivacaine, without or with intrathecal morphine, vs. intrathecal bupivacaine and morphine after caesarean section. Anaesthesia. 2017;72:1225–9.
25. Jeong HW, Kim CS, Choi KT, Jeong SM, Kim DH, Lee JH. Preoperative versus postoperative rectus sheath block for acute postoperative pain relief after laparoscopic cholecystectomy: a randomized controlled study. J Clin Med. 2019;8:1018.
26. Karaarslan E, Topal A, Avcı O, Tuncer US. Research on the efficacy of the rectus sheath block method. Agri. 2018;30:183–8.
27. Cockrell R, Bonzo J, Lee D. Robot-assisted simple prostatectomy. J Endourol. 2018;32:S33–s8.
28. Du Y, Long Q, Guan B, Mu L, Tian J, Jiang Y, et al. Robot-assisted radical prostatectomy is more beneficial for prostate cancer patients: a system review and meta-analysis. Med Sci Monit. 2018;24:272–87.
29. Stein C. New concepts in opioid analgesia. Expert Opin Investig Drugs. 2018;27:765–75.
30. Yanagidate F, Strichartz GR. Local anesthetics. Handb Exp Pharmacol. 2007: 95–127.
31. Ljungqvist O. ERAS--enhanced recovery after surgery: moving evidence-based perioperative care to practice. JPEN J Parenter Enteral Nutr. 2014;38: 559–66.
32. Kang R, Chin KJ. Bilateral single-injection erector spinae plane block versus intrathecal morphine for postoperative analgesia in living donor laparoscopic hepatectomy: a randomized non-inferiority trial; 2019.
33. Jun JH, Kim GS, Lee JJ, Ko JS, Kim SJ, Jeon PH. Comparison of intrathecal morphine and surgical-site infusion of ropivacaine as adjuncts to intravenous patient-controlled analgesia in living-donor kidney transplant recipients. Singap Med J. 2017;58:666–73.
34. De Pietri L, Siniscalchi A, Reggiani A, Masetti M, Begliomini B, Gazzi M, et al. The use of intrathecal morphine for postoperative pain relief after liver resection: a comparison with epidural analgesia. Anesth Analg. 2006;102: 1157–63.
35. Motamed C, Bouaziz H, Franco D, Benhamou D. Analgesic effect of low-dose intrathecal morphine and bupivacaine in laparoscopic cholecystectomy. Anaesthesia. 2000;55:118–24.
36. Koju RB, Gurung BS, Dongol Y. Prophylactic administration of ondansetron in prevention of intrathecal morphine-induced pruritus and post-operative nausea and vomiting in patients undergoing caesarean section. BMC Anesthesiol. 2015;15:18.

37. Kumar K, Singh SI. Neuraxial opioid-induced pruritus: an update. J Anaesthesiol Clin Pharmacol. 2013;29:303–7.
38. Szarvas S, Chellapuri RS, Harmon DC, Owens J, Murphy D, Shorten GD. A comparison of dexamethasone, ondansetron, and dexamethasone plus ondansetron as prophylactic antiemetic and antipruritic therapy in patients receiving intrathecal morphine for major orthopedic surgery. Anesth Analg. 2003;97:259–63 table of contents.
39. Nguyen M, Vandenbroucke F, Roy JD, Beaulieu D, Seal RF, Lapointe R, et al. Evaluation of the addition of bupivacaine to intrathecal morphine and fentanyl for postoperative pain management in laparascopic liver resection. Reg Anesth Pain Med. 2010;35:261–6.
40. Girgin NK, Gurbet A, Turker G, Aksu H, Gulhan N. Intrathecal morphine in anesthesia for cesarean delivery: dose-response relationship for combinations of low-dose intrathecal morphine and spinal bupivacaine. J Clin Anesth. 2008;20:180–5.
41. Kim SC, Hauser S, Staniek A, Weber S. Learning curve of medical students in ultrasound-guided simulated nerve block. J Anesth. 2014;28:76–80.
42. Baranauskas MB, Margarido CB, Panossian C, Silva ED, Campanella MA, Kimachi PP. Simulation of ultrasound-guided peripheral nerve block: learning curve of CET-SMA/HSL anesthesiology residents. Rev Bras Anestesiol. 2008;58:106–11.
43. Leo S, Sng BL, Lim Y, Sia AT. A randomized comparison of low doses of hyperbaric bupivacaine in combined spinal-epidural anesthesia for cesarean delivery. Anesth Analg. 2009;109:1600–5.
44. Álvarez NER, Ledesma RJG, Hamaji A, Hamaji MWM, Vieira JE. Continuous femoral nerve blockade and single-shot sciatic nerve block promotes better analgesia and lower bleeding for total knee arthroplasty compared to intrathecal morphine: a randomized trial. BMC Anesthesiol. 2017;17:64.

6

Adding dexmedetomidine to morphine-based analgesia reduces early postoperative nausea in patients undergoing gynecological laparoscopic surgery

Huai Jin Li[1†], Shan Liu[2†], Zhi Yu Geng[1*] and Xue Ying Li[3]

Abstract

Background: Few studies have investigated the effect of dexmedetomidine on postoperative nausea and vomiting (PONV) in patients underwent gynecological laparoscopic surgery. We investigated if adding dexmedetomidine to a morphine-based patient-controlled analgesia (PCA) could decrease the incidence of PONV in this high-risk patient population.

Methods: In this prospective, randomized, double-blind and placebo-controlled study, 122 patients underwent gynecological laparoscopic surgery were assigned into two groups. Patients in the dexmedetomidine group (Group Dex) received a loading dose of dexmedetomidine 0.4 μg/kg before the end of surgery, followed by morphine 0.5 mg/ml plus dexmedetomidine 1 μg/ml for postoperative i.v. PCA. Patients in the control group (Group Ctrl) received normal saline before the end of surgery, followed by morphine 0.5 mg/ml alone for postoperative i.v. PCA. PCA pump was programmed as followed: bolus dose 2 ml, lockout interval 8 min and background infusion at a rate of 1 ml/h. The primary outcome was the incidence of nausea and vomiting within the first postoperative 24 h.

Results: Although there were no significant differences in regard to the total incidence of PONV (41.0% vs 52.5%, $P = 0.204$), PONV score, time to first onset of PONV, or the need for rescue antiemetics within the first postoperative 24 h between the two groups, the incidence of nausea and total PONV during the first 2 h period was significantly lower in the Group Dex than in the Group Ctrl (9.8% vs 24.6%, $P = 0.031$ and 0.031, respectively). More patients in Group Dex were over sedated or had bradycardia during the PACU compared with Group Ctrl ($P = 0.040$ and 0.036, respectively).

Conclusion: Our protocol in which dexmedetomidine was administered postoperatively – after a loading dose – to intravenous PCA morphine in patients undergoing gynecological laparoscopic surgery, had only early antiemetic effects, while no clinically meaningful antiemetic effect could be evidenced within the first 24 h after surgery.

Keywords: Dexmedetomidine, Gynecological, Laparoscopic surgery, Patient-controlled analgesia, Postoperative nausea and vomiting

* Correspondence: gengzhiyu2013@163.com
†Huai Jin Li and Shan Liu contributed equally to this work.
[1]Department of Anesthesiology, Peking University First Hospital, Beijing, China

Background

Postoperative nausea and vomiting (PONV) is an unpleasant experience and distressing adverse events after general anesthesia, especially in the first 24 h postoperatively [1].Patients after gynecological surgery are at particularly high risk and the incidence of PONV could even be as high as 80%in this population [2, 3].The Society for Ambulatory Anesthesia consensus guidelines recommended combination antiemetic therapy in high-risk patients population and adoption of prophylactic strategies to reduce the baseline risk of PONV [1]. Opioid-sparing technique is an integral part of enhanced recovery after major gynecological surgery protocol, because it not only reduces PONV but also decreases other opioid-related side effects that can have an influence onpatients' recovery, such as sedation and postoperative ileus [4].

Dexmedetomidine is a highly selective α2-adrenoreceptor agonist which has sedative, anxiolytic, analgesic, sympatholytic properties and minimal depression of respiratory function. Due to benefits such as maintaining haemodynamic stability, reducing opioid consumption and improving the quality of recovery, it has been widely used in clinical anesthesia, postoperative analgesia and sedation in the intensive care unit [5]. Two meta-analyses demonstrated that intraoperative dexmedetomidine significantly lowered postoperative pain score and opioid consumption, and this could lead to a reduced opioid-related adverse events including PONV [6, 7].

In our previous study, we demonstrated that intraoperative supplemental use of dexmedetomidine resulted in a lower incidence of nausea during the first 2 h postoperatively for patients undergoing gynecological laparoscopic surgery [8]. Intraoperative use of dexmedetomidine was investigated in other other studies about susceptible patients who underwent gynecological laparoscopic surgery [9–12]. Few studies evaluated the effect of postoperative use of dexmedetomidine as patient-controlled analgesia (PCA) regimen in preventing PONV.

A recent study found that adding dexmedetomidine to a fentanyl-based PCA reduced the frequency and severity of postoperative nausea during the time interval 1to 3 h postoperatively in patients underwent lumbar spinal surgery [13].

Thus, in this prospective, randomized, double-blind study, we aimed to evaluate the efficacy of adjunctive dexmedetomidine to morphine-based analgesia for PONV prophylaxis in women undergoin gelective gynecological laparoscopic surgery. Our primary hypothesis was that adding dexmedetomidine to a morphine-based PCA would reduce PONV in this patient population in comparison to only morphine-based PCA.

Methods

This prospective,randomized, double-blind clinical trial was performed between August 2018 to December 2018 at Peking University First Hospital. The trial was registered at Chictr.org.cn, Number ChiCTR1800017172, on July 162,018, http://www.chictr.org.cn/usercenter.aspx. Ethical approval for this study was provided by the Ethics Committee of Peking University First Hospital, Peking, China (Number 2018–130, principal investigator: Zhi Yu Geng) on 25 July 2018. Written informed content was obtained from all patients before enrollment.

Participants selection

We used the methodology previously described by our recent study [8].Participant screening was performed the day before surgery. The inclusion criteria were: (1) female patients; (2) age between 18 and 65 years old; (3) scheduled for elective laparoscopic myomectomy or laparoscopy-assisted vaginal hysterectomy. Patients who met any of the following criteria were excluded: (1) American Society of Anesthesiologists physical status >II before surgery, (2) previous history of schizophrenia, Parkinson's Disease, epilepsy and myasthenia gravis, (3) unable to communicate due to coma, dementia and other diseases, (4) obesity defined as BMI (body mass index) > 30 kg m^{-2}, (5) known sick sinus syndrome, severe bradycardia (heart rate < 50 beats per minute), or severe atrioventricular block without pacemaker before surgery, (6) pre-existing of severe hepatic disease (Child-Pugh class C), (7) pre-existing of chronic renal failure (receive renal replacement therapy preoperatively), (8) Neo-adjuvant chemoradiotherapy before surgery, (9) alcoholism or drug abuse, (10) any regimen of antiemetic, glucocorticoids or psychotropic drugs which are known to have an influence on the occurrence of PONV within 24 h before surgery.

Randomisation and drug administration

Random numbers were generated by computer software in a 1:1 ratio. Patients were randomized to receive morphine 0.5 mg ml^{-1} with or without dexmedetomidine 1 μg ml^{-1}. Study drugs were prepared according to the randomization results by a study coordinator. Anesthesiologist and the investigator responsible for the study outcomes assesssment were blinded.

For patients in the dexmedetomidine group (Group Dex), an initial loading dose of 0.4 μg kg^{-1} dexmedetomidine was given by intravenous infusion 0.5 h before the end of surgery. PCA was begun with 0.5 mg ml^{-1} morphine plus 1 μg ml^{-1} dexmedetomidine in 100 ml normal saline. While for patients in the control group (Group Ctrl), normal saline was given 0.5 h before the end of surgery, and PCA was begun with 0.5 mg ml^{-1} morphine in 100 ml normal saline. For all patients, PCA was programmed to deliver a 2 ml bolus on-demand with a lockout time of 8 min and a background infusion at a rate of 1 ml h^{-1}.

The investigator assessing patients outcomes was blinded to group assignment and blinding was maintained throughout the study period.

Anesthesia and perioperative care

No pre-medication was administered before induction. Routine monitoring included non-invasive blood pressure, pulse oximetry, electocadiogram, Bispectral index and end-tidal carbon dioxide partial pressure were applied intraoperatively.

All patients received dexamethasone 5 mg before induction. General anesthesia was induced intravenously with 0.03 mg kg^{-1} midazolam, 2 mg kg^{-1} propofol, and target controlled infusion of remifentanil with an effect-site concentration of 3 ng ml^{-1}. Rocuronium was administered to facilitate laryngeal mask airway insertion. Total intravenous anesthesia was provided with propofol and remifentanil. Bispectral index was maintained between 40 and 60 during surgery and blood pressure was adjusted within ±20% from baseline. Mechanical ventilation was maintained with a mixture of oxygen and air (FiO_2 0.5) and an end-tidal carbon dioxide partial pressure was adjusted between 35 and 55 mmHg intraoperatively. Lactated Ringer's solution was infused at a rate of 6 ml kg^{-1} h^{-1} throughout the surgery.

Morphine 0.1 mg kg^{-1} and parecoxib sodium 40 mg were administered 0.5 h before the end of surgery. Residual neuromuscular block was reversed with neostigmine (0.04 mg kg^{-1}) and atropine (0.02 mg kg^{-1}) at the end of the surgery.

Upon completion of surgery, laryngeal mask airway was removed and the patient was transferred to the post-anesthesia care unit (PACU) for 1 hour monitoring. The patient-controlled analgesia pump was started and continued until 24 h after surgery.

Data collection

Data were collected by research personnel who were blinded to the randomization and not involved in the clinical care. The 24 h observation period started at the time of removal of the laryngeal mask airway. The researcher assessed the patients at 2, 6 and 24 h postoperatively. Baseline characteristics of patientssuch as previous history of PONV, chronic smoking, primary risk score for PONV, co-existing systemic diseases and concurrent medication were recorded. Intra-operative parameters including duration of anesthesia and surgery, doses of anesthetics and analgesics, and total fluid administered were collected. Postoperative data including presence and severity of nausea and vomiting, visual analogue scale (VAS) pain scores, the cumulative dose of PCA morphine, requirement for rescue antiemetics, vital signs, sedation scores, and any adverse events were documented.

Outcome measures

The primary outcome was the incidence of PONV over the first 24 h postoperative hours. Patients who experienced at least one episode of nausea, vomiting or retching or any combination of these during the first 24 h after surgery were considered to have PONV. Patients were asked to rate their degree of nausea using a four-point scale (0 = none, 1 = mild, 2 = moderate, 3 = severe) [14, 15]. Postoperative vomiting was defined as at least one episode of vomiting or retching and the PONV score was rated as 4. Tropisetron 5 mg was used as the rescue antiemetic. If tropisetron failed to relieve the symptom, metoclopramide was administered. Rescue antiemetics were administered on the following conditions: two or more episodes of vomiting or retching, any nausea lasting for more than 30 min, a 'severe' degree of nausea or whenever treatment was requested by the patient.

The secondary outcomes included the VAS scores at 2, 6 and 24 h after surgery, the total 24 h morphine consumption, and the occurrence of adverse events during PACU stay. Pain intensity was assessed at PACU, 2 h, 6 h and 24 h postoperatively using an 11-point VAS on which 0 indicated no pain and 10 indicated the worst pain imaginable. In the PACU, supplemental morphine bolus of 2 mg i.v. was administered for moderate pain (VAS ≥4). Sedation levels were assessed using the Ramsay sedation scale (1 = agitated and uncomfortable, 2 = co-operative and orientated, 3 = can follow simple directions, 4 = asleep but strong response to stimulation, 5 = asleep and slow response to stimulation and 6 = asleep and no response to stimulation). Over sedation was defined as a sedation score ≥ 4 [16].Agitation was evaluated using the Ricker sedation-agitation scale and emergence agitation was defined as a sedation-agitation score ≥ 5 [17].

Sample size calculation

Study sample size was calculated according to our previous studies [3, 8]. In order to detect a 50% reduction in the incidence of PONV (i.e. from 50 to 25%) in the dexmedetomidine group for this patient population, which we considered as clinically meaningful, with a 5% type-I error and power of 80%, we estimated that 55 patients in each group were needed. To allow for a possible dropout rate of 10%, we aimed to enroll 61 patients in each group.

Statistical analysis

Categorical data are expressed as number (percentage) and were analysed using the χ^2 test or the Fisher's exact test as appropriate. Continuous data are expressed as means (standard deviation [SD]) or medians (interquartile range [IQR]) and were analyzed with the unpaired Student's t-test or Mann–Whitney U test as appropriate. A two-sided P value less than 0.05 was considered statistically significant.

Statistical analysis was performed using the SPSS 22.0 software (SPSS, Inc., Chicago, Illinois, USA).

Results

Between August 2018 and December 2018, a total of 128 patients were enrolled and six patients were excluded from the analysis. As a result, 122 patients completed the study: 61 in each group, a flowchart is shown in Fig. 1. There were no significant differences with regard to patient's baseline characteristics and perioperative data including risk scores of PONV, durations of anesthesia and surgery, propofol and remifentanil doses, and intraoperative fluids between the two groups (Table 1).

The primary outcome was the incidence of PONV over the first 24 h postoperative hours and we found no difference between the two groups (Group Dex vs. Group Ctrl, 25(41.0%) and 32(52.5%), $P = 0.204$) (Table 2).

We found that the incidence of nausea and total PONV during the first 0-2 h after surgery was significantly lower in the Group Dex compared with the Group Ctrl (6(9.8%) and 15(24.6%), $P = 0.031$). We did not find any differences in the incidence of nausea, vomiting and total PONV during the 2-6 h and 6-24 h, PONV score, time to first PONV and the requirement of rescue antiemetics between two groups (Table 2).

The total consumption of morphine during 6-24 h after surgery was significantly less in the Group Dex than in the Group Ctrl ($P = 0.009$), but the cumulative consumption of morphine for the total 24 h after surgery was not significantly different between the groups. The percentage of over sedation and bradycardia during the

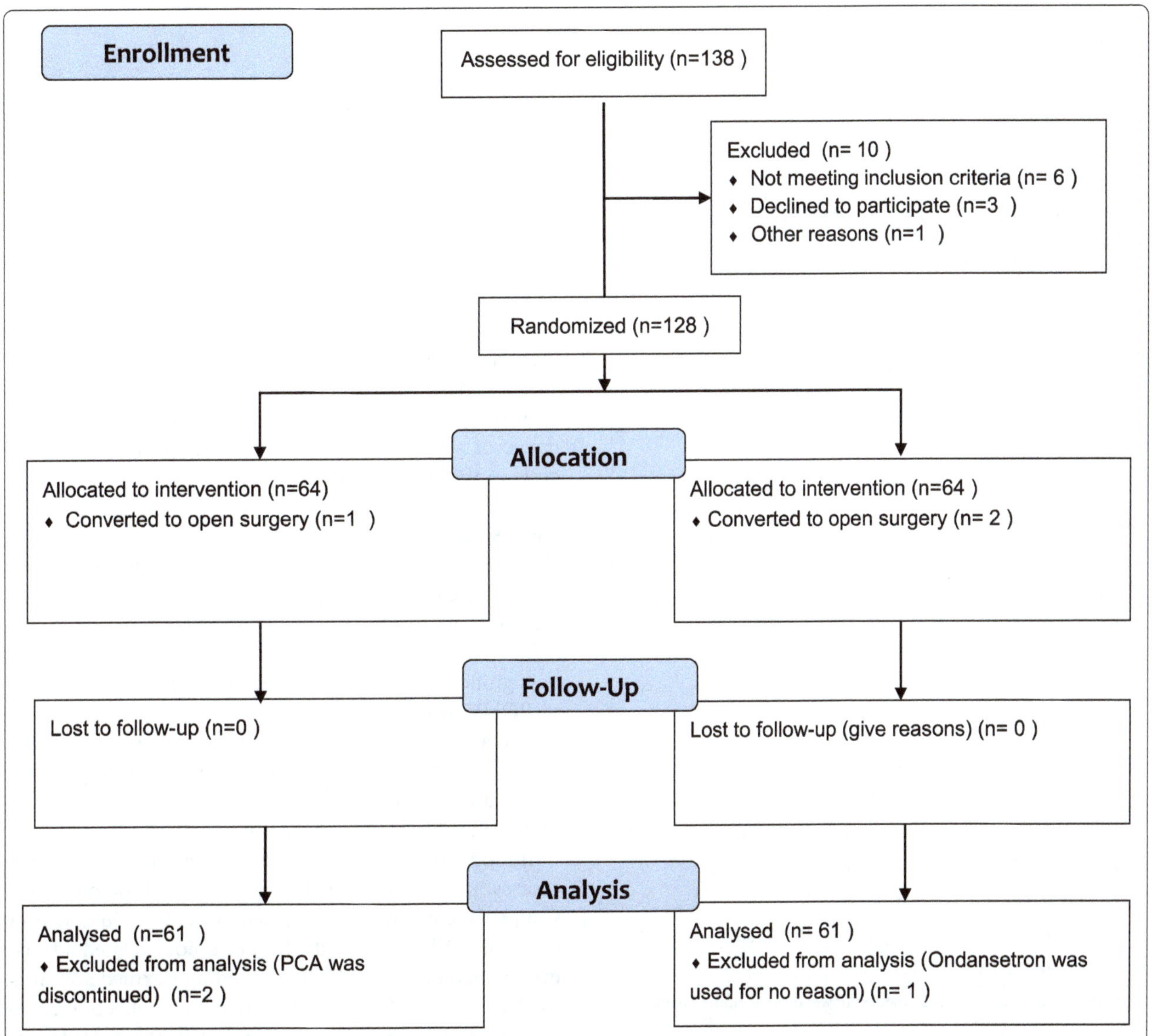

Fig. 1 Consort flow diagram

Table 1 Clinical characteristics and intraoperative variables ($n = 61$)

	Group Dex	Group Ctrl	*P* value
Age (years)	44.0 (8.1)	44.2 (8.4)	0.896
Height (cm)	161.3 (5.8)	160.6 (5.5)	0.503
Weight (kg)	61.0 (8.8)	60.8 (8.8)	0.885
BMI (kgm^{-2})	23.5 (3.1)	23.5 (2.8)	0.872
ASA status I/II (n)	34/27	31/30	0.586
Smoking (n/%)	3 (4.9)	3 (4.9)	1.000
History of motion sickness (n/%)	19 (31.1)	22 (36.1)	0.565
History of PONV (n/%)	4 (6.6)	7 (11.5)	0.343
Apfel score for PONV risk (n/%)			0.492
1	0	0	
2	3 (4.9)	1 (1.6)	
3	38 (62.3)	36 (59.0)	
4	20 (32.8)	24 (39.3)	
Average number of risk scores	3.3 (0.6)	3.4 (0.5)	0.679
Duration of anesthesia(min)	133 (59)	131 (52)	0.837
Duration of surgery(min)	112 (59)	112 (49)	0.969
Intraoperative propofol(mg·kg^{-1}·h^{-1})	5.4 (1.2)	5.4 (0.8)	0.784
Intraoperative remifentanil (μg·kg^{-1}·h^{-1})	7.3 (1.4)	7.1 (1.2)	0.367
Intraoperative fluids (ml)	1285 (433)	1239 (417)	0.545

Data are presented as mean (SD) or n (%). *BMI* body mass index
PONV postoperative nausea and vomiting
Dex dexmedetomidine, *Ctrl*control

Table 2 Comparison of overall postoperative nausea and vomiting outcomes ($n = 61$)

	Group Dex	Group Ctrl	*P* value
Nausea (n/%)			
0-2 h	6(9.8)	15(24.6)	0.031
2-6 h	7(11.5)	11(18.0)	0.307
6-24 h	21(34.4)	17(27.9)	0.434
Vomiting (n/%)			
0-2 h	3(4.9)	6(9.8)	0.488
2-6 h	3(4.9)	5(8.3)	0.715
6-24 h	8(13.1)	7(11.5)	0.809
PONV(n/%)			
0-2 h	6 (9.8)	15 (24.6)	0.031
2-6 h	7 (11.5)	13 (21.3)	0.142
6-24 h	20 (32.8)	17 (27.9)	0.555
Total 24 h PONV (n/%)	25 (41.0)	32 (52.5)	0.204
PONV score	0 (0, 2.5)	1 (0, 4)	0.226
Time to first PONV (hr)	0(0,4)	0.5(0,3)	0.430
Rescue antiemetics (n/%)	7(11.5)	10(16.4)	0.433

Data are presented as mean (SD), median (lower quartile, upper quartile) or n (%)
Dex dexmedetomidine, *Ctrl* control
PONV postoperative nausea and vomiting

PACU stay was significantly higher in the Group Dex than in the Group Ctrl ($P = 0.040$ and 0.036, respectively). There were no differences between the two groups regarding VAS score at everytime point, the incidence of shivering, agitation and requiring rescue analgesic in the PACU (Tables 3,4).

Discussion

Our study showed that for patients who underwent gynecological laparoscopic surgery, adding dexmedetomidine to a morphine-based PCA only decreased the incidence of early nausea during the recovery. There were no significant differences in regard to the total incidence of PONV, time to first onset of PONV, or the need for rescue antiemetics within the first postoperative 24 h between the two groups. Thus, only early antiemetic effects was found when dexmedetomidine was used as an adjunctive analgesic with morphine.

Intraoperative dexmedetomidine administration decreases postoperative pain intensity and opioids consumption compared with placebo. This opioid-sparing effect might lead to a reduction of opioid-related adverse events including PONV [6, 7]. Adding dexmedetomidine to PCA seemed to have some beneficial effects on preventing PONV as well. Du and colleagues [18] used intravenous 0.5 μg kg^{-1} dexmedetomidine as a loading

Table 3 Comparison of PCA morphine consumption and adverse events in PACU (*n* = 61)

	Group Dex	Group Ctrl	*P*value
VAS at PACU	2(1,3)	2(2,3)	0.442
VAS at 2 h	2(1,3)	2(1,3)	0.498
VAS at 6 h	1(0,1)	1(0,1)	0.800
VAS at 24 h	0 (0,1)	0 (0,1)	0.191
Total morphine consumption (mg)			
0-2 h	2.8 (1.5)	2.8 (1.5)	0.907
2-6 h	2.3 (0.6)	2.2 (0.6)	0.280
6-24 h	9.0 (0.1)	9.3 (1.3)	0.009
0-24 h	14.1 (1.8)	14.3 (2.1)	0.524
Use of rescue analgesic (n/%)	10 (16.4)	9(14.8)	0.803

Data are presented as mean (SD) or n (%)
Dex dexmedetomidine, *Ctrl* control
PCA patient controlled analgesia, *PACU* postanesthesia care unit

dose and followed by continuous infusion as an adjunct to butorphanol PCA in patients undergoing total laparoscopic hysterectomy. Their result showed that the administration of dexmedetomidine provided effective analgesia, significant butorphanol sparing and less nausea and vomiting. Another study investigated the effect of dexmedetomidine alone for intravenous PCA after gynecological laparoscopic operation. The result showed that dexmedetomidine alone was effective for postoperative pain control and the incidence of PONV was significant lower in the Dex group [19].

In our present study, we chose the incidence of first 24 h PONV as primary endpoint and demonstrated that dexmedetomidine combined with morphine only reduced early nausea of the first 2 h postoperatively. During the 24 h postoperative period, the cumulative PCA morphine consumption was 14.1 (1.8) mg and 14.3 (2.1) mg respectively in this minimally invasive surgery. In Lin and colleagues' study [20], they also investigated the effect of combining dexmedetomidine and morphine PCA in patients undergoing total abdominal hysterectomy. Patients

Table 4 Adverse events in PACU (n = 61)

	Group Dex	Group Ctrl	*P*value
Hypertension (n/%)	2 (3.3)	2 (3.3)	0.611
Hypotension (n/%)	0(0.0)	1 (1.6)	1.000
Respiratory depression (n/%)	0(0.0)	0(0.0)	
Bradycardia (n/%)	6(9.8)	0(0.0)	0.036
Agitation (n/%)	1(1.6)	3(4.9)	0.611
Over sedation (n/%)	10 (16.4)	3 (4.9)	0.040
Shivering (n/%)	7 (11.5)	10 (16.4)	0.433

Data are presented as n (%)
Dex dexmedetomidine, *Ctrl* control
PACU postanesthesia care unit

receiving dexmedetomidine consumed 29% less PCA morphine and the 4–24 h incidence of nausea was significantly lower in dexmedetomidine group (34% vs 56.3%). Since laparotomy surgery is more painful than laparoscopic surgery, the total morphine consumption and dexmedetomidine dose were much higher than in our study. We speculate this may be the reason for different result.

In our previous research about this PONV susceptible patient population, we found that intraoperative use of dexmedetomidine reduced the incidence of early nausea but not vomiting within 24 h after gynecological laparoscopic surgery [8]. While in this subsequent trial, we focused on the preventive efficacy of postoperative dexmedetomidine when added to morphine PCA and obtained a similar result. The consistent result might be attributed to the initial loading dose of dexmedetomidine before the end of the surgery, since its terminal half-life is about 2 h.

Song and colleagues [13] investigated the effect of combining dexmedetomidine and fentanyl analgesia in patients undergoing lumbar spinal surgery. They found that the Dex group experienced less nausea during 1 to 3 h postoperatively and the intensity of nausea was similar between groups during the first 48 h. Although less PCA fentanyl was required in the Dex groupup to 12 h, there was no statistical significance in the incidence of vomiting between the groups. In addition, in our study, although the cumulative consumption of morphine during 6-24 h after surgery was statistically greater in the Group Ctrl, the incidence of nausea and vomiting was not significantly different between the groups. Since postoperative opioid is one of the primary drivers of PONV, it appears that the intensity of opioid-sparing effect of dexmedetomidine might be crucial to decreasing nausea and vomiting.

The stimulation of nausea and vomiting originates from the inputs of visceral, vestibular and chemoreceptor trigger areas, which are mediated by serotonin, dopamine, histamine and acetylcholine, respectively. Nauseogenic stimulus activates nucleus suchas amugdala, putamen and locus coeruleus, which converted into fear conditioning and emotional triggering. This eventually leads to a strong sensation of nausea [21]. In our study, dexmedetomidine showed some weak and short-lived anti-nausea effect that maybe explained by the properties of α2 agonist. As PONV may be triggered by high catecholamine concentration, it may produce a direct anti-nausea effect through activating the α2-adrenoceptor and decreasing sympathetic tone. Furthermore, dexmedetomidine has concentrate dependent sedative and hypnotic effects that mediated through activation of central α2-receptors in the locus coeruleus. The sedative property mightbe involved in reduing nausea just as benzodiazepines since in our research more patients in the Group Dex were over sedated during the PACU stay.

Dexmedetomidine may increase the risk of postoperative bradycardia [6].When dexmedetomidine combined with sufentanil PCA was used in patient undergoing radical gastrectomy, the incidences of oversedation and bradycardia increased significantly and these side effects were dose-dependent [22]. Despite the low dose regimen of dexmedetomidine in our study, the percentage of patients who experienced bradycardia and over sedation in PACU was significantly higher in the Group Dex. Thus, when determine the optimal dose of dexmedetomidine for postoperative analgesia, the potential increased risk of significant hypotension, bradycardia, respiratory depression and over sedation should be balanced against the maximal beneficial analgesic effect.

There are several limitations of this study. First, in our study PCA was programmed to deliver bolus with a background basal infusion of morphine with or without dexmedetomidine. This continuous infusion dose of morphine might have masked the difference of opioid demands between groups. Second, we only chose one dose and the concentration of dexmedetomidine (1 μg ml^{-1}) was relatively small in PCA. Further dose finding studies of dexmedetomidine are required to confirm the optimal efficacy and safety outcomes for these PONV susceptible patients.

Conclusions

In conclusion, our protocol in which dexmedetomidine was administered postoperatively – after a loading dose – to intravenous PCA morphine in patients undergoing gynecological laparoscopic surgery, had only early antiemetic effects, while no clinically meaningful antiemetic effect could be evidenced within the first 24 h after surgery.

Abbreviations

PACU: Post-anesthesia care unit; PCA: Patient-controlled analgesia; PONV: Postoperative nausea and vomiting; VAS: Visual analogue scale

Acknowledgements

We thank Ms. Gui-Ying Guan (Department of Anesthesiology, PekingUniversity First Hospital, Beijing, China) for her help in preparing the study drugs.

Authors' contributions

Study design and supervision: ZYG, HJL. Data collection: SL. Data analysis:ZYG, XYL. Drafting/writing paper: HJL. Revising manuscript: ZYG. Final approval of manuscript: all authors.

Author details

[1]Department of Anesthesiology, Peking University First Hospital, Beijing, China. [2]Department of Anesthesiology, Beijing Shangdi Hospital, Beijing, China. [3]Department of Biostatics, Peking University First Hospital, Beijing, China.

References

1. Gan TJ, Diemunsch P, Habib AS, et al. Society for Ambulatory Anesthesia consensus guidelines for the management of postoperative nausea and vomiting. Anesth Analg. 2014;118:85–113.
2. Apfel CC, Läärä E, Koivuranta M, Greim CA, Roewer N. A simplified risk score for predicting postoperative nausea and vomiting: conclusions from cross-validations between two center. Anesthesiology. 1999;91:693–700.
3. Geng ZY, Hu X. Clinical observation of postoperative nausea and vomiting in patient undergone gynecological laparoscopy under total intravenous anesthesia. Chin J Min InvSurg. 2009;9:892–5.
4. Bauchat JR, Habib AS. Evidence-based anesthesia for major gynecologic surgery. Anesthesiol Clin. 2015;33:173–207.
5. Weerink MAS, Struys MMRF, Hannivoort LN, Barends CRM, Absalom AR, Colin P. Clinical pharmacokinetics and pharmacodynamics of Dexmedetomidine. Clin Pharmacokinet. 2017;56:893–913.
6. Blaudszun G, Lysakowski C, Elia N, Tramèr MR. Effect of perioperative systemic α2 agonists on postoperative morphine consumption and pain intensity. Anesthesiology. 2012;116:1312–22.
7. Schnabel A, Meyer-Frießem CH, Reichl SU, Zahn PK, Pogatzki-Zahn EM. Is intraoperative dexmedetomidine a new option for postoperative pain treatment? A meta-analysis of randomized controlled trials. Pain. 2013;154:1140–9.
8. Geng ZY, Liu YF, Wang SS, Wang DX. Intra-operative dexmedetomidine reduces early postoperative nausea but not vomiting in adult patients after gynaecological laparoscopic surgery: a randomised controlled trial. Eur J Anesthesiol. 2016;33:761–6.
9. Elvan EG, Oç B, Uzun S, Karabulut E, Coşkun F, Aypar U. Dexmedetomidine and postoperative shivering in patients undergoing elective abdominal hysterectomy. Eur J Anesthesiol. 2008;25:357–64.
10. Ge DJ, Qi B, Tang G, Li JY. Intraoperative Dexmedetomidine promotes postoperative analgesia and recovery in patients after abdominal hysterectomy: a double-blind. Randomized Clinical Trial Sci Rep. 2016;23:21514.
11. Bulow NMH, Barbosa NV, Rocha JBT. Opioid consumption in total intravenous anesthesia is reduced with dexmedetomidine: a comparative study with remifentanil in gynecologic video laparoscopic surgery. J Clin Anesth. 2007;19:280–5.
12. Lee C, Kim YD, Kim JN. Antihyperalgesic effects of dexmedetomidine on high-dose remifentanil-induced hyperalgesia. Korean J Anesthesiol. 2013;64:301–7.
13. Song Y, Shim JK, Song JW, Kim EK, Kwak YL. Dexmedetomidine added to an opioid-based analgesic regimen for the prevention of postoperative nausea and vomiting in highly susceptible patients. Eur J Anaesthesiol. 2015;33:75–83.
14. McKeen DM, Arellano R, O'Connell C. Supplemental oxygen does not prevent postoperative nausea and vomiting after gynecological laparoscopy. Can J Anesth. 2009;56:651–7.
15. Torup H, Hansen EG, Bøgeskov M, et al. Transversus abdominis plane block after laparoscopic colonic resection in cancer patients: a randomised clinical trial. Eur J Anaesthesiol. 2016;33:725–30.
16. Gurbet A, Basagan-Mogol E, Turker G, Ugun F, Kaya FN, Ozcan B. Intraoperative infusion of dexmedetomidine reduces perioperative analgesic requirements. Can J Anesth. 2006;53:646–52.
17. Kim SY, Kim JM, Lee JH, Song BM, Koo BN. Efficacy of intraoperative dexmedetomidine infusion on emergence agitation and quality of recovery after nasal surgery. Br J Anaesth. 2013;111:222–8.
18. Du J, Li JW, Jin J, Shi CX, Ma JH. Intraoperative and postoperative infusion of dexmedetomidine combined with intravenous butorphanol patient-controlled analgesia following total hysterectomy under laparoscopy. Exp Ther Med. 2018;16:4063–9.
19. Wang X, Liu W, Xu Z, et al. Effect of Dexmedetomidine alone for intravenous patient-controlled analgesia after gynecological laparoscopic surgery: a consort-prospective, randomized, controlled trial. Medicine (Baltimore). 2016;95:e3639.
20. Lin TF, Yeh YC, Lin FS, et al. Effect of combining dexmedetomidine and morphine for intravenous patient-controlled analgesia. Br J Anaesth. 2009; 102:117–22.
21. Singh P, Yoon SS, Kuo B. Nausea: a review of pathophysiology and therapeutics. Ther Adv Gastroenterol. 2016;9:98–112.
22. Shang Y, Long XH, Gao GJ, Xu YY, Yu Y, Hou X. Dosage study of dexmedetomidine-assisted sufentanil administration on vein analgesia after gastric cancer surgery. J Clin Anesth. 2013;29:247–50.

7

The analgesic efficacy compared ultrasound-guided continuous transverse abdominis plane block with epidural analgesia following abdominal surgery

Chaosheng Qin[1], Yuanming Liu[2], Jijun Xiong[1], Xiaogang Wang[1], Qinghua Dong[1], Tingshi Su[3] and Jingchen Liu[1*]

Abstract

Background: This review and meta-analysis aims to evaluate the analgesic efficacy of continuous transversus abdominis plane (TAP) block compared with epidural analgesia (EA) in adults after abdominal surgery.

Methods: The databases PubMed, Embase and Cochrane Central Register were searched from inception to June 2019 for all available randomized controlled trials (RCTs) that evaluated the analgesic efficacy of continuous TAP block compared with EA after abdominal surgery. The weighted mean differences (WMDs) were estimates for continuous variables with a 95% confidence interval (CI) and risk ratio (RR) for dichotomous data. The pre-specified primary outcome was the dynamic pain scores 24 h postoperatively.

Results: Eight trials including 453 patients (TAP block:224 patients; EA: 229 patients) ultimately met the inclusion criteria and seven trials were included in the meta-analysis. Dynamic pain scores after 24 h were equivalent between TAP block and EA groups (WMD:0.44; 95% CI: 0.1 to 0.99; $I^2 = 91\%$; $p = 0.11$). The analysis showed a significant difference between the subgroups according to regularly administering (4 trials; WMD:-0.11; 95% CI: − 0.32 to 0.09; $I^2 = 0\%$; $p = 0.28$) non-steroidal anti-inflammatory drugs (NSAIDs) or not (3 trials; WMD:1.02; 95% CI: 0.09 to 1.96; $I^2 = 94\%$; $p = 0.03$) for adjuvant analgesics postoperatively. The measured time of the urinary catheter removal in the TAP group was significantly shorter (3 trials, WMD:-18.95, 95% CI:-25.22 to − 12.71; $I^2 = 0\%$; $p < 0.01$), as was time to first ambulation postoperatively (4 trials, WMD:-6.61, 95% CI: − 13.03 to − 0.19; $I^2 = 67\%$; $p < 0.05$).

Conclusion: Continuous TAP block, combined with NSAIDs, can provide non-inferior dynamic analgesia efficacy compared with EA in postoperative pain management after abdominal surgery. In addition, continuous TAP block is associated with fewer postoperative side effects.

Keywords: TAP block, Epidural analgesia, Abdominal surgery, Meta-analysis

* Correspondence: 44483316@qq.com
[1]Department of Anesthesiology, The First Affiliated Hospital of Guangxi Medical University, Nanning, Guangxi 530021, People's Republic of China

Background

Epidural analgesia (EA) has long been recognized as the gold-standard technique for analgesia after abdominal surgery [1]. However, the benefits of EA are accompanied by a number of potential side effects, such as hypotension and urinary retention, which has led professionals to seek other analgesic methods [2, 3].

The transversus abdominis plane (TAP) block provides an analgesic effect on the anterolateral abdominal wall [4, 5]. Growing evidence supports the effectiveness of TAP blocks for various types of abdominal surgeries. In addition, with the advancements in ultrasound technology, the safety of TAP block has greatly improved; there has been a surge of interest in ultrasound-guided TAP blocks as an adjunct for analgesia following abdominal operations [6, 7]. However, the effect of a single TAP block is not durable, and its analgesic efficacy lasts less than 24 h [5, 8]. Thus, continuous TAP block by placing the catheter into the transverse abdominal plane and infusing local anaesthetic drugs continuously or intermittently through the catheter were used [9–11]. Continuous infusion of different doses of local anaesthetics in different regions of the TAP is complicated, and researchers have reported different and even conflicting outcomes compared with EA [12–15]. However, there has been no systematic assessment comparing the analgesic effect of continuous TAP block with traditional EA following several abdominal surgeries. Therefore, this review and meta-analysis aimed to systematically evaluate the analgesic efficacy of continuous TAP block compared with EA in adults after abdominal surgery, as well as its clinical safety and its impact on patient recovery.

Methods

Search strategy and selection criteria

We used the recommendations of PRISMA for this systematic review and meta-analysis. We searched the online databases PubMed, Embase and Cochrane Central Register for all relevant studies. Search terms included: epidural anaesthesia OR epidural analgesia OR epidural injection OR epidural administration. The results of this search subsequently combined the following terms: continuous TAP block OR continuous transversus abdominis plane block OR transversus abdominis plane catheters OR TAP block catheters OR abdominal wall block OR transversus abdominal wall block OR nerve block. The search strategy was limited to randomized controlled trials (RCTs) and those performed on humans. No language restriction was applied. The most recent electronic search was completed in June of 2019. We also manually checked the bibliographies of relevant articles for other potentially eligible trials.

Population

This systematic review and meta-analysis is only aimed at female and male adults (18 years or older) who have undergone different types of abdominal surgery.

Intervention and control

Ultrasound-guided continuous TAP blocks adopting various approaches (subcostal, oblique subcostal, lateral, or posterior [5, 16]) compared with EA following abdominal surgeries were included in this study.

Outcomes

The pre-specified primary outcome was dynamic pain scores (upon movement) 24 h after abdominal surgery. Secondary outcomes were pain scores at rest after 24 h and pain scores, at rest and dynamic, after 12 h, 48 h and 72 h. Postoperative opioid consumption was measured at 24 h, 48 h, and 72 h following surgery. Meanwhile, we addressed function-related outcomes including time of removal of the urinary catheter, time to first flatus, time to first ambulation, and length of hospital stay. Outcomes of side effects were also evaluated, including hypotension and block complications within the first 24 h postoperatively.

Data extraction

We extracted independent data using established standard data collection forms by two authors (QCS and LYM). Disagreements were resolved by discussion with another author (LJC). If needed, we contacted the corresponding authors of selected articles to obtain the mean and standard deviation of the data. If there was no response, we used the median and quartile ranges to approximate the estimation [17, 18]. Different pain scores assessed with verbal, visual, or numeric rating scales were all converted to a standardized number (on a 10-point scale) for analysis. All opioid analgesic drug usages were converted to equianalgesic doses of intravenous morphine for quantitative evaluations (10 mg of IV morphine = 1.5 mg of IV hydromorphone = 0.1 mg of IV fentanyl = 75 mg of IV pethidine = 100 mg of IV tramadol = 30 mg of oral morphine = 7.5 mg of oral hydromorphone = 20 mg of oral oxycodone) [19].

Assessment of trial quality

The quality of the reviewed trials was assessed independently by two authors (QCS and LYM) following the Cochrane Collaboration Risk of Bias Tool for randomized controlled trials [20]. Disagreements were resolved by discussion with another author (LJC). The Cochrane Risk of Bias Tool measured the following: adequacy of sequence generation, allocation concealment, blinding of participants, blinding of outcome assessment, incomplete outcome data, selective outcome reporting, and other potential sources of bias.

Statistical analysis

All statistical analyses were performed with the assistance of Review Manager software (RevMan version 5.3.5; The Cochrane Collaboration 2014). For continuous data, when measuring methods were different, the standardized mean difference (SMD) with 95% confidence interval (CI) was calculated; otherwise, the weight mean difference (WMD) with 95% CI was calculated. A risk ratio (RR) with a 95% CI was calculated for dichotomous data. The I^2 statistic, used for evaluating heterogeneity, was predefined using the following three scales: low ($I^2 < 50\%$), moderate ($I^2 = 50–74\%$), and high ($I^2 > 75\%$) [21]. We pooled outcome data using a fixed effects model in the case of low heterogeneity; otherwise, we chose a random effects model. Predetermined subgroup analysis was conducted according to the type of surgical operation (open surgery or laparoscopy), the method of local anesthetic administration (continuous or intermittent), and whether other anti-inflammatory drugs were regularly used postoperatively. A P-value of < 0.05 was considered statistically significant.

Results

Search results

In total, 977 potentially eligible studies were identified through the literature search. We excluded 217 records that were duplicates and a further 738 records for other reasons. After review of the remaining 22 articles in full, 8 RCTs [13, 15, 22–27] ultimately met the inclusive criteria and 7 RCTs [13, 15, 22–26] were included in the meta-analysis. A flowchart of this process, including the reasons for excluding studies, is shown in Fig. 1.

Characteristics of trials

Ultimately included trials in this review were published between 2011 and 2017, totaling 453 patients (224 in the TAP block group and 229 in the EA group). Six trials [13, 22–25, 27] were published in English and the other 2 trials [15, 26] were published in Chinese. The detailed characteristics of the included trials (8 RCTs) are presented in Table 1.

Risk of bias in included studies

According to our assessment of the Cochrane Collaboration Risk of Bias tool (Fig. 2), most trials have a high risk of bias, which is mainly related to the blindness of

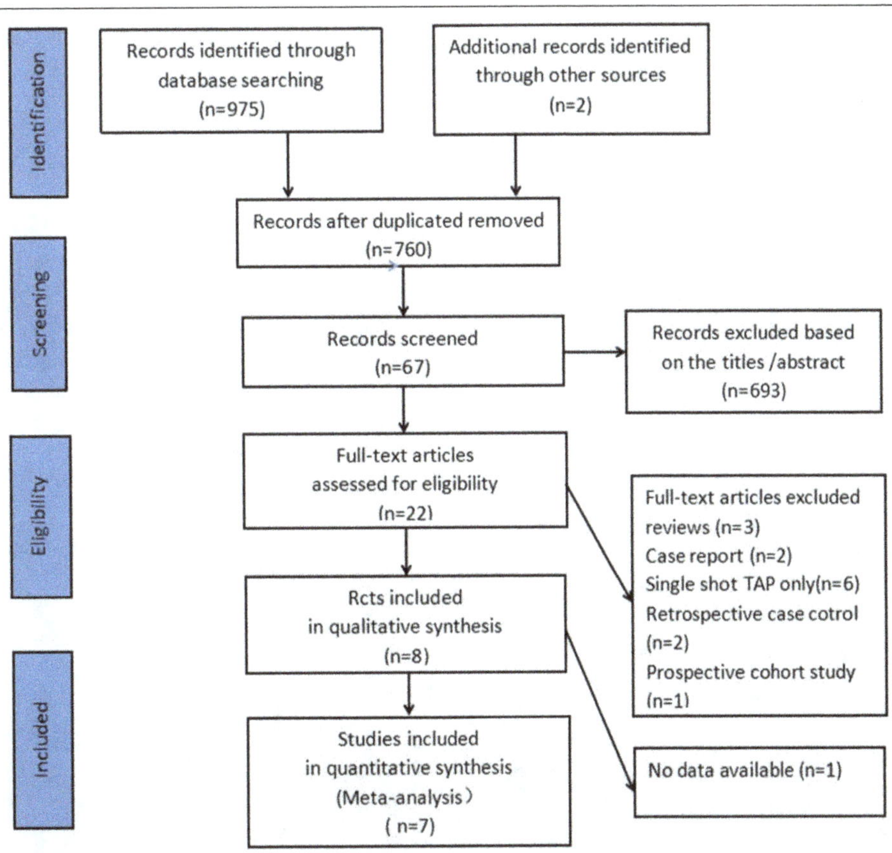

Fig. 1 Flow diagram showing results of search and reasons for exclusion of studies

Table 1 Characteristics of included randomized controlled studies

Author /Year	Group(n)	Types of surgery	Surgical approach	TAP block technique	Catheter site	Local anesthetic administered for TAP block	Local anesthetic administered for Epidural analgesia	Anesthetic strategy	Additional NSAIDs drugs for TAP block	Postoperative opioid analgesia required
Kadam 2013 [23]	TAP group(22) EA group(19)	Colorectal Upper gastrointestinal Urological	laparotomy	US-guided, single injection followed by continuous infusion	Bilateral Posterior	0.375% ropivacaine 20 ml single-injection bilaterally, followed by 0.2% ropivacaine at 8 mL/h through each catheter for 72 h	0.2% ropivacaine(8-15 ml) bolus followed by 0.2% ropivacaine at 5–15 ml/h	GA	paracetamol 1.0 g every 8 h	PCA using fentanyl 10 to 40 μg bolus per press with a lockout time of 6 min and no basal infusion
Niraj 2011 [22]	TAP group(27) EA group(31)	Partial hepatectomy Pancreatic surgery Radical nephrectomy Biliary bypass	laparotomy	US-guided, single injection followed by continuous infusion	Bilateral Subcostal	0.375% bupivacaine (1 mg/kg) single-injection bilaterally, followed a bolus of 0.375% bupivacaine(1 mg/kg) very 8 h through each catheter for 72 h	0.25% bupivacaine(20 ml) followed by 0.125% bupivacaine with 2 μg/ml Fentanyl at 6-12 mL/h for 72 h (2 ml bolus, lockout 30mins)	GA	paracetamol 1 g every 6 h	intravenous tramadol as required
Niraj 2014 [13]	TAP group(30) EA group(31)	Right hemicolectomy Left hemicolectomy Anterior resection Sigmoid colectomy Ileocolic resection	laparoscope	US-guided, single injection followed by continuous infusion	Bilateral Posterior	0.375% levobupivacaine (1.25 mg/kg)single-injection bilaterally,followed by 0.25% levobupivacaine at 8–10 mL/h through both catheters for 72 h	0.25% Bupivacaine 20 mL followed by 0.125% bupivacaine with 2 μg/mL fentanyl at 8–12 mL/h (2 ml bolus, lockout 30mins)	GA	paracetamol 1 g every 6 h, diclofenac 150 mg/day	intravenous tramadol as required
Ganapathy 2015 [25]	TAP group(26) EA group(24)	Small bowel surgery Large bowel surgery Ostomy reversal Whipples'operation	laparotomy	US-guided, single injection followed by continuous infusion	Bilateral Subcostal Inferior	0.2% ropivacaine 30 ml single-injection bilaterally followed by 0.35% ropivacaineat 4–5 ml/h for 72 h	0.25% bupivacaine 5 ml followed by 0.1% bupivacaine with hydromorphone(10 mg/mL) at 8 ml/h for 72 h	GA	naproxen 500 mg twice daily, paracetamol 650 mg every 6 h	PCA using hydromorphone 0.2 mg bolus per press with a lockout time of 6 min and no basal infusion
Lyer 2017 [27]	TAP group(33) EA group(36)	lower abdominal surgery	laparotomy	US-guided, single injection followed by continuous infusion	Bilateral Posterior	0.125% bupivacaine 20 ml single-injection bilaterally followed by 15 ml bolus every 8 h through each catheter for 48 h	0.125% bupivacaine 10 ml followed by 0.125% bupivacaine 10 ml every 8 h for 48 h	GA	Paracetamol 1 g was given to patients if their VAS scores were > 3/10	intravenous tramadol as required
Qin 2016 [26]	TAP group(35) EA group(36)	laparoscopic colorectal surgery	laparoscope	US-guided, single injection followed by continuous infusion	Bilateral Posterior	0.375% ropivacaine 1.25 mg/kg single-injection bilaterally followed by 0.2% ropivacaine at 6–8 ml/h through both catheters for 48 h	0.375% ropivacaine 10 ml followed by 0.15% ropivacaine with fentanyl 2 μg/ml at 3–6 mL/h for 48 h (3 ml bolus, lockout 15mins)	GA	/	Intravenous tramadol as required
Wahba 2014 [24]	TAP group(22) EA group(22)	Large bowel surgery Small bowel surgery Gastrectomy Abdominal Hernia	laparotomy	US-guided, single injection followed by continuous infusion	Bilateral Subcostal	0.25% bupivacaine 20 ml single-injection bilaterally followed by 15 ml bolus every 8 h through each catheter for 48 h	0.125% bupivacaine 10 ml followed by 0.125% bupivacaine at 6–8 ml/h for 48 h	GA	/	PCA 1 mg morphine bolus per press with a lockout interval of 10 min
Dai 2017 [15]	TAP group(27) EA group(30)	laparoscopic colorectal surgery	laparoscope	US-guided, single injection followed by continuous infusion	Bilateral Posterior	0.375% ropivacaine 0.15 ml/kg single-injection bilaterally followed by 0.2% ropivacaine at 0.1 ml/kg/h through both catheters for 48 h	0.375% ropivacaine 8-10 ml followed by 0.15% ropivacaine at a 3–4 ml/h for 48 h (3 ml bolus, lockout 15mins)	GA	/	intravenous tramadol as required

IV **intravenous,** ***PCA*** **patient controlled analgesia,** ***TAP*** **transverse abdominis plane,** ***US*** **ultrasound,** ***GA*** **General anesthesia**

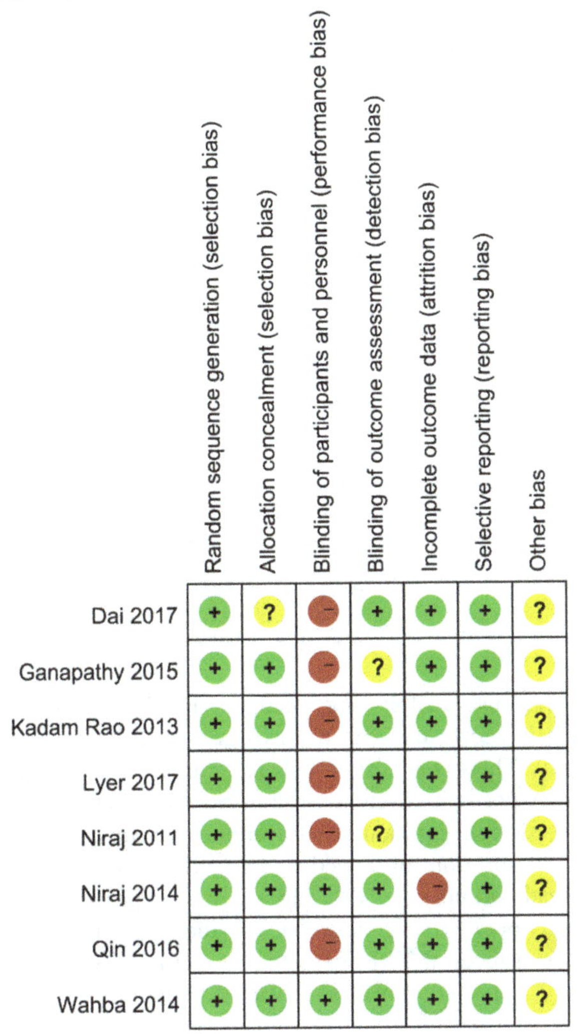

Fig. 2 Cochrane collaboration risk of bias summary: evaluation of bias risk items for each included study. Green circle = low risk of bias; red circle = highrisk of bias; yellow circle = unclear risk of bias

participants and evaluators. However, in these trials, it was extremely difficult to blind patients and clinicians.

Primary outcome

Seven studies [13, 15, 22–26], including the meta-analysis with a total of 384 patients (TAP block group: 191 patients; EA group: 193 patients), reported dynamic pain scores 24 h postoperatively (Fig. 3). Dynamic pain scores after 24 h were overall equivalent between TAP block and EA groups (7 trials [13, 15, 22–26]; WMD: 0.44; 95% CI: 0.1 to 0.99; I^2 = 91%; $p = 0.11$). No significant difference was found in the subgroup analysis of open surgery (4 trials [23–26]; WMD:0.58; 95% CI: − 0.52 to 1.69; I^2 = 95%; $p = 0.3$) and laparoscopic surgery (3 trials [13, 15, 26]; WMD:0.29; 95% CI: − 0.18 to 0.77; I^2 = 79%; $p = 0.22$) (Fig. 3), and no difference was found between the continuous local anesthetics subgroup (5 trials [13, 15, 23, 25, 26]; WMD:0.23; 95% CI: − 0.1 to 0.57; I^2 = 68%; $p = 0.17$) and intermittent local anesthetics subgroup (2 trials [22, 24]; WMD:0.85; 95% CI: − 1.41 to 3.31; I^2 = 98%; $p = 0.46$) (Fig. 4). However, there was a significant difference between the subgroups of regularly administering NSAIDs (4 trials [13, 22, 23, 25]; WMD:-0.11; 95%CI: − 0.32 to 0.09; I^2 = 0%; $p = 0.28$) or not (3 trials [15, 24, 26]; WMD:1.02; 95%CI: 0.09 to 1.96; I^2 = 94%; $p = 0.03$) for adjuvant analgesics postoperatively (Fig. 5). The pain score in the subgroup not administering NSAIDs was significantly higher. We also performed sensitivity analysis by omitting one study each time, which did not alter the overall combined WMD, and the pooled result was still robust ($P > 0.05$).

Secondary outcomes

The pain scores at rest showed no significant difference between the two groups 12 h (3 trials [15, 24, 26]; WMD: 0.67; 95%CI: − 0.14 to 1.48; I^2 = 95%; $p = 0.1$), 24 h (6 trials [15, 22–26]; WMD:-0.07; 95% CI: − 0.21 to 0.06; I^2 = 90%; $p = 0.3$), or 48 h (5 trials [15, 22–24, 26]; WMD:0.82; 95% CI: − 0.04 to 1.21; I^2 = 91%; $p = 0.06$) postoperatively.

With movement, there were no significant differences in pain scores 12 h (3 trials [15, 24, 26], WMD:0.99; 95%CI: − 0.10 to 2.09; I^2 = 92%; $p = 0.07$), 48 h (5 trials [15, 22–24, 26];WMD:0.52; 95% CI: − 0.16 to 1.21; I^2 = 91%; $p = 0.14$), or 72 h (2 trials [22, 23]; WMD:-0.21; 95% CI:-0.69 to 0.28; I^2 = 72%; $p = 0.4$) postoperatively. There was also no significant difference in morphine consumption postoperatively after 24 h (3 trials [23–25]; WMD:1.99; 95%CI: − 4.86 to 8.84; I^2 = 90%; $p = 0.57$), 48 h (5 trials [13, 23–26]; WMD:4.12; 95% CI: − 3.13 to 11.16; I^2 = 93%; $p = 0.27$) (Fig. 6), and 72 h (3 trials [22, 23, 25]; WMD:7.67; 95% CI: − 3.40 to 18.73; I^2 = 90%; $p = 0.17$) compared with the EA group.

Recovery outcomes

Regarding functional recovery, time to first flatus was no different between the two groups (5 trials [13, 15, 24–26]; WMD:1.57; 95% CI: − 4.7 to 7.84; I^2 = 52%; $P = 0.62$). However, time of removal of the urinary catheter measured in the TAP group was significantly shorter (3 trials [13, 15, 26], WMD:-18.95, 95%CI:-25.22 to − 12.71; I^2 = 0%; $p < 0.01$), as was time to first ambulation postoperatively (4 trials [13, 15, 24, 26], WMD:-6.61, 95%CI: − 13.03 to − 0.19; I^2 = 67%; $p < 0.05$). Meanwhile, length of hospital stay revealed no difference between the TAP and EA groups (4 trials [13, 15, 23, 26], WMD:-0.02; 95%CI: − 0.28 to 0.23; I^2 = 0%; $p = 0.85$).

Complications

The incidence of hypotension was significantly higher postoperatively in the EA group than in the TAP group (5 trials [15, 23–26]; RR: 0.16; 95%CI: 0.06 to 0.42; I^2 = 0%;

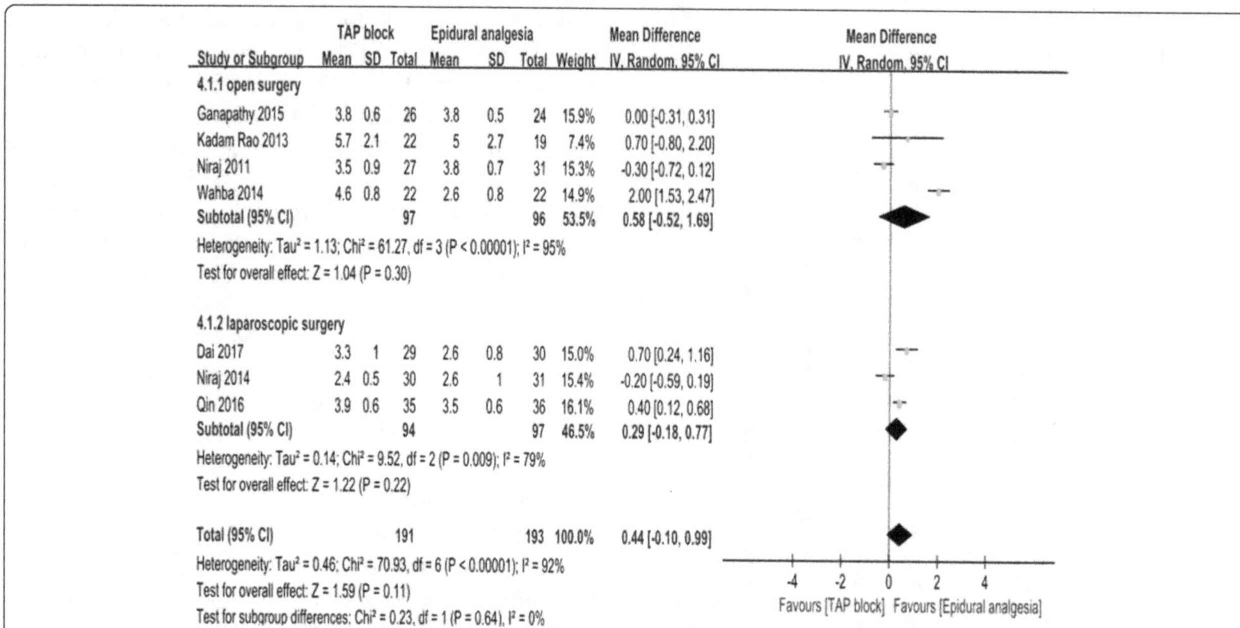

Fig. 3 pain scores at dynamic at 24 h postoperatively according to type of operation (open surgery VS laparoscopic surgery)

$P = 0.0002$). One trial reported that a patient in the TAP group developed a unilateral abdominal wall hematoma immediately after surgery. However, the author was unclear whether this was due to a trauma caused by the insertion of the TAP catheter or surgical puncture.

Discussion

This review and meta-analysis, comparing continuous TAP block with EA in adults after abdominal surgery, included 8 RCTs with a total of 453 patients. The result of the meta-analysis suggested no significant difference in pain scores between the two groups 24 h postoperatively. There was also no significant difference in pain scores postoperatively, as well as no difference in equianalgesic consumption of intravenous morphine.

The location of injection into the TAP alters the spread and effect of TAP blocks. It is proposed that the range of TAP injections be classified as follows [16]: upper subcostal TAP (deep to the rectus, mainly covering T7 and T8), lower subcostal TAP (lateral to rectus,

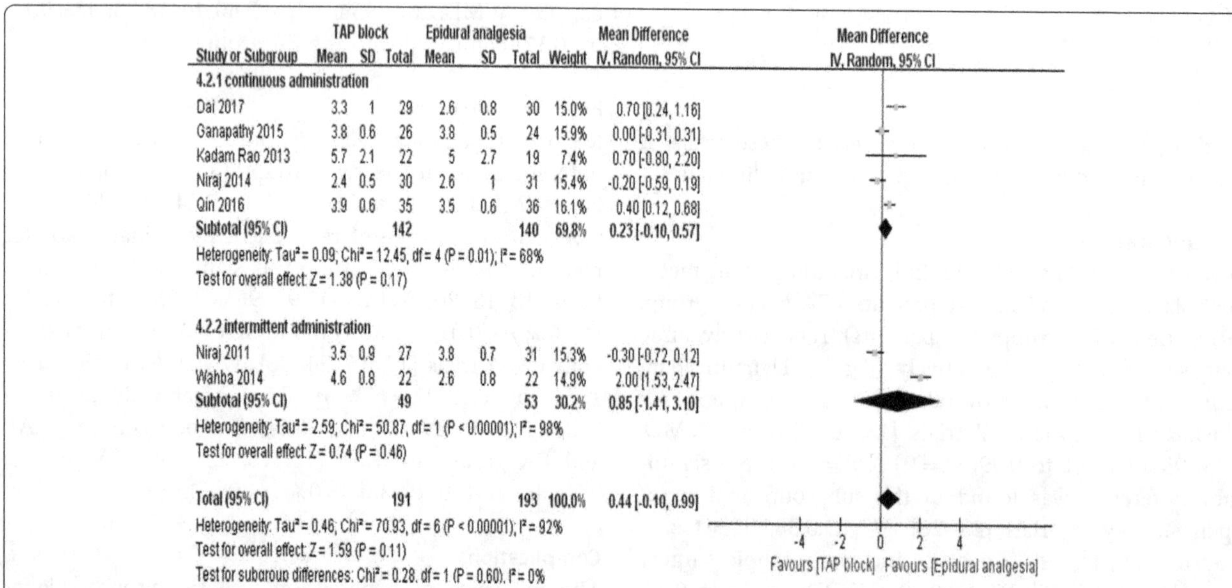

Fig. 4 pain scores at dynamic at 24 h postoperatively according to the way of local anesthetic administration (sustaining administration VS intermittent administration)

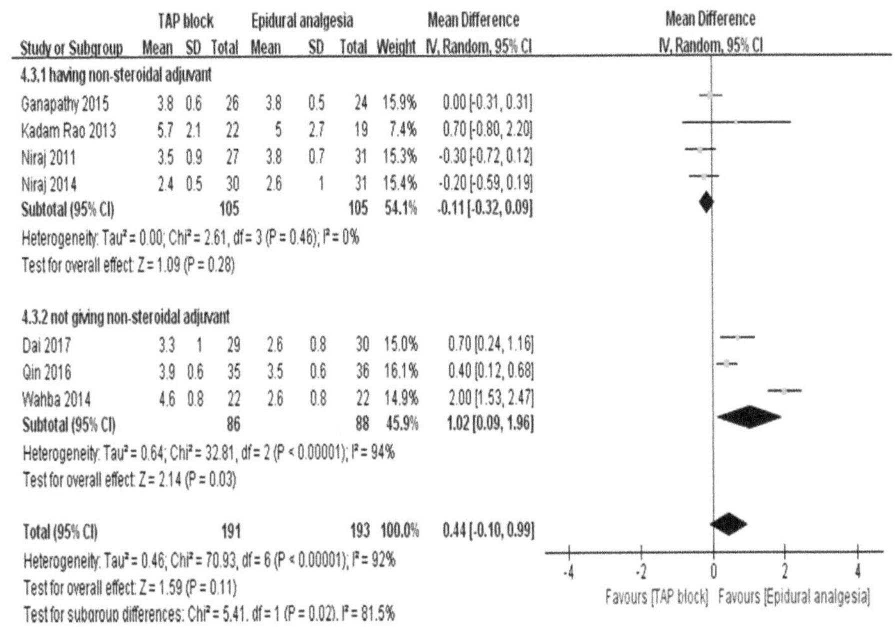

Fig. 5 pain scores at dynamic at 24 h postoperatively according to the using regularly non-steroidal drugs postoperatively (giving regularly the non-steroidal adjuvant analgesics VS not giving)

mainly covering T11), lateral TAP (midway between the costal margin and iliac crest in the mid-clavicular line, mainly covering T11 and T12), ilio-inguinal TAP (near the iliac crest lateral to the anterior superior iliac spine, mainly covering T12 and L1), and posterior TAP (in the triangle of Petit). A previous meta-analysis comparing TAP block with EA suggested that TAP block can provide equivalent analgesic effect at rest 24 h after abdominal surgery [28]. However, studies have shown that the analgesic effect of a single TAP block lasts less than 24 h [29, 30]. This review included both single TAP block and continuous TAP block. For this reason, choosing a timepoint of 24 h after surgery as the endpoint for the primary outcome might increase the bias of analysis. Therefore, in our review, we excluded the single TAP block variable and chose the dynamic pain score at 24 h after surgery as our primary outcome, which can adequately reflect the efficacy and duration of continuous TAP block.

In addition, the subgroup analysis of laparotomy and laparoscopic surgery showed no significant difference,

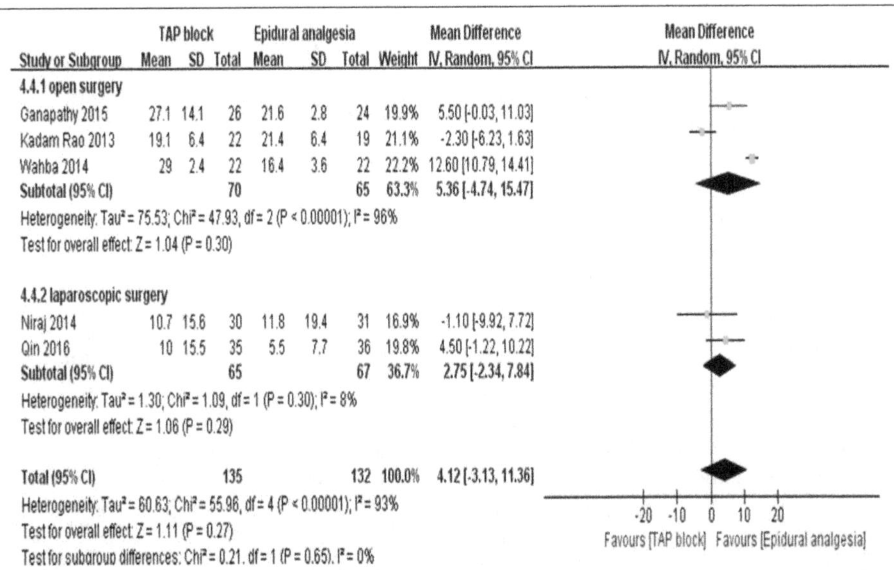

Fig. 6 Opioid consumption in 48 h postoperatively according to type of operation (open surgery VS laparoscopic surgery)

and a similar result was found in the subgroups comparing the mode of local anesthetic administration. However, the heterogeneity between trails should be noted. Laparoscopic surgery is considered minimally invasive compared with open surgery in the clinical setting [31, 32]. Various types of abdominal surgery were included in this meta-analysis, which easily explains why the heterogeneity of the laparotomy group was significantly higher than in the laparoscopy group. According to the mode of local anesthetic administration, only two trials were included in the intermittent administration group, and there was a relatively small sample size. We also analyzed those who took NSAIDs postoperatively as a separate subgroup. However, there was a significant difference between the subgroups. Meanwhile, the heterogeneity in the NSAIDs group was significantly reduced. This suggested that TAP block combined with NSAIDs can provide more relief for patients after abdominal surgery. The NSAIDs would better treat the visceral pain and reduce the usage of opioids postoperatively [33]. Therefore, TAP block is usually combined with NSAIDs to participate in multimodal analgesia [13, 34].

Continuous TAP block analgesia does not cause urinary retention compared with EA postoperatively. On the contrary, patients who received EA used the urinary catheter for significantly longer. Due to limited reports on the outcomes of the complications between the two groups, we cannot draw more evidential results about the relative benefits of the two technologies. However, it should be noted that the episodes of postoperative hypotension associated with EA were significantly higher than those of the TAP group.

Limitations

There are several limitations that must be taken into consideration when interpreting the results of this review. Firstly, because of different surgical procedures, the location of TAP blocks and local anesthetic infusion strategies may be individualized. There are many factors that affect the procedure of continuous TAP block, including puncture location, catheter size, depth of catheter insertion, and various local anesthetic dosage, which will increase the heterogeneity between trails. Secondly, the protocols of anti-inflammatory drugs in the included trials were significantly different (including the type of drug, dosage and delivery speed), which may lead to increased heterogeneity. Such anti-inflammatory drugs may interfere with the overall evaluation of the pain score (somatic and visceral pain). Furthermore, the success of the TAP catheter also depends on the surgeon's level of experience. Moreover, it was extremely difficult to blind patients and clinicians, when we were conducting a TAP block performance, but we judge that this lack of blindness is unlikely to affect our primary outcomes. In addition, specific criteria for removing the urinary catheter and specific ambulation protocols were not defined in the same way in the included trials. Therefore, more structured and standardised continuous TAP blocking protocols should be developed to compare with EA.

Conclusion

This systematic review and meta-analysis suggests that the technique of continuous TAP block, combined with NSAIDs, can provide non-inferior dynamic analgesia efficacy compared with epidural infusion in adults after abdominal surgery. Continuous TAP block presents another option for effective and safe extended analgesia postoperatively. However, additional higher-quality RCTs would better define the comparable efficacy before supporting a stronger recommendation for continuous TAP block, which causes less hypotension and allows for a significantly shorter duration of urinary catheter use postoperatively compared with EA after abdominal surgery.

Abbreviations

CI: Confidence interval; EA: Epidural analgesia; NSAIDs: Non-steroidal antiinflammatory drugs; PRISMA: Preferred reporting items for systematic reviews and meta-analyses; RCTs: Randomized controlled trials; RR: Risk ratio; SMD: Standardized mean difference; TAP: Transversus abdominis plane block; VAS: Visual analogue scale; WMD: Weighted mean difference

Acknowledgements

Not Applicable.

Authors' contributions

Study conception and design – QCS and LJC; Extraction of data – QCS and LYM; interpretation and analysis of data – QCS, WXG and STS; writing manuscript – QCS, XJJ and DQH. All authors read and approved the final manuscript.

Author details

[1]Department of Anesthesiology, The First Affiliated Hospital of Guangxi Medical University, Nanning, Guangxi 530021, People's Republic of China. [2]Department of Ultrasound, Affiliated Hospital of Guilin Medical University, Guilin, Guangxi 541001, People's Republic of China. [3]Department of radiotherapy, Affiliated Tumor Hospital of Guangxi Medical University, Nanning, Guangxi 530021, People's Republic of China.

References

1. Rodgers A, Walker N, Schug S, McKee A, et al. Reduction of postoperative mortality and morbidity with epidural or spinal anaesthesia: results from overview of randomised trials. BMJ. 2000;321(7275):1493.
2. Popping DM, Elia N, Van Aken HK, et al. Impact of epidural analgesia on mortality and morbidity after surgery: systematic review and meta-analysis of randomized controlled trials. Ann Surg. 2014;259(6):1056–67.
3. Bos EME, Hollmann MW, Lirk P. Safety and efficacy of epidural analgesia. Curr Opin Anaesthesiol. 2017;30(6):736–42.
4. Jakobsson J, Wickerts L, Forsberg S, et al. Transversus abdominal plane (TAP) block for postoperative pain management: a re view. F1000Res. 2015;4.
5. Tsai HC, Yoshida T, Chuang TY, Yang SF, et al. Transversus Abdominis plane block: an updated review of anatomy and techniques. Biomed Res Int. 2017;2017:8284363.
6. Chin KJ, McDonnell JG, Carvalho B, et al. Essentials of our current understanding: abdominal wall blocks. Reg Anesth Pain Med. 2017;42(2):133–83.

7. Kim AJ, Yong RJ, Urman RD. The Role of Transversus Abdominis Plane Blocks in Enhanced Recovery after Surgery Pathways for Open and Laparoscopic Colorectal Surgery. J Laparoendosc Adv Surg Tech. 2017;27(9): 909–14.
8. Maeda A, Shibata SC, Kamibayashi T, et al. Continuous subcostal oblique transversus abdominis plane block provides more effective analgesia than single-shot block after gynaecological laparotomy: a randomised controlled trial. Eur J Anaesthesiol. 2015;32(7):514–5.
9. Gomez-Rios MA, Paech MJ. Continuous posterior TAP analgesia after laparoscopic colorectal surgery. Anaesthesia. 2014;69(9):1054–5.
10. Niraj G, Kelkar A, Hart E, et al. Four quadrant transversus abdominis plane block and continuous transversus abdominis plane analgesia: a 3-year prospective audit in 124 patients. J Clin Anesth. 2015;27(7):579–84.
11. Bakes D, Littlejohn C, Frenk V. Effectiveness of adding transverse abdominus plane (TAP) catheters to patient-controlled analgesia (PCA) in laparoscopic colon resections: Aretrospective chart review. Dis Colon Rectum. 2016;59(5):e310.
12. Heil JW, Nakanote KA, Madison SJ, et al. Continuous transversus abdominis plane (TAP) blocks for postoperative pain control after hernia surgery: a randomized, triple-masked, placebo-controlled study. Pain Med. 2014;15(11): 1957–64.
13. Niraj G, Kelkar A, Hart E, et al. Comparison of analgesic efficacy of four-quadrant transversus abdominis plane (TAP) block and continuous posterior TAP analgesia with epidural analgesia in patients undergoing laparoscopic colorectal surgery: an open-label, randomised, non-inferiority trial. Anaesthesia. 2014;69(4):348–55.
14. Cowlishaw PJ, Kotze PJ, Gleeson L, et al. Randomised comparison of three types of continuous anterior abdominal wall block after midline laparotomy for gynaecological oncology surgery. Anaesth Intensive Care. 2017;45(4): 453–8.
15. Dai Y, Sun XD, Liu JC. A comparative study of the analgesic effect of transverse abdominal block and thoracic epidural block after colorectal surgery. J Guanxi Med Univ. 2017;34(08):1213–6.
16. Hebbard P. TAP block nomenclature. Anaesthesia. 2015;70(1):112–3.
17. Wan X, Wang W, Liu J, et al. Estimating the sample mean and standard deviation from the sample size, median, range and/or interquartile range. BMC Med Res Methodol. 2014;14:135.
18. Collaboration, TC: Cochrane Handbook for systematic reviews of interventions version 5.1.0. Available at: http://ims.cochrane.org/revman. Accessed 20 Sept 2017.
19. Shaheen PE, Walsh D, Lasheen W, et al. Opioid equianalgesic tables: are they all equally dangerous? J Pain Symptom Manag. 2009;38(3):409–17.
20. Higgins JP, Altman DG, Gotzsche PC, et al. The Cochrane Collaboration's tool for assessing risk of bias in randomised trials. BMJ. 2011;343:d5928.
21. Melsen WG, Bootsma MC, Rovers MM, et al. The effects of clinical and statistical heterogeneity on the predictive values of results from meta-analyses. Clin Microbiol Infect. 2014;20(2):123–9.
22. Niraj G, Kelkar A, Jeyapalan I, et al. Comparison of analgesic efficacy of subcostal transversus abdominis plane blocks with epidural analgesia following upper abdominal surgery. Anaesthesia. 2011;66(6):465–71.
23. Rao Kadam V, Van Wijk RM, Moran JI, et al. Epidural versus continuous transversus abdominis plane catheter technique for postoperative analgesia after abdominal surgery. Anaesth Intensive Care. 2013;41(4):476–81.
24. Wahba SS, Kamal SM. Analgesic efficacy and outcome of transversus-abdominis plane block versus low thoracic-epidural analgesia after laparotomy in ischemic heart disease patients. J Anesth. 2014;28(4):517–23.
25. Ganapathy S, Sondekoppam RV, Terlecki M, et al. Comparison of efficacy and safety of lateral-to-medial continuous transversus abdominis plane block with thoracic epidural analgesia in patients undergoing abdominal surgery: a randomised, open-label feasibility study. Eur J Anaesthesiol. 2015; 32(11):797–804.
26. Qin CS, Lin YN, Liu JC. Clinical study of ultrasound-guided continuous transversus abdominis plane block on thefficacy of postoperative analgesia in patients undergoing laparoscopic colorectal surgery. J Minim Invasive Med. 2016;11(05):664–8.
27. Lyer SS, Bavishi H, Mohan CV, et al. Comparison of epidural analgesia with Transversus Abdominis plane analgesia for postoperative pain relief in patients undergoing lower abdominal surgery: a prospective randomized study. Anesth Essays Res. 2017;11(3):670–5.
28. Baeriswyl M, Zeiter F, Piubellini D, et al. The analgesic efficacy of transverse abdominis plane block versus epidural analgesia: a systematic review with meta-analysis. Medicine (Baltimore). 2018;97(26):e11261.
29. Stoving K, Rothe C, Rosenstock CV, et al. Cutaneous sensory block area, muscle-relaxing effect, and block duration of the Transversus Abdominis plane block: a randomized, blinded, and placebo-controlled study in healthy volunteers. Reg Anesth Pain Med. 2015;40(4):355–62.
30. Abdallah FW, Laffey JG, Halpern SH, et al. Duration of analgesic effectiveness after the posterior and lateral transversus abdominis plane block techniques for transverse lower abdominal incisions: a meta-analysis. Br J Anaesth. 2013; 111(5):721–35.
31. Trejo-Avila ME, Valenzuela-Salazar C, Betancourt-Ferreyra J, et al. Laparoscopic versus open surgery for abdominal trauma: a case-matched study. J laparoendosc Adv Surg Tech A. 2017;27(4):383–7.
32. Arsalani-Zadeh R, Ullah S, Khan S, et al. Oxidative stress in laparoscopic versus open abdominal surgery: a systematic review. J Surg Res. 2011;169(1): e59–68.
33. Choi YM, Byeon GJ, Park SJ, et al. Postoperative analgesic efficacy of single-shot and continuous transversus abdominis plane block after laparoscopic cholecystectomy: a randomized controlled clinical trial. J Clin Anesth. 2017; 39:146–51.
34. Jadon A, Jain P, Chakraborty S, et al. Role of ultrasound guided transversus abdominis plane block as a component of multimodal analgesic regimen for lower segment caesarean section: a randomized double blind clinical study. BMC Anesthesiol. 2018;18(1):53.

8

Antinociceptive effects of magnesium sulfate for monitored anesthesia care during hysteroscopy

Peng-fei Gao[1], Jing-yan Lin[1,2*], Shun Wang[1], Yun-feng Zhang[1], Guo-qiang Wang[1], Qi Xu[1] and Xiao Guo[1]

Abstract

Background: Opioids are the most effective antinociceptive agents, they have undesirable side effects such as respiratory depressant and postoperative nausea and vomiting. The purpose of the study was to evaluate the antinociceptive efficacy of adjuvant magnesium sulphate to reduce intraoperative and postoperative opioids requirements and their related side effects during hysteroscopy.

Methods: Seventy patients scheduled for hysteroscopy were randomly divided into 2 groups. Patients in the magnesium group (Group M) received intravenous magnesium sulfate 50 mg/kg in 100 ml of isotonic saline over 15 min before anesthesia induction and then 15 mg/kg per hour by continuous intravenous infusion. Patients in the control group (Group C) received an equal volume of isotonic saline as placebo. All patients were anesthetized under a BIS guided monitored anesthesia care with propofol and fentanyl. Intraoperative hemodynamic variables were recorded and postoperative pain scores were assessed with verbal numerical rating scale (VNRS) 1 min, 15 min, 30 min, 1 h, and 4 h after recovery of consciousness. The primary outcome of our study was total amount of intraoperative and postoperative analgesics administered.

Results: Postoperative serum magnesium concentrations in Group C were significantly decreased than preoperative levels (0.86 ± 0.06 to 0.80 ± 0.08 mmol/L, $P = 0.001$) while there was no statistical change in Group M (0.86 ± 0.07 to 0.89 ± 0.07 mmol/L, $P = 0.129$). Bradycardia did not occur in either group and the incidence of hypotension was comparable between the two groups. Total dose of fentanyl given to patients in Group M was less than the one administered to Group C [100 (75–150) vs 145 (75–175) μg, median (range); $P < 0.001$]. In addition, patients receiving magnesium displayed lower VNRS scores at 15 min, 30 min, 1 h, and 4 h postoperatively.

Conclusions: In hysteroscopy, adjuvant magnesium administration is beneficial to reduce intraoperative fentanyl requirement and postoperative pain without cardiovascular side effects. Our study indicates that if surgical patients have risk factors for hypomagnesemia, assessing and correcting magnesium level will be necessary.

Keywords: Hysteroscopy, Magnesium sulphate, Monitored anesthesia care, Opioid, Pain

* Correspondence: 419931094@qq.com
[1]Department of Anesthesiology, North Sichuan Medical College, Nanchong 637000, Sichuan, China
[2]Department of Anesthesiology, Affiliated Hospital of North Sichuan Medical College, Nanchong 637000, Sichuan, China

Background

Hysteroscopy is currently one of the most common procedures for patients with cervical or endometrial disorders [1]. Although the development of new techniques and equipment has made hysteroscopy a minimally invasive procedure, it's still believed to be a painful experience which needs effective analgesia to achieve maximum patient comfort and cooperation [2, 3]. Fentanyl is generally the preferred agent administered as analgesics during hysteroscopy because of its low price and powerful analgesic effect. However, serious side effects such as respiratory depressant and postoperative nausea and vomiting (PONV) restrict its dosage in clinical practice [4].

Multimodal analgesia is a strategy that involves the use of two or more analgesic agents and techniques to provide adequate analgesia, and aims to reduce opioid consumption and minimize opioid-related adverse effects [5]. When compared with opioid-free anaesthesia, strong evidence shows that opioid-inclusive anaesthesia does not reduce postoperative pain, but is associated with more PONV [6]. As the fourth most plentiful cation in the body, magnesium (Mg) acts as a non-competitive N-methyl-D-aspartate (NMDA) receptor antagonist and calcium channel blocker. It has antinociceptive stimulus property [7]. Hypomagnesemia is a common entity occurring in up to 12% of hospitalized patients [8] and has been reported in many kinds of surgeries such as thyroidectomy, cardiac surgery, and kidney transplantation. A recent study indicated that serum magnesium level was also significantly decreased after hysteroscopy [9] and magnesium deficiency produces hyperalgesia that can be reversed by NMDA antagonists [10]. In consequence, magnesium administration may be beneficial to patients undergoing hysteroscopy.

We hypothesize that intravenous magnesium sulphate as an adjuvant drug to fentanyl analgesia during hysteroscopy as monitored by Bispectral Index Scale (BIS) could reduce intraoperative and postoperative analgesics requirements and their related side effects.

Methods

Ethics and registration

This randomized controlled study adheres to CONSORT guideline. The study was approved by the Ethics Committee of Affiliated Hospital of North Sichuan Medical College [2019ER(R) 074–01] and was registered at the Chinese Clinical Trials Registry (ChiCTR1900024596). Written informed consent was obtained from each patient.

Patient inclusion and exclusion criteria

Inclusion criteria were patients aged 18–55 years old, with American Society of Anesthesiologists (ASA) physical status I or II, scheduled for hysteroscopy between July 2019 and October 2019 in Affiliated Hospital of North Sichuan Medical College. Exclusion criteria were patients with cardiovascular disease (ejection fraction < 40%, atrioventricular conductance disturbance, hypertension, coronary heart disease, or cerebrovascular disease), liver dysfunction (transaminases above the normal level), renal failure (creatine > 150 μmol/L), preoperative opioids use, neurological disorder, diabetes, body mass index > 30 kg/m^2, history of neuromuscular disease, history of chronic pain, drugs or alcohol abuse. We also excluded patients when they face serious intraoperative hypoxemia and need endotracheal intubation.

Randomization and blinding

Patients were randomly assigned into the control group (Group C, n = 35) and the magnesium group (Group M, n = 35) by computer-generated randomization Web-based, random number generator (available at http://www.random.org). Patients in the Group M received IV magnesium sulfate (Brilliant Pharmaceutical Co., Ltd.) 50 mg/kg in 100 ml of isotonic saline over 15 min before anesthesia induction and then 15 mg/kg per hour by continuous IV infusion until the end of the procedure, whereas patients in the Group C received an equal volume of isotonic saline as a placebo. An anesthetic technician who did not participate in the study was provided with group assignment and prepared the Infusions in pharmacy. Anesthesia provider, patients, and all investigators were blinded to group assignment until completion of the study.

Anesthesia

On arrival in the operating room, ECG, noninvasive blood pressure (NIBP), and pulse oximetry (SpO_2) monitoring were commenced. Electrodes were placed on the forehead to monitor bispectral index (BIS). After a 20-G intravenous cannula was inserted, 100 ml of study medicine was started to infusion. Four minutes before the start of procedure, all patients received 1.5 μg/kg bolus doses of fentanyl (Yichang Humanwell Pharmaceutical Co., Ltd.). Sedation was initiated with propofol (Corden Pharma Latina S.p.A) 1.5 mg/kg and then maintained at a rate of 4–12 mg/kg per hour. The speed of propofol infusion was adjusted to maintain a BIS value of 50 to 60. Inadequate analgesia was defined as body movement or an increase in mean blood pressure (MBP) or heart rate (HR) by more than 15% of baseline [4]. A 0.5 μg/kg bolus dose of fentanyl was administered if signs of inadequate analgesia occurred with a BIS value in the recommended range contemporarily. When inadequate analgesia occurred and BIS value simultaneously increased upon 60 or even 70, the speed of propofol infusion was enhanced and a 0.5 μg/kg bolus dose of fentanyl was administered. The infusions of propofol and study medicine were ceased when gynecologists pronounced the completion of the procedure.

During the procedures, all patients were allowed to breathe spontaneously with oxygen 2 L/min via face mask. When SpO_2 < 95% were observed, patients were managed by jaw thrust and when SpO_2 < 90% by assisted ventilation. At the same time, ephedrine or atropine was administered if hypotension (SBP ≤ 90 mmHg) or bradycardia (HR ≤ 45bmp) was observed.

Data collection

After the procedures, patients were transferred to the postanesthesia care unit (PACU) if modified Aldrete score ≥ 9 [11]. Respiratory depression (defined as SpO_2 less than 95 and 90%), time for recovery of consciousness (time between disconnection of propofol infusion and ability for the patient to provide her name) were recorded. Postoperative pain score was assessed with verbal numerical rating scale (VNRS; 0 = no pain; 4–6 = moderate pain; 10 = worst pain). The VNRS scores were recorded 1 min, 15 min, 30 min, 1 h, and 4 h after recovery of consciousness. If VNRS scores ≥4, bolus doses of dezocine (Yangtze River Pharmaceutical Co., Ltd.) 10 mg used for rescue analgesics were administered intravenously. Patients with PONV were treated with intravenous ondansetron (Qilu Pharmaceutical Co., Ltd.) 4 mg. Gynecologists and Patients' global satisfaction levels regarding fluency of procedures or comfort level were assessed immediately and 4 h after procedures respectively using a satisfaction scale (0 = complete dissatisfaction; 10 = best satisfaction). Serum magnesium concentrations were collected one day before and one day after the procedure. In addition, PONV and other adverse effects were also recorded during the study period.

Outcomes

The primary outcome of our study was total amount of intraoperative and postoperative analgesics administered. The following data were collected as secondary outcomes of interest: serum magnesium concentrations, duration of procedure, variations of HR and MBP during procedures, respiratory depression, time for recovery of consciousness, PONV, satisfaction score from gynecologists and patients, VNRS scores after procedures.

Sample size and statistical analysis

The sample size of this study was based on the total dose of fentanyl requirement. Sample size calculations based on 10 subjects per group were required to achieve a power of 90% with a type 1 error of 0.05. Preliminary data revealed that a total sample size of 62 was required (31 per group) to detect 0.5 μg/kg reduction in fentanyl requirement [12]. In consideration of possible dropout, we enrolled 35 subjects per group.

Data were analyzed using SPSS for Windows version 19.0 (SPSS Inc., Chicago, IL, USA). Normality assessment of distribution was performed with Kolmogorov-Smirnov. Data were set out in the form of mean ± standard deviation, median (range), or the number of patients (proportion). The Student's t-test was employed in the analysis of the parametric data. Nonparametric data were analyzed by using the Mann-Whitney U test. Categorical data were analyzed using Fisher's exact test or the chi-square test, if appropriate. Two-way repeated measures ANOVA was used to compare HR and MBP at each point of time. A P-value of less than 0.05 was accepted as statistically significant.

Results

Flow diagram of the study was presented in Fig. 1: A total of 70 patients participated in our study without exclusion. They were randomly divided into two groups: the control group (Group C, n = 35) and the magnesium group (Group M, n = 35). One patient in Group C and two patients in Group M were lost to follow up, thus 34 patients in Group C and 33 patients in Group M were analyzed. The patients' demographic characteristics and satisfaction scores are described in Table 1. Age, height, weight, BMI, and ASA physical status were statistically similar between the two groups. There were no significant differences in the duration of procedure and recovery of consciousness. Gynecologists showed higher satisfaction scores in Group M (P = 0.026) while patients displayed similar satisfaction scores between two groups (P = 0.057).

Normal range of serum magnesium level in our institution is 0.75–1.02 mmol/L. Preoperative serum magnesium concentrations were similar between the two groups (0.86 ± 0.06 vs 0.86 ± 0.07 mmol/L in Group C and Group M, respectively). Postoperative serum magnesium concentrations in Group C were significantly declined than preoperative levels (0.86 ± 0.06 to 0.80 ± 0.08 mmol/L, P = 0.001) while there was no statistical change in Group M (0.86 ± 0.07 to 0.89 ± 0.07 mmol/L, P = 0.129).

The total dose and number of times fentanyl given to patients in Group M was less than these administered to Group C [100 (75–150) vs 145 (75–175) μg, median (range); P < 0.001], [2 (1–4) vs 3 (1–5), median (range); P < 0.001], meanwhile, propofol consumption was similar between the two groups (P = 0.157). Thus, IV magnesium sulphate allowed a 31% reduction in the total dose of fentanyl used during the procedure (Table 2). There was no statistically significant difference for patients who needed rescue analgesic between the two groups [14 vs 6 subjects in Group C and Group M, RR = 0.44 (0.19 to 1.01), P = 0.052, NNT 4.349]. All patients' postoperative pain can be well controlled when they received rescue analgesic for only one time. VNRS scores at 1 min after recovery of consciousness were statistically similar between the two groups but were statistically

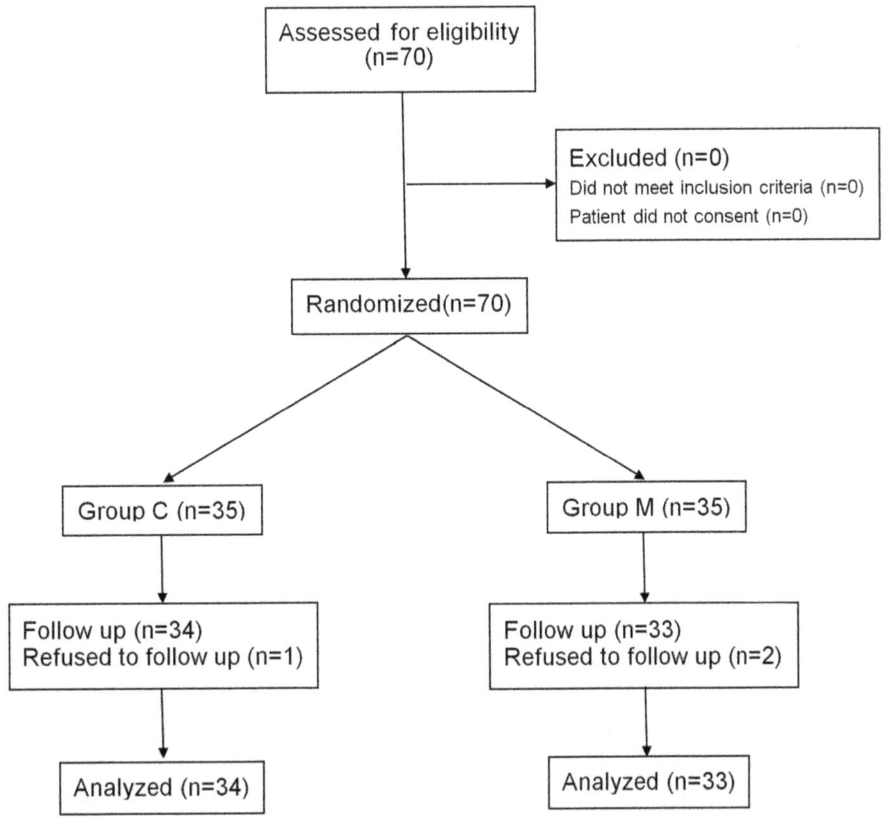

Fig. 1 Flow diagram representing patient enrollment, group assignment, and analysis. A total of 70 patients participated in our study without exclusion. They were randomly divided into two groups: the control group (Group C, n = 35) and the magnesium group (Group M, *n* = 35). One patient in Group C and two patients in Group M were lost to follow up, thus 34 patients in Group C and 33 patients in Group M were analyzed

lower in the Group M at 15 min, 30 min, 1 h, and 4 h postoperatively than in Group C ($P < 0.05$, Table 3). In this study, there was no patient who experienced a VNRS score ≥ 7.

Hemodynamic variables during the procedure at each point of time are shown in Fig. 2. A similar trend of heart rate was observed in Group C and Group M, but it was significantly lower in Group M at 5 min, 10 min, 15 min after propofol administration, the end of the procedure, and arrive in PACU. ($P < 0.05$, Fig. 2a). Mean blood pressures at 1 min and 5 min after propofol administration were significantly lower in Group M ($P < 0.05$,

Table 1 Demographic characteristics and satisfaction scores between two groups

	Group C (*n* = 34)	Group M (*n* = 33)	*p* value
Age (years)	37.0 ± 8.8	37.3 ± 8.9	0.900
Weight (kg)	52.5 (44–70)	53.0 (47–65)	0.782
Height (cm)	157.5 ± 4.3	158.1 ± 4.4	0.575
BMI(Kg/m^2)	22.2 ± 2.5	21.9 ± 2.1	0.618
ASA Physical status (I/II) (n)	13/21	14/19	0.727
Duration of procedure (min)	24.7 ± 12.0	20.4 ± 9.6	0.116
Recovery of consciousness (min)	4 (3–6)	4 (3–5)	0.530
Satisfaction score from gynecologists	8 (7–10)	9 (8–10) [a]	0.026
Satisfaction score from patients	9 (8–10)	10 (8–10)	0.057

Values are presented as mean ± standard deviation or median (range)
Group C Control group, *Group M* Magnesium group
ASA American Society of Anesthesiologists
[a] The difference was significant at 0.05 level

Table 2 Anesthetic requirements and frequencies of perioperative adverse events

	Group C ($n = 34$)	Group M ($n = 33$)	p value
Propofol (mg)	31.2 ± 10.8	28.0 ± 7.0	0.157
Fentanyl (μg)	145(75–175)	100(75–150) [a]	< 0.001
Total number of times fentanyl needs	3(1–5)	2(1–4) [a]	< 0.001
Need for rescue analgesics	14 (41%)	6 (18%)	0.052
Hypertension (SBP > 150 mmHg)	0 (0%)	0 (0%)	
Hypotension (SBP < 90 mmHg)	7 (21%)	5 (15%)	0.562
Tachycardia (HR > 110 bpm)	2 (6%)	0 (0%)	0.157
Bradycardia (HR < 50 bpm)	0 (0%)	0 (0%)	
Respiratory depression			
SpO_2 < 95%	18 (53%)	12 (36%)	0.172
SpO_2 < 90%	12 (35%)	7 (21%)	0.201
PONV	4 (12%)	3 (9%)	0.721

Values are presented as mean ± standard deviation, number (proportion) or median (range)
Group C Control group, *Group M* Magnesium group
PONV Postoperative nausea and vomiting
[a] The difference was significant at 0.05 level

Fig. 2b). Hypertension or bradycardia did not occur in either group. Incidence of hypotension was comparable between the two groups and patients were treated with ephedrine when hypotension was observed. However, there was no case of tachycardia in Group M, while two cases were observed in Group C (Table 2). The numbers of patients who experienced oxygen desaturation below 95% (18 vs 12 subjects in Group C and Group M, respectively) or below 90% (12 vs 7 subjects in Group C and Group M, respectively) were statistically insignificant between the two groups (Table 2). No patient experienced a serious adverse event related to the infusion of magnesium sulphate.

Discussion

In the present study, we evaluated the antinociceptive effects of intravenous magnesium sulphate by reducing perioperative analgesics requirements during hysteroscopy in patients under monitored anesthesia care. We demonstrate, in hysteroscopy, that adding intravenous magnesium sulphate to propofol-fentanyl anesthesia results in a reduction in intraoperative fentanyl needs. Patients receiving magnesium displayed slower heart rate and less postoperative pain.

Table 3 Postoperative pain profiles during 4 h

	Group C ($n = 34$)	Group M ($n = 33$)	p value
VNRS scores			
1 min	2 (0–4)	1 (0–4)	0.074
15 min	3 (1–6)	2 (1–5) [a]	0.001
30 min	3 (2–6)	2 (1–6) [a]	< 0.001
1 h	2 (1–5)	1 (0–5) [a]	0.001
4 h	2 (1–4)	1 (0–4) [a]	0.003
VNRS ≥4	14 (41%)	6 (18%)	0.052

Values are presented as median (range) or number (proportion)
Group C Control group, *Group M* Magnesium group
VNRS Verbal numerical rating scale
[a] The difference was significant at 0.05 level

Propofol is an intravenous sedative drug and exerts its effects through potentiation of the inhibitory neurotransmitter, γ-aminobutyric acid (GABA). It has gained widespread use due to its favorable drug effect profile such as rapid and smooth induction with nearly no excitation phenomena and fast terminal half-life time [13]. Fentanyl is an agonist of the μ-opioid receptor which is known to be 100 times more potent than morphine. Analgesic effect occurs as soon as 1 to 2 min and lasts 2 to 4 h [14]. Propofol and fentanyl is metabolized mainly via the liver and excreted in the urine.

Nowadays, hysteroscopic surgeries are frequently performed in ambulatory surgery settings, which benefit the patients for shorter hospital stays and reduction of costs [15]. This procedure has been considered a less invasive treatment, combine short operative time with early discharge, postoperative analgesia is always underestimated and ignored. However, severe pain is caused by uterine cervical dilatation and intrauterine tissue extraction, thus effective pain management is the key point for patients' comfort and satisfaction. While opioids are the most effective antinociceptive agents, they have undesirable side effects, including respiratory depression, nausea, vomiting, urinary retention, constipation, ileus, and pruritus. Another problem is opioid addiction, a 4.8–6.5% incidence of persistent opioid use after surgery in older children and adults in the United States [16]. With this in mind, opioid-free anesthesia (OFA) was introduced to avoid current crisis. This can be achieved with alpha-2-agonists, ketamine, lidocaine, nonsteroidal

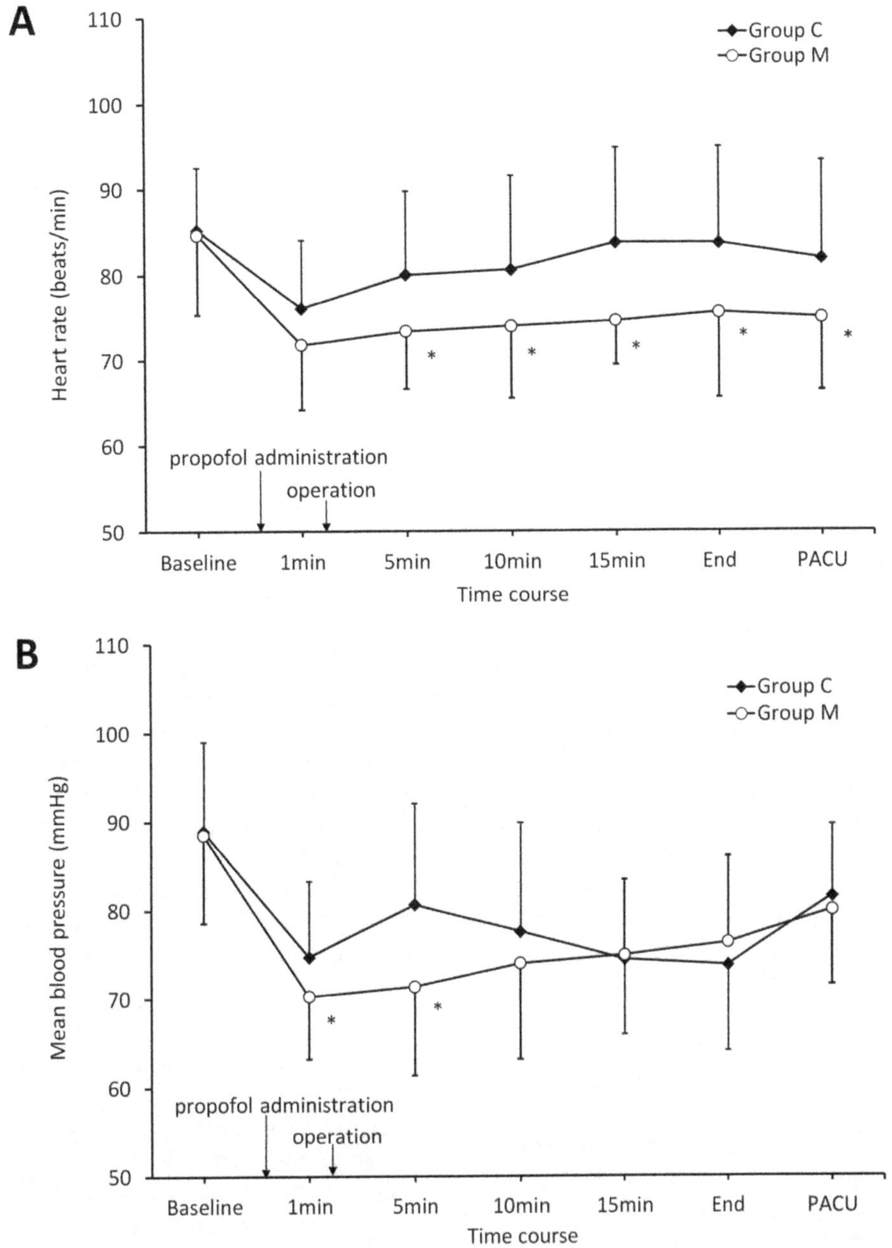

Fig. 2 Hemodynamic variables during the procedure. **a** Heart rate in the control group (Group C, $n = 34$) and the magnesium group (Group M, $n = 33$) at each point of time. **b** Mean blood pressure in the control group (Group C, $n = 34$) and the magnesium group (Group M, $n = 33$) at each point of time

anti-inflammatory drugs (NSAIDs) and magnesium, each working on a different target and therefore described as multitarget anesthesia [17]. In hysteroscopy, non-opioid analgesics such as NSAIDs and dexmedetomidine had been evaluated. Although both of these drugs could reduce the pain after hysteroscopy, NSAIDs fail to eliminate the discomfort occurring during the procedure [18] and dexmedetomidine may cause prolonged hypotension and bradycardia [19].

A case report indicated that there is a close connection between hypomagnesaemia and pain. Séamus et al. [20] reported two patients with hypomagnesaemia suffer from severe cancer pain. Their pain was well controlled after treating with intravenous magnesium. During hysteroscopy, distending media is essential to allow for optimal uterine visualization. Nevertheless, excess absorption of large volumes of electrolyte-free, low-viscosity fluid can result in volume overload with hyponatremia and water intoxication [21]. In our study, patients' postoperative serum magnesium level was consistent with recent research [9] which significantly decreased. The use of diuretics is advocated to treat volume overload in hysteroscopy [21], but diuretics can reduce renal magnesium reabsorption. In the meantime, perioperative inadequate dietary intake of magnesium makes patients undergoing hysteroscopy more susceptible to hypomagnesaemia.

Magnesium has antinociceptive effect in animal and human models of pain [22]. As a matter of fact, noxious stimuli activate the release of glutamate in the dorsal horn, which then activates the NMDA receptors, causing intracellular calcium influx, neuronal excitation, and central sensitization and hyperalgesia [23]. Therefore, NMDA receptor antagonists play an important role in perioperative pain control. Furthermore, compared with acute cutaneous pain sensation, NMDA receptor antagonists provide better pain control for acute visceral pain [24].

Less opioid consumption and better analgesia were observed when patients' magnesium deficiency was corrected. These observations support both the opioid-sparing effect and co-analgesic properties of magnesium. There are two major mechanisms by which hypomagnesemia can be induced: gastrointestinal or renal losses [8]. As diet is the only source of magnesium, the most common cause of hypomagnesemia in surgical patients is prolonged NPO. Other risk factors include diarrhea, alcoholism, acute pancreatitis, uncontrolled diabetes mellitus, and medication such as a proton pump inhibitor and diuretics [25]. Our results indicate that if patients have these risk factors with complex pain, assessing and correcting magnesium level will be necessary. There is a declining trend for the risk of oxygen desaturation and PONV in the magnesium group, although it did not reach statistically significant. This probably due to short operating time and propofol's antiemetic effect. Moreover, the recovery of consciousness was not delayed in Group M, while Altan et al. [26] reported that magnesium sulphate caused a delay in recovery for patients undergoing spinal surgery. Magnesium sulphate is known to prolong and potentiate neuromuscular block by non-depolarizing neuromuscular blocking agents [27]. Patients in our study did not receive muscle relaxant and they keep breathe spontaneously. Different surgical model may explain the diverse results on the time of recovery of consciousness between the present study and the result of Altan et al.

Intravenous administration of magnesium generally is associated with minor side effects. Common magnesium-related side effects include flushing, dizziness, and cardiovascular events. Nevertheless, a meta-analysis indicated that magnesium did not have a statistically significant effect on the incidence of dizziness, hypotension, or bradycardia [28]. On the contrary, it was beneficial to reduce postoperative shivering. Hypomagnesaemia can produce numerous symptoms such as pain, weakness, tetany, hallucinations, and arrhythmias [8, 20]. A stable serum magnesium concentration might be helpful for patients' comfort and postoperative recovery. Jee et al. [29] found that magnesium administration can reduce the release of catecholamine and vasopressin during laparoscopic cholecystectomy. Its antinociceptive effect and direct vasodilatory effect through a calcium channel blockade might explain the lower HR and MBP in Group M. Although there was no significant difference of hypotension between the two groups in our study, relatively lower MBP might be helpful to reduce intraoperative bleeding and stress response. Even though we did not record the specific reasons for adding bolus doses of fentanyl in our study, less fentanyl consumption can reflect fewer times of body movement. These advantages of magnesium sulphate may create good conditions for operation, shorten the duration of procedure, and eventually improve the satisfaction of gynecologists.

Some limitations of the present study should be noted. First, it was a single-center study, and the relatively small number of patients limited the ability to detect statistically significant differences in adverse events of fentanyl between two groups. Second, we only applied magnesium to propofol-fentanyl anesthesia in hysteroscopy. The combination of magnesium with some other medicine in different targets such as lidocaine, ketamine, and dexmedetomidine may be more effective to reduce opioids consumption, even achieve opioid-free anesthesia. Last, we didn't record magnesium level when we assess postoperative pain scores, so it's difficult to draw an accurate conclusion on the relationship between magnesium and pain. In further research, magnesium level and pain scores should be assessed dynamically and simultaneously.

Conclusion

In hysteroscopy, adjuvant magnesium administration is beneficial to reduce intraoperative fentanyl requirement and postoperative pain without cardiovascular side effects. Our study indicates that if surgical patients have risk factors for hypomagnesemia, assessing and correcting magnesium level will be necessary.

Abbreviations

PONV: Postoperative nausea and vomiting; BIS: Bispectral Index Scale; ASA: American Society of Anesthesiologists; NIBP: Noninvasive blood pressure; SpO2: Pulse oximetry; MBP: Mean blood pressure; HR: Heart rate; PACU: Post anesthesia care unit; VNRS: Verbal numerical rating scale; OFA: Opioid-free anesthesia

Acknowledgments

We thank all the patients, their families, and the institutions for supporting this study.

Authors' contributions

JYL and PFG were resposible for conceived, designed this study and collected the data. SW and YFZ were responsible for study execution and manuscript writing. GQW was responsible for data analysis. QX and XG were responsible interpretation of results and manuscript writing. All authors have read and approved the final version of the manuscript.

References

1. Sutton C. Hysteroscopic surgery. Best Pract Res Clin Obstet Gynaecol. 2006; 20:105–37.
2. Gupta JK, Clark TJ, More S, Pattison H. Patient anxiety and experiences associated with an outpatient "one-stop" "see and treat" hysteroscopy clinic. Surg Endosc. 2004;18:1099–104.
3. Emanuel MH. New developments in hysteroscopy. Best Pract Res Clin Obstet Gynaecol. 2013;27:421–9.
4. Ryu JH, Kim JH, Park KS, Do SH. Remifentanil-propofol versus fentanyl-propofol for monitored anesthesia care during hysteroscopy. J Clin Anesth. 2008;20:328–32.
5. Munro A, Sjaus A, George RB. Anesthesia and analgesia for gynecological surgery. Curr Opin Anaesthesiol. 2018;31:274–9.
6. Frauenknecht J, Kirkham KR, Jacot-Guillarmod A, Albrecht E. Analgesic impact of intra-operative opioids vs. opioid-free Anaesthesia: a systematic review and meta-analysis. Anaesthesia. 2019;74:651–62.
7. Shin HJ, Na HS, Do SH. Magnesium and pain. Nutrients. 2020;12:E2184.
8. Agus ZS. Mechanisms and causes of hypomagnesemia. Curr Opin Nephrol Hypertens. 2016;25:301–7.
9. Ting WH, Lin HH, Hsiao SM. Manual versus pump infusion of distending media for hysteroscopic procedures: a randomized controlled trial. Sci Rep. 2019;9:14943.
10. Dubray C, Alloui A, Bardin L, et al. Magnesium deficiency induces an hyperalgesia reversed by the NMDA receptor antagonist MK801. Neuroreport. 1997;8:1383–6.
11. Aldrete JA. The post-anesthesia recovery score revisited. J Clin Anesth. 1995;7:89–91.
12. Küçük M, Uğur B, Oğurlu M. Comparing the Administration of Fentanyl 1 μg kg^{-1} and fentanyl 0.5 μg kg^{-1} in dilation and curettage procedures. Gynecol Endocrinol. 2012;28:736–9.
13. Sahinovic MM, Struys MMRF, Absalom AR. Clinical pharmacokinetics and pharmacodynamics of propofol. Clin Pharmacokinet. 2018;57:1539–58.
14. Stanley TH. The fentanyl story. J Pain. 2014;15:1215–26.
15. Brix LD, Thillemann TM, Nikolajsen L. Local anesthesia combined with sedation compared with general anesthesia for ambulatory operative hysteroscopy: a randomized study. J Perianesth Nurs. 2016;31:309–16.
16. Franz AM, Martin LD, Liston DE, Latham GJ, Richards MJ, Low DK. In pursuit of an opioid-free pediatric ambulatory surgery center: a quality improvement initiative. Anesth Analg. 2020. https://doi.org/10.1213/ANE.0000000000004774.
17. Mulier JP. Is opioid-free general anesthesia for breast and gynecological surgery a viable option? Curr Opin Anaesthesiol. 2019;32:257–62.
18. Sharma JB, Aruna J, Kumar P, Roy KK, Malhotra N, Kumar S. Comparison of efficacy of oral drotaverine plus mefenamic acid with paracervical block and with intravenous sedation for pain relief during hysteroscopy and endometrial biopsy. Indian J Med Sci. 2009;63:244–52.
19. Tanriverdi TB, Koceroglu I, Devrim S, Celik MG. Comparison of sedation with dexmedetomidine vs propofol during hysteroscopic surgery: single-Centre randomized controlled trial. J Clin Pharm Ther. 2019;00:1–6.
20. Séamus C, Daniel M. Improved analgesia by correction of hypomagnesaemia? BMJ Support Palliat Care. 2018;8:294–6.
21. Witz CA, Silverberg KM, Burns WN, Schenken RS, Olive DL. Complications associated with the absorption of hysteroscopic fluid media. Fertil Steril. 1993;60:745–56.
22. Mentes O, Harlak A, Yigit T, Balkan A, Balkan M, et al. Effect of intraoperative magnesium sulphate infusion on pain relief after laparoscopic cholecystectomy. Acta Anaesthesiol Scand. 2008;52:1353–9.
23. Jabbour HJ, Naccache NM, Jawish RJ, et al. Ketamine and magnesium association reduces morphine consumption after scoliosis surgery: prospective randomised double-blind study. Acta Anaesthesiol Scand. 2014; 58:572–9.
24. Strigo IA, Duncan GH, Bushnell MC, Boivin M, Wainer I, et al. The effects of racemic ketamine on painful stimulation of skin and viscera in human subjects. Pain. 2005;113:255–64.
25. Chen KC, Chu P. The case | Hypomagnesemia with knee pain. Kidney Int. 2017;91:1261–2.
26. Altan A, Turgut N, Yildiz F, Türkmen A, Ustün H. Effects of magnesium sulphate and clonidine on propofol consumption, haemodynamics and postoperative recovery. Br J Anaesth. 2005;94:438–41.
27. Telci L, Esen F, Akcora D, Erden T, Canbolat AT, Akpir K. Evaluation of effects of magnesium sulphate in reducing intraoperative anaesthetic requirements. Br J Anaesth. 2002;89:594–8.
28. De Oliveira GS Jr, Castro-Alves LJ, Khan JH, McCarthy RJ. Perioperative systemic magnesium to minimize postoperative pain: a meta-analysis of randomized controlled trials. Anesthesiology. 2013;119:178–90.
29. Jee D, Lee D, Yun S, Lee C. Magnesium sulphate attenuates arterial pressure increase during laparoscopic cholecystectomy. Br J Anaesth. 2009;103:484–9.

9

Postoperative analgesic efficacy of ear acupuncture in patients undergoing abdominal hysterectomy

Hamdy A. Hendawy[1] and Mohamed E. Abuelnaga[2*]

Abstract

Background: Numerous studies have revealed that acupuncture can increase the somatic pain threshold. Electro-acupuncture (EA) can help pain-relieving with minimal physiologic disturbance. Various painful disorders, as well as pain following various surgeries, like cesarean section, gastrostomy, and enterectomy were managed properly with acupuncture. Therefore we studied the postoperative analgesic effect of EA in patients undergoing abdominal hysterectomy.

Methods: A randomized, prospective clinical trial study was carried out on 56 women undergoing hysterectomy under spinal anesthesia. Patients were allocated randomly to receive either spinal anesthesia and electric ear acupuncture (EEA group) or spinal anesthesia alone (control group). EEA was done by fine needles to anatomically defined 4 points of the ear: Shen Men Point, thalamus Point 26, Analgesia Point 3, and Uterus Point 58, and connected to EA therapeutic apparatus. After finishing surgery, the fine needles were substituted by permanent press needles to be removed after 24 hours. The primary outcome was the postoperative 24 h morphine consumption by patient-controlled analgesia, while secondary outcomes included Post-operative pain scores and postoperative 1st request of analgesia.

Results: Total morphine consumption in the first 24 postoperative hours was obviously reduced in the EEA group versus the control group (mean ± SD:6.214± 2.1319 mg vs 15.714 ± 3.3428 mg, d = − 3.3886, 95% Confidence interval = − 4.2061,-2.5712, *p*-value =0.000). The postoperative pain scores were significantly reduced in the EEA group in comparison to the control group, with delayed 1st request of postoperative analgesia.

Conclusions: Electric ear acupuncture provides postoperative analgesia, reducing morphine requirement and consequently its side effects.

Keywords: Electric ear acupuncture, Post-operative pain relief, Abdominal hysterectomy

* Correspondence: Mohamed_abuelnga@med.suez.edu.eg
[2]Department of Anesthesia, Intensive Care and Pain Management, Faculty of Medicine, Suez Canal University, P.O. Box: 41522, Ard Elgameiat, Ismailia City, Egypt

Background

Acupuncture is considered as a traditional therapeutic technique with a long history of 4000 years. Electro-acupuncture (EA) is a new type of hand acupuncture that can deliver effective analgesia with a minute physiological disturbance [1, 2]. It was used effectively for pain management in different disorders including post-surgical pain following cesarean section, gastrostomy, and enterectomy [1, 3, 4]. Acupuncture and Transcutaneous electrical nerve stimulation (TENS) were showed to have valuable efficacy in increasing the somatic pain threshold [5]. Kitade and Hyodo [6] investigated the effect of auricular acupuncture stimulation on the threshold of somatic pain. They found the Shen-Men, lungs, sympathicus, and kidney points showed a significant pain threshold rise when compared to non-acupuncture auricular points. Even though the results differ greatly depending on the individual and body region, to some degree they elucidated that auricular acupuncture points had parallels in specific body regions and the authors concluded that auricular acupuncture stimulation can achieve an analgesic effect. It is believed that the human body encompasses energy pathways or channels representing the internal organs. Energy is thought to stream continuously through these pathways ending to the body surface with acupuncture points that work as gateways to these channels. Stimulation of these acupoints is claimed to activate the body's inherent healing power [7].

Generally, acupuncture can boost physical and emotional health through the release of certain neurochemicals from the nervous system, as well as affecting cerebral areas responsible for reducing pain and anxiety [7, 8]. Acupuncture can help in postoperative pain reduction by altering the brain's chemistry, increasing endorphins and neuropeptide Y levels, and reducing serotonin levels [7]. Systematic reviews revealed the effectiveness of acupuncture as a useful adjuvant for post-surgical pain relief. Randomized controlled trials have found that acupuncture can ameliorate postoperative pain, reduce the use of patient-controlled analgesia (PCA), and postoperative nausea and vomiting [8]. Several publications have found the analgesic effectiveness of body acupuncture in gynaecologic surgery including hysterectomy [9–12]. Tsang et al. reported that a single session of auricular TENS delivered 24 hours after surgery was effective in reducing post-hysterectomy pain for at least 30 min [13]. This study aims to investigate the role of preoperative electric ear acupuncture (EEA) in reducing post-operative pain in patients undergoing hysterectomy by fine acupuncture needles (10 mm × 30 gauge) for four points of ear acupuncture. We hypothesize that EAA will reduce the required postoperative analgesia following abdominal hysterectomy.

Methods

The current study is a single-blinded randomized controlled clinical trial. After Obtaining approval by the Hospital Ethics Committee, and Written informed patient consent with an explanation regarding the purpose, methods, effects, and complications of techniques, 56 patients were randomly allocated into two equal groups using simple random tables generated from a computer software program (http://www.randomizer.org). The allocation sequence was concealed in opaque numbered envelopes. The outcome assessor was another anesthesiologist who was blind to the study group. Inclusion criteria included patients aged between 21-60 years old and have an American society of anaesthesiologist (ASA) physical status I & II. Patients who have contraindications for spinal anesthesia as (infection at the site of puncture, coagulopathy, platelet abnormalities, and concurrent treatment with anticoagulant drugs), allergy to morphine, and/or bupivacaine, morbid obesity (body mass index (BMI) > 35 Kg/m^2), psychological disease, narcotic abuse, prolonged use of sedatives or opioid drug use, contraindications for ear acupuncture (infection at the acupuncture site) and patients refused to participate in the study were excluded. The primary objective was to assess the influence of auricular acupuncture regarding the postoperative analgesic requirement in patients scheduled for abdominal hysterectomy, while secondary objectives were intraoperative hemodynamic parameters, Post-operative pain scores, and Postoperative 1st request of analgesia.

The 56 patient were randomized into two equal groups:-

Group I (EEA group): 28 females received electric ear acupuncture after spinal anesthesia.
Group II (control group): 28 females received spinal anesthesia without ear acupuncture.

Preoperative visit to the chosen patients was done where

Explanation of the whole procedure including the expected benefits and complications was done. All Patients were instructed preoperatively for the use of the PCA apparatus.

A) Pre-operative assessment

The patient's age, ASA status, and BMI were recorded. Medical history was reviewed to rule out excluded patients from the study. General examination, vital signs: heart rate (HR), blood pressure (BP), temperature, chest, heart, abdominal examination, and airway evaluation were done. Investigations done were complete blood count, random blood sugar, bleeding profile as prothrombin time, International Randomized Ratio, and partial thromboplastin time.

B) Intra-operative measures

The patient was reassured and the procedure was explained to her. Airway devices and anesthesia machines, ventilators, flowmeters, and equipment were checked promptly.

Routine Monitoring equipment (Datex-Ohmeda®) was attached to the patient including 3 leads electrocardiogram (ECG), non-invasive BP, and pulse oximetry. An 18- gauge intravenous cannula was inserted into the patient's forearm and 500 mills of intravenous (I.V.) fluid (ringer acetate) were administrated. No premedications were given. All patients in both groups were given spinal anesthesia by 25 G needle with hyperbaric bupivacaine 0.5% (15-20 mg) according to the patient's height, in the L4- L5 intervertebral space. During spinal injection, no supplementary opioids were given; the level of anesthesia was assessed by pin-prick every 5 min in the first 20 min till it reached T4-T6 which would be considered sufficient to start the surgery.

The procedure of acupuncture

Acupuncture was done based on our institutional experience. EEA was done by fine needles (10 mm x 30guage) to the anatomically defined 4 points of ear acupuncture which are called; Shen Men Point (Divine Gate Point) or point 55 which is a sedative analgesic anti-inflammatory point, thalamus Point 26 which is an analgesic point in acute and chronic severe pain, Analgesia Point 3, and Uterus Point 58 [7, 8].

Then four pre-sterilized single-use acupuncture needles were inserted in the predetermined acupoints and connected to clamps of electrode cords that were connected to the electro-acupuncture therapeutic apparatus (KWD-808I MULTIPURPOSE HEALTH DEVICE, Changzhou Yingdi Electronic Medical Device Co., China. (Fig. 1).

The EA device was switched on and adjusted according to the instruction manual for use to provide continuous-wave with a frequency of 2 Hz and output impulse amplitude of 6-10 V according to the patient's ability. At the end of the surgery, the electro-acupuncture device was switched off and the fine needles were replaced by press needles in the same acupoints to be removed after 24 hours.

Measurements and postoperative care

All intraoperative and postoperative recordings were done by another anesthesiologist who was blind to the allocation group. Vital signs (BP, HR, respiratory rate) and oxygen saturation were recorded and analyzed every 5 min in the first 20 min, then every 20 min for the rest of the surgery. At the end of the operation, the duration of surgery and spinal level were recorded for both groups, and Diclofenac potassium 75 mg was administered to all patients by intramuscular injection. Postoperative BP and HR were recorded immediately after transfer to the post-anesthesia care unit (PACU), then after 1, 3,6,12, and 24 hours. Post-operative pain assessment was done by visual analog scale .when the reported visual analog scale (VAS) was 3 or more, a loading dose of morphine 0.05 mg/kg was administered via slow I.V. route. Then, a PCA was administered. The PCA pump was loaded with 1 mg / ml of morphine and set to deliver on-demand doses of 2 ml with 10 min lockout intervals and 4 h limit of 20 mg. No background infusion was allowed. The pain score was reassessed at the end of the 1st postoperative 24 hours. The time to the 1st postoperative request of analgesia was recorded using the PCA delivery system. The total amount of morphine consumption over the 1st 24 hours postoperatively was recorded. Side effects associated with morphine consumption as nausea, vomiting, and over sedation were recorded. Nausea and vomiting were assessed using a 5 point scale from zero to four, where 0 is no nausea or vomiting, 1 = mild nausea, 2 = severe nausea, 3 = vomiting once, 4 = vomiting more than one. These assessments were performed in the PACU immediately

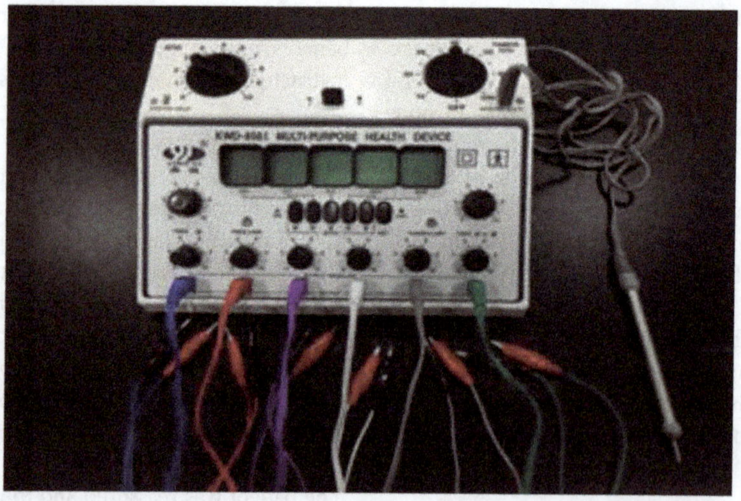

Fig. 1 KWD-808I MULTIPURPOSE HEALTH DEVICE is connected to grey acupoint detecting pen for acupoint detection APD and six electrode cords with 6 different colors for electro-acupuncture

after discharge and after 1, 3, 6, 12, and 24 h postoperatively. Side effects associated with auricular acupuncture-like bleeding, excessive pain, fainting, broken needles, and local infection were recorded.

Statistical analysis

The statistical analysis was performed using IBM SPSS Statistics® 22 for Windows 10 operating system. Normality was assessed using the Kolmogorov–Smirnov test and visual inspection of histograms. For demographic and baseline comparison, the standardized difference was calculated using a web-based effect-size calculator [14]. 2-tailed t-test was used to analyze the continuous variables (hemodynamic parameters, pain score, 1st request of analgesia, 24 hours analgesic consumption) between the two studied groups while chi-square test was used for categorical and dichotomous variables (incidence of nausea, vomiting and level of the block at end of surgery). Values were expressed as mean ± standard deviation (SD) for continuous variables or as a percentage of the group from which they were derived (categorical variables). P-value < 0.05 was considered significant. Presentation of the statistical outcomes in the form of tables and graphs was performed using the "Microsoft Office Excel® 2010" program.

24 patients per group were needed to detect 5.39 mg difference between the means of total 24 hours postoperative morphine consumption in patients undergoing cesarean section between electro-acupuncture and control groups, at a standard deviation of 5.18 [15], with 95% power and a level of significance 5%. After considering a 20% dropout rate, the required sample size was 56 patients (28 patients/group).

Results

Fifty-six patients were randomly assigned for two equal groups EEA group and the control group (Fig. 2)

The two groups were comparable in age, BMI, ASA status, history of chronic illness, duration of surgery, and level of the block at end of surgery. The duration of surgery was about 80 min in both groups. (Table 1) no statistically significant difference was found between the 2 groups as regard intraoperative hemodynamics.

The time to the 1st request of analgesia was much delayed in the EEA group versus the control group (mean ± SD: 268.893 ± 31.6044 vs 52.036 ± 9.5316 min) in both groups respectively with statistically significant difference (d = 9.2905, 95% CI = 7.4919, 11.089, p-value =0.000). Total post-operative 24 hours morphine consumption was markedly reduced in favor of the EEA group (6.214± 2.1319 mg) versus (15.714 ± 3.3428 mg) in

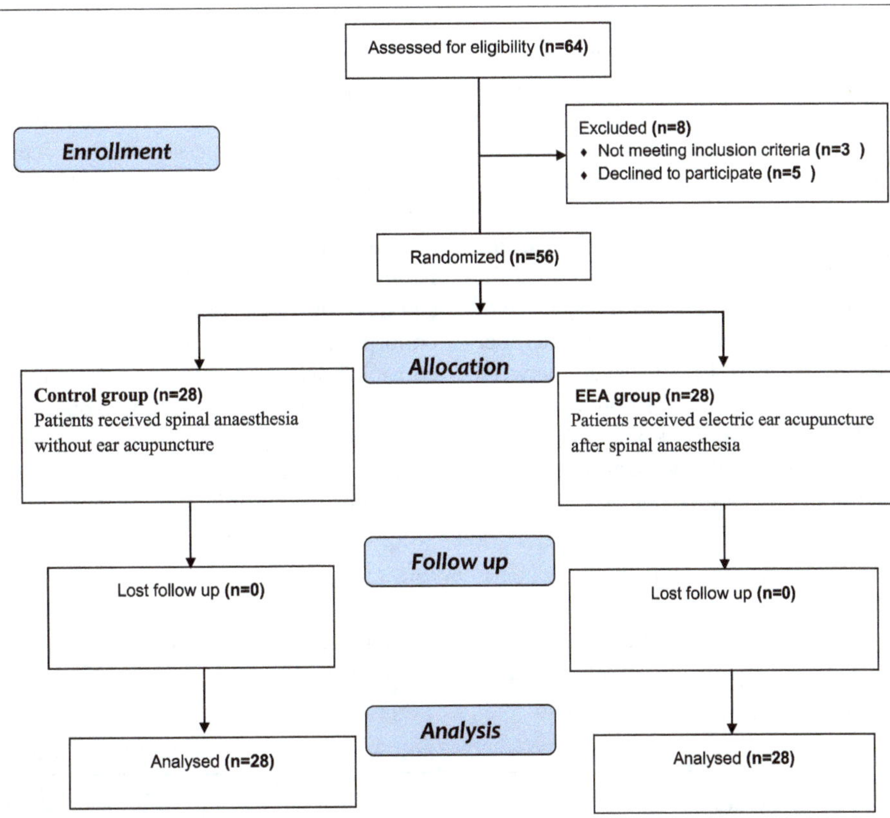

Fig. 2 Flow chart of patient's participation progress throughout the study

Table 1 Demographic characteristics among the studied patients

Demographic characteristics			EEA group (*n* = 28)	control group (*n* = 28)	*d*	95% C.I.	p
Age	Mean ± SD		49.857 ± 3.9320	49.643 ± 3.8318	0.0551	− 0.4688,0.579	0.837 (NS)
BMI	Mean ± SD		27.02 ± 3.401	28.38± 2.794	− 0.437	− 0.967,0.0931	0.108(NS)
ASA I ASA II	N (%)		16 (57.1%) 12 (42.9%)	16 (57.1%) 12 (42.9%)	0	−0.5292,0.5292	1.0(NS)
Chronic illness	Hypertension	N (%)	5 (17.9%)	4 (14.3%)	−0.0981	−0.6222,0.4261	0.716(NS)
	Diabetes mellitus	N (%)	7 (25.0%)	8 (28.6%)	0.0813	−0.4427,0.6054	0.763(NS)
Duration of surgery	Mean ± SD		79.96 ± 8.113	80.61 ± 6.190	−0.0901	−0.6142,0.434	0.74(NS)
Level of the block at end of surgery	T4 T6	N (%)	15 (53.6%) 13 (46.4%)	14 (50%) 14 (50%)	−0.0721	−0.5961,0.4519	0.789 (NS)

NS Non-significant difference ($P > 0.05$)
p *p*-value for comparing between the two groups
d standardized mean-difference effect size
C.I confidence interval

the control group with statistically significant difference (d = – 3.3886, 95% CI = -4.2061,-2.5712,*p*-value =0.000). postoperative VAS score after 24 hours was lower in the favor of the EEA group in comparison to the control group (mean ± SD: 2.536 ± 1.1380VS 5.036 ± 1.3467) in both groups respectively with statistically significant difference (d = – 2.0053, 95%CI = - 2.6474, – 1.3631, *p*-value =0.000). (Table 2).

There was a statistically significant difference(*p*-value < 0.05) between the two groups regarding the incidence of nausea at 1 h, 3 h, 6 h, and 12 h in the favor of the EEA group. (Table 3).

Vomiting occurred in 4 patients of the control group at 6 h time point while it was not noted to occur in the EAA group with a significant difference between both groups (*p*-value =0.038). (Table 3). Over-sedation was not noted in both groups of the study. No complications were recorded from auricular acupuncture.

Statistically, a significant difference was noted regarding postoperative systolic blood pressure changes between the two studied groups after 6 h and 12 h of surgery in favor of the EEA group. There was also a significant difference regarding the post-operative diastolic BP changes between the two groups after 3 h, 6 h, 12 h, and 24 hours after surgery in the favor of the EEA group. No statistically significant difference was noted as regards the postoperative HR between both groups at all time points. (Fig. 3).

Discussion

Acupuncture and TENS were proven to increase the threshold of somatic pain. Ishimaru and colleagues examined how low flow electric acupuncture (LFEA) can influence pain threshold in the abdominal area; they advocated that LFEA can be helpful for analgesia following abdominal surgery [16].

The effect of LFEA and TENS on the deep pain threshold at the skin surface and deeper layers has been examined by a few studies [17, 18]. Kitade and colleagues found an increased pain threshold for 50 min following LFEA, with no identified increase in the levels of plasma β-endorphin or adrenocorticotropic hormone in the cerebrospinal fluid [19]. These results eliminate the role of β-endorphin in the analgesic effect of acupuncture. Because acupuncture analgesia was offset by naloxone, there is a probability that some types of endogenous opioid peptides are responsible for the analgesic effect of acupuncture. Ishimaru et al. showed that 30 min of LFEA produced analgesia [20]. They found increased levels of plasma β-endorphin [20, 21], with no change in plasma adrenocorticotropic hormone level [21]. This result matches what has been found in patients with post-operative pain [21].

Several mechanisms for acupuncture pain have been reported as the release of spinal natural opioids like dynorphin, endorphin, and encephalin, which are potent

Table 2 Postoperative time for the first analgesic request (mins), VAS at 24 hours postoperatively, and total analgesic consumption in the 1st 24 hours (mgs)

	EEA group (*n* = 28)	Control group (*n* = 28)	*d*	95% C.I.	*p*
First analgesic request (Mean ± SD)	268.893 ± 31.6044	52.036 ± 9.5316	9.2905	7.4919,11.089	0.000*
24 hours morphine consumption (mean ± SD)	6.214± 2.1319	15.714 ± 3.3428	−3.3886	−4.2061,-2.5712	0.000*
VAS at 24 hours (Mean ± SD)	2.536 ± 1.1380	5.036 ± 1.3467	-2.0053	-2.6474, −1.3631	0.000*

*statistically significant at $p \leq 0.05$
p *p*-value for comparing between the two groups
d standardized mean-difference effect size
C.I confidence interval

Table 3 Post-operative incidence of nausea and vomiting

		post-operative nausea			post-operative vomiting		
		EEA group (*n* = 28)	Control group (*n* = 28)	*p*	EEA group (*n* = 28)	Control group (*n* = 28)	*p*
PACU	N (%)	0	0	.	0	0	.
After 1 h	N (%)	0	7 (25%)	0.005*	0	0	.
After 3 h	N (%)	0	6 (21.4%)	0.01*	0	0	.
After 6 h	N (%)	0	8 (28.6%)	0.002*	0	4 (14.3%)	0.038*
After 12 h	N (%)	0	20 (71.4%)	0.000*	0	0	.
After 24 hr	N (%)	0	0	.	0	0	.

*statistically significant at $p \leq 0.05$
p *p*-value for comparing between the two groups

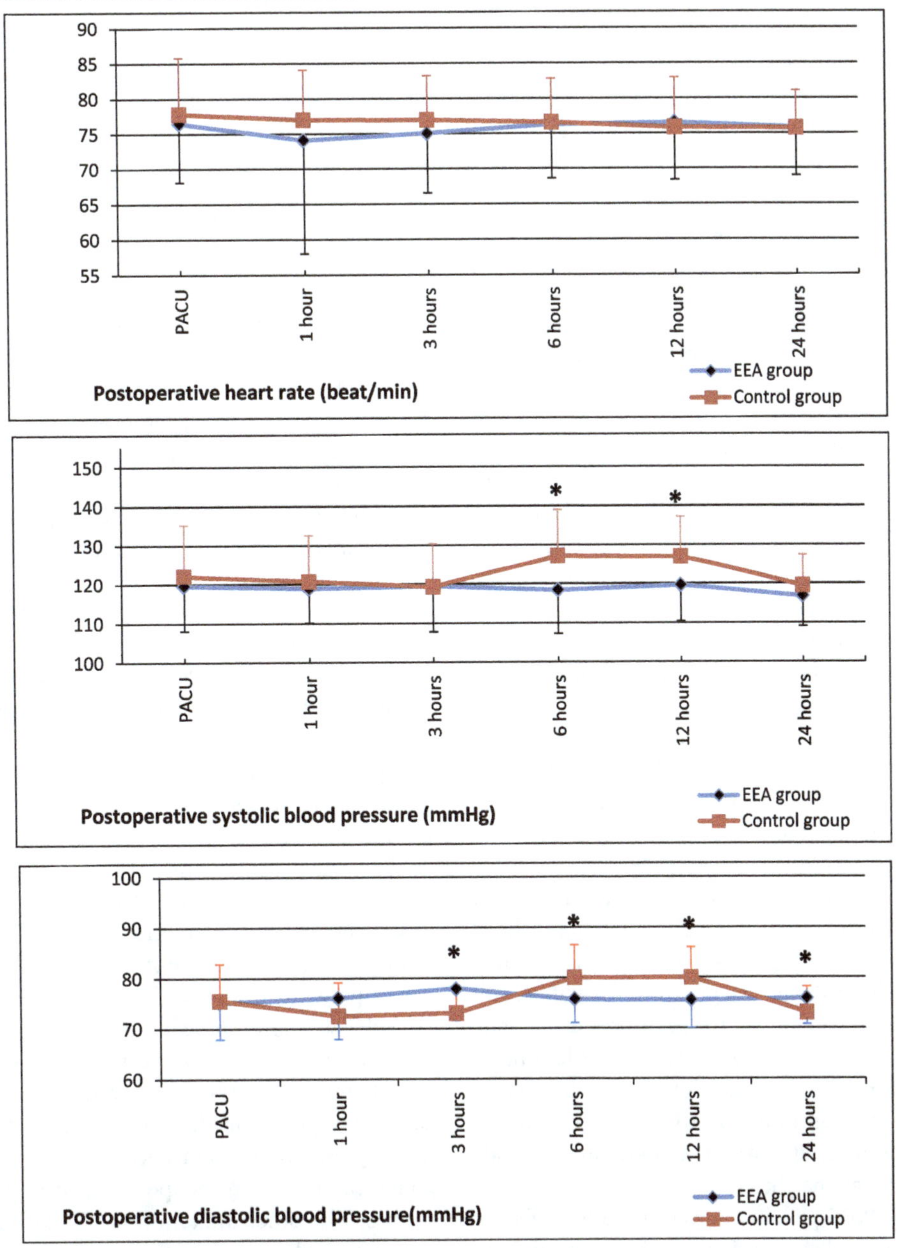

Fig. 3 Postoperative hemodynamics in the study groups

pain suppressors, increase in local blood flow that encourages the process of healing, gate control theory of pain, the endogenous release of adrenocorticotrophic hormones, myofibrillary entanglement relaxation, and creating a balance in the mesolimbic neural pain pathway [22].

In 2016, De Freitas et al., have reported in an animal study that acupuncture has a pre-emptive analgesic effect [23]. Sim et al. 2002 compared preoperative versus postoperative body EA for lower abdominal gynaecologic surgery. Preoperative acupuncture was found to be more effective in reducing postoperative morphine consumption in these patients [11].

In the current study, we decided to use preoperative EEA along with continuous postoperative acupoint stimulation by press needles to achieve the maximum analgesic effect. Our study demonstrated that the total postoperative PCA morphine consumption in the first 24 hours was reduced in the EEA group versus the control group; also the time of the first request for supplemental analgesia was delayed in the EEA group when compared with the control group.

Similar to our findings: In a prospective, randomized study done by WU Hung-Chien et al. [15] and conducted for 60 primigravida women scheduled for cesarean section under spinal anesthesia. Patients were allocated to one of three groups: control group, acupuncture group, and electro-acupuncture group. Acupuncture was started postoperatively after recovery from anesthesia and was applied for San yin Jiao (Sp6) body acupoint for 30 min. The results showed delayed first analgesic request in both the electro-acupuncture group (39.5 ± 16.9 min) and the acupuncture group (40.3 ± 13.8 min) versus the control group (29.0 ± 15.0 min). The total PCA morphine consumption during the first 24 postoperative hours was much reduced in the acupuncture group (10.66 ± 4.68) mg, and the electroacupuncture was (9.89 ± 5.18) mg than in the control group was (15.28 ± 4.99) mg [15]..

In our study, we had a delayed first morphine request and less total morphine dose which may be due to our usage of diclofenac potassium by intramuscular injection, the pre-emptive effect of acupuncture, and also acupuncture needles were replaced in the EEA group by press needles.

In our study, the VAS pain scores were lower in the EEA group versus the control group. Similarly, WU Hung-Chien, et al. [15] found that VAS pain scores were significantly lower in the auricular acupuncture group versus the control group at 0.5, 1, 1.5, and 2 hours in the postoperative period.

Similarly, Iacobone,m et al. 2014 [24], found less postoperative pain scores and reduced postoperative acetaminophen consumption in acupuncture treated groups versus the control group in patients undergoing thyroidectomy under general anesthesia.

Chen, C. C et al., 2015 [25], have investigated the effect of acupuncture on Pain Relief following total knee arthroplasty in a randomized controlled trial. The total amount of postoperative fentanyl consumption was found much reduced in the acupuncture group in comparison with the control group [mean (SD), 620.7 (258. 2) vs. 868.6 (319.3) μg, respectively, as well as delayed first request for fentanyl [median time, 89 vs. 37 min], in the acupuncture group and the control group respectively. Postoperative pain scores were much reduced in the acupuncture group versus the control groups at 2, 4, 8, 12, and 24 hours. Dingmann, J et al. 2017 [26], have found in their study the efficacy of acupuncture in reducing postoperative swallowing pain scores following tonsillectomy in patients aged 16 years or more.

In our study, there was a statistical difference between both groups as regards the incidence of nausea at some time points in the favor of the EEA group; also we found a significant difference between both study groups concerning the incidence of vomiting after 6 h in the favor of acupuncture group. This may be explained by a reduced total amount of 24 hours of morphine consumption in the acupuncture group in comparison to the control group.

Usichenk et al. 2004 [27] found that auricular acupuncture (AA) is effective in the treatment of various pain conditions. They conducted a blinded study to assess the analgesic effect of AA for pain management following total hip arthroplasty. The patients were randomly assigned to receive either true AA or sham acupuncture, with press acupuncture needles kept in place for 3 postoperative days. Thirty-six hours of analgesic requirement following surgery was lower in the AA group versus the control group. No difference was found between both groups as regard VAS Pain scores or analgesia-related adverse effects.

Chang et al. 2012 [28] have conducted a randomized controlled study to investigate the potential benefits of auricular acupressure for postoperative pain relief and ameliorating the passive range of motion in patients who underwent total knee replacement (TKR). Sixty-two patients were randomly allocated to either the acupressure group or the control group. The acupressure was performed three times a day for 3 days. The patients in both groups were found to have a comparable high level of postoperative pain scores. However, analgesic drug consumption was markedly reduced in the acupressure group versus the control group ($P < 0.05$), with markedly improved passive knee motion by the third postoperative day in patients treated with acupressure ($P < 0.05$) [28].

Lastly, we have some limitations. The analgesic effect found in the current study can be the result of either preoperative EEA, continuous post-operative acupoint stimulation by press needles, or combined effect of both techniques. Comparison between EEA and pressure acupuncture in the same acupoints is recommended in future studies. The other limitation in the current study was the use of a single postoperative non-opioid analgesic. In future studies, at least two non-opioid analgesics should be used to determine the real influence of acupuncture on postoperative analgesia requirements.

Conclusion

Auricular acupuncture is a useful analgesic adjuvant as it reduced postoperative analgesic requirements following abdominal hysterectomy. It provided more patient satisfaction regarding postoperative pain control without any hazard.

Abbreviations

EA: Electroacupuncture; EEA: Electric ear acupuncture; PCA: Patient controlled analgesia; TENS: Transcutaneous electrical nerve stimulation; ASA: American society of anesthesiologist; BMI: Body mass index; HR: Heart rate; BP: Blood pressure; PACU: Postanesthesia care unit; VAS: Visual analog scale

Acknowledgments

We would like to thank all participant patients in our study, our colleagues, and the nursing staff in Suez Canal university hospital.

Authors' contributions

Hamdy A. Hendawy, MD: This author helped in preparing the Concept of the research, Design, Clinical work, Data acquisition, Manuscript review, and editing, and final editing of the paper. Mohamed E. Abuelnaga, MD: This author helped in Literature search, Clinical work, Manuscript preparation, Data Acquisition, and Manuscript review. The author(s) read and approved the final manuscript.

Author details

[1]Faculty of Medicine, Suez Canal University, Ismailia, Egypt. [2]Department of Anesthesia, Intensive Care and Pain Management, Faculty of Medicine, Suez Canal University, P.O. Box: 41522, Ard Elgameiat, Ismailia City, Egypt.

References

1. Haltrecht H. Veterinary acupuncture. Can Vet J. 1999;40:401–3.
2. Taguchi R. Acupuncture anesthesia and analgesia for clinical acute pain in Japan. Evid Based Complement Alternat Med. 2008;5:153–8.
3. Inoue M, Kitakoji H, Yano T, Ishizaki N, Itoi M, Katsumi Y. Acupuncture treatment for low back pain and lower limb symptoms the relation between acupuncture or electroacupuncture stimulation and sciatic nerve blood flow, Evid Based Complement Alternat Med. 2008;5:133–43.
4. Chen CL. Traditional Chinese veterinary medicine. Chin Agric Encyclopedia. 1991:57–8.
5. Hyodo M, Nakamura N, Yukimati T, Sugasawa T, Oki J. The experience of acupuncture anesthesia. Jap J Anesthesiol. 1973;22:251–8.
6. Kitade T, Hyodo M. The effects of stimulation of ear acupuncture points on the body's pain threshold. Am J Chin Med. 1979;7:241–52.
7. Vadivelu N, Mitra S, Narayan D. Recent advances in postoperative pain management. Yale J Biol Med. 2010;83:11.
8. Rubach A. Principles of ear acupuncture—microsystem of the auricle, hippokrates; 2001.
9. Lin JG, Lo MW, Wen YR, Hsieh CL, Tsai SK, Sun WZ. The effect of high and low frequency electroacupuncture in pain after lower abdominal surgery. Pain. 2002;99:509–14.
10. Kim KS, Nam YM. The analgesic effects of capsicum plaster at the Zusanli point after abdominal hysterectomy. Anesth Analg. 2006;103:709–13.
11. Sim CK, Xu PC, Pua HL, Zhang G, Lee TL. Effects of electroacupuncture on intraoperative and postoperative analgesic requirement. Acupunct Med. 2002;20:56–65.
12. Chen L, Tang J, White PF. The effect of location of transcutaneous electrical nerve stimulation on postoperative opioid analgesic requirement: acupoint versus nonacupoint stimulation. Anesth Analg. 1998;87:1129–34.
13. Tsang HC, Lam CS, Chu PW, Yap J, Fung TY, Cheing GL. A randomized controlled trial of auricular transcutaneous electrical nerve stimulation for managing posthysterectomy pain. Evid Based Complement Alternat Med. 2011:1–9.
14. Wilson DB. Practical meta-analysis effect size calculator 2016. URL: http:// www.Campbellcollaboration org/escalc/HTML/EffectSizeCalculator-SMD1 PHP [accessed 2020-04-25] [WebCite Cache ID 6MqcuP70x].
15. Wu H, Liu YC, Ou KL, Chang YH, Hsieh CL, HCT A, et al. Effects of acupuncture on post-cesarean section pain. Chin Med J. 2009;122:1743–8.
16. Ishimaru K, Shinohara S, Kitade T, Morioka T, Kudou D, Umeki N. Effect on pain threshold of low frequency electrical acupuncture and silver spike point electrical stimulation. Meiji Shinkyu Igaku. 1990;6:61–7.
17. Ishimaru K, Shinohara S, Iwa M, Kawakita K, Higuchi J, Watanabe S. Effects of electrical acupuncture on deep pain threshold in human subjects. Meiji Shinkyu Igaku. 1991;8:27–33.
18. Ishimaru K, Kawakita K, Sakita M. Analgesic effects induced by TENS and electroacupuncture with different types of stimulating electrodes on deep tissues in human subjects. Pain. 1995;63:181–7.
19. Kitade T, Minamikawa M, Hyodo M, Nakao K, Oki S, Imura H. β-Endorphin and ACTH concentrations in plasma and cerebrospinal fluid during acupuncture analgesia in human subjects. Orient Med Pain Clinic. 1980;10:116–20.
20. Ishimaru K, Sekido R, Sakita M. Association between endogenous analgesia and meridians in LI4 (Hegu, Gokoku) point electro-acupuncture. J Jap Soc Acupunct Moxibust. 2003;53:184–9.
21. Ishimaru K. Effects of acupuncture analgesia on postoperative pain after abdominal surgery and the relationship of endogenous analgesic substances. Meiji Shinkyu Igaku. 2000;26:11–22.
22. Vickers AJ, Cronin AM, Maschino AC, Lewith G, MacPherson H, Foster NE. Acupuncture for chronic pain: individual patient data meta-analysis. Arch Intern Med. 2012;172:1444–53.
23. De Freitas ATG, Lemonica L, De Faveri J, Pereira S, Henao MDB. Preemptive analgesia with acupuncture monitored by c-Fos expression in rats. J Acupunct Meridian Stud. 2016;9(1):16–21.
24. Iacobone M, Citton M, Zanella S, Scarpa M, Pagura G, Tropea S, et al. The effects of acupuncture after thyroid surgery: a randomized controlled trial. Surgery. 2014;156:1605–13.
25. Chen CC, Yang CC, Hu CC, Shih HN, Chang YH, Hsieh PH. Acupuncture for pain relief after total knee arthroplasty: a randomized controlled trial. Reg Anesth Pain Med. 2015;40:31–6.
26. Dingemann J, Plewig B, Baumann I, Plinkert PK, Sertel S. Acupuncture in post-tonsillectomy pain. Hno. 2017;65:73–9.
27. Usichenko T, Dinse M, Hermsen M, Witstruck T, Pavlovic D, Lehmann C. Auricular acupuncture for pain relief after total hip arthroplasty–a randomized controlled study. Pain. 2005;114:320–7.
28. Chang L, Hsu CH, Jong GP, Ho S, Tsay SL, Lin KC. Auricular acupressure for managing postoperative pain and knee motion in patients with total knee replacement:a randomized sham control study. Evid Based Complement Alternat Med. 2012;2012:1–7.

10

Using four different clinical tools as predictors for pain after total hip arthroplasty

Anja Geisler[1,2*], Josephine Zachodnik[1], Jens Laigaard[1], Laura S. Kruuse[1], Charlotte V. Sørensen[3], Magnus Sandberg[2], Eva I. Persson[2] and Ole Mathiesen[1,4]

Abstract

Background: Treatment of postoperative pain remains a significant clinical problem, and prediction of patients with a risk of higher postoperative pain levels is an important focus. We aimed to identify patients undergoing total hip arthroplasty (THA) with risk of higher pain levels at 24 h postoperatively by using four simple and easily available clinical tools.

Methods: This prospective observational cohort study included 102 patients having THA at Zealand University Hospital in Denmark. The following predictive tools were investigated for identifying patients with higher postoperative pain levels at 24 h postoperatively, both at rest and during mobilization: preoperative pain by peripheral venous cannulation (PVC) (dichotomized according to numerical rating scale pain ≤ 2/> 2 (PVC-Low/PVC-High) (primary outcome); the post anesthesia care unit (PACU) nurses' expectations of patients pain levels; patients early pain levels at the PACU; and patients own forecast of postoperative pain levels. The Mann-Whitney U test was used to analyze comparisons between prediction groups. For the primary outcome we considered a p-value < 0.01 as statistically significant and for other outcomes a p-value of 0.05.

Results: We found no significant differences between the PVC groups for pain during mobilization at 24-h postoperatively: PVC-Low: 6 (4–8) (median, (IQR)) versus PVC-High: 7 (5–8) (median, (IQR)), $p = 0.10$; and for pain at rest: PVC-Low 2 (0–3) (median, (IQR)) versus PVC-High 3 (2–5) (median, (IQR)), $p = 0.12$. Other comparisons performed between predictive groups did not differ significantly.

Conclusions: In this prospective cohort study of 102 THA patients, we did not find that preoperative pain by PVC, when using a cut-off point of NRS ≤ 2, were able to predict postoperative pain at 24 h postoperatively. Neither did PACU nurses' prediction of pain, patients forecast of pain, nor did maximum pain levels at the PACU.

Keywords: Postoperative pain, Prediction, Total hip arthroplasty

Background

Despite considerable efforts in optimizing postoperative pain, this clinically important symptom remains a major challenge [1]. It is therefore important to identify individuals at risk of developing high postoperative pain levels, but clinically useful predictive tools are virtually absent [2].

A newer study indicated that pain intensity by preoperative peripheral venous cannulation (PVC), using a grouping according to numerical rating scale pain (NRS) ≤ 2 and > 2, was associated with pain levels at the post anesthesia care unit (PACU) [3]. This study, however, did not investigate the prediction of pain later at the surgical ward, which is particularly relevant, since sufficient pain treatment is a cornerstone for optimal rehabilitation [4].

* Correspondence: agei@regionsjaelland.dk
[1]Department of Anesthesiology, Zealand University Hospital, Lykkebækvej 1, 4600 Koege, Denmark
[2]Department of Health Sciences, Faculty of Medicine, Lund University, Lund, Sweden

Nurse's prediction of patient outcomes has been investigated in different settings but with varying results [5, 6]. Therefore, it is relevant to investigate if experienced nurses at the PACU can predict which patients will suffer from higher levels of pain after PACU discharge.

As patients may be predisposed to certain levels of postoperative pain due to e.g. sex, preoperative pain, genetic variations [7], anxiety, or type of surgery [8, 9], it could be relevant to investigate if patient's pain levels at the PACU, using moderate to severe pain (NRS > 3) as an indicator, can predict pain levels after PACU discharge.

A recent study reported that 47% of patients correctly predicted their pain levels 2 weeks after hand surgery, but they did not investigate the prediction of acute postoperative pain [10]. A subsequent commentary pointed out, that further prospective studies are needed regarding patient's ability to forecast their disability and pain [11].

Total hip arthroplasty (THA) is a surgical procedure of which patients' have reported moderate to severe postoperative pain [12]. Therefore, this population is relevant for investigating which patients are high pain responders including a particular focus on pain during recovery at the surgical ward. With this study, we hypothesized that different clinical parameters, nursing staff impressions and patients forecast could be used to predict postoperative pain. This study aimed to investigate if preoperative pain by PVC could be used to identify groups of THA patients with higher levels of pain during mobilization at 24 h postoperatively (primary outcome). Additionally, that PACU nurses' capability of predicting patients with higher pain levels at the ward, pain levels at the PACU, and patients' forecast preoperatively, could be used to identify patients with higher postoperative pain levels at 24 h after THA (secondary outcomes).

Methods

This prospective observational cohort study was approved by the Danish Data Protection Agency (REG-158-2017) and first posted at ClinicalTrials.gov (NCT03439566) on 20th February 2018. The Research Ethics Committee of the Capital Region was consulted, but approval was not needed according to Danish law (Reg. nr. J.nr. 17–000048). Consecutive data was collected at Zealand University Hospital, Koege (ZUHK) in the period from January 2018 to February 2019. The head nurse and chief physician from the orthopaedic department at ZUHK accepted departmental participation in the study, including the collection of patient data. The manuscript follows the STrengthening the Reporting of Observational Studies in Epidemiology (STROBE) statement guidelines [13]. The participants were enrolled after giving verbal and written informed consent when attending the pre-scheduled surgical and anesthetic information meeting about 2 weeks before to surgery.

Participants

The participants were enrolled after giving verbal and written informed consent when attending the pre-scheduled surgical and anesthetic information meeting about 2 weeks before to surgery.

Inclusion criteria were: age ≥ 18 years old, speaking Danish and/or English, and scheduled for primary elective THA in spinal anesthesia. Exclusion criteria were: not able to-cooperate according to investigators judgement, alcohol or drug abuse, or if correct placement of the PVC was impossible. No investigational intervention was initiated during the study. The department followed the usual local protocols for postoperative pain treatment and standard of care. Two surgical specialists performed all the THA procedures. The lateral surgical approach was used for all patients.

Outcomes

Primary outcome was: numeric rating scale (NRS) pain (0–10) during mobilization at 24 h postoperatively.

Secondary outcomes were: NRS-pain at rest at 24 h postoperatively, and 24 h intravenous morphine equivalent consumption, mg.

A correctly placed PVC was defined as a cannula placed in a vein on the dorsum part of the dominant hand. The NRS score was performed during the first attempt otherwise the patients were excluded. The allowed cannula sizes were 20G or 22G.

Anesthesia and analgesic treatment

All patients received spinal anesthesia (10–15 mg bupivacaine). The standard analgesic treatment that was provided for patients at the hospital was: perioperative methylprednisolone IV 125 mg (after induction of anesthesia). At the POTA patients were supplied with opioids as needed, according to usual practice. At the ward, postoperatively, paracetamol 1000 mg OR every 6 h, and slow-release oxycodone 10 mg OR administrated twice a day, supplemented with oxycodone IV as needed.

Psychological profile

Patients' psychological profile and relation to pain were tested using the validated self-administered questionnaire, Pain Catastrophizing Scale (PCS). The scale includes 13 items and assesses the extent of the patient's catastrophizing thoughts and emotions associated with pain. Such thoughts or feelings are rated from zero (not at all) to five (all the time). The PCS has a maximum score of 52. A clinically relevant cut off for being a pain catastrophizer was considered as numbers above 30 [14].

Supplemental data regarding PACU nurses'prediction

When PACU nurses were asked to state if they predicted a patient to be a high pain responder or not, they were also asked to tick a box with the following statements underpinning their choice: patients' appearance, patients' pain intensity, my own intuition, patients' need of opioids, the patient's expression of concern and anxiety, or optional additional information – described in their own words.

Collection of data

For evaluation of pain, the NRS-scale was used, 0 to 10 (0 = no pain and 10 = worst imaginable pain). All patients were instructed preoperatively in how to use the NRS tool [15]. The patients stated their own pain. All data were entered directly into the patient Case Report Form (CRF). All opioids were converted to IV morphine equivalents (eqv) (Additional file 1).

At inclusion, patients completed the PCS questionnaire and provided information about years of education after high school, civil status, employment, as well as their forecast of pain levels. The anesthesia nurse at the operation theater, who performed the peripheral cannulation, asked patients' about the levels of NRS pain after placement of the PVC. The nurses on the PACU collected data on NRS pain after the spinal anesthesia had ceased, as well as performed a prediction of which patients they believed would experience moderate or severe pain at 24 h during mobilization. The primary investigator, a project nurse or research assistants performed the data collection at the ward at 24 h +/– 2 h postoperatively for pain and opioid consumption.

The following information was registered from the electronic patient records. Preoperative data: height, weight, sex, American Society of Anesthesiologists physical score (ASA), usual preoperative analgesic consumption and premedication. Perioperative data: analgesic and antiemetic treatment, duration of surgery. Postoperative data: analgesics used from 0 h to 24 h postoperatively, and length of stay (LOS). All data were registered in the CRF, imported to the statistical package IBM SPSS version 25, and the final data set was double-checked for errors.

The patients also filled out a diary from postoperative day one to five at home regarding pain, side effects, use of analgesics and quality of sleep. These data will be reported elsewhere.

Sample size and statistics

A sample size estimation was performed for NRS pain during mobilization based on data from a prior study that investigated a similar patient population [12]. To reduce the risk of spurious significant findings, we choose an alfa = 0.01 and a power of 0.9. Furthermore, we used a standard deviation (SD) of 2.5. We found 93 patients were needed to detect a minimal clinically important difference (MCID) of NRS-pain at 1.0. To compensate for the uncertainty of SD we aimed to include 100 consecutive patients undergoing THA.

For comparisons we defined groups based on the following:

1) Pain by preoperative PVC dichotomized to NRS ≤ 2 (PVC-Low) or NRS > 2 (PVC-High)
2) PACU nurses' prediction of patients being a high pain responder or not (Nurse-Low, or Nurse-High)
3) Maximum NRS pain at the PACU dichotomized to NRS ≤ 3 / > 3 (when spinal anesthesia has ceased, Bromage score 0—1) (PACU-NRS ≤ 3, or PACU-NRS > 3)
4) Patients reporting of being a high pain responder or not (Forecast-Low, or Forecast-High)

Normal distribution was tested visually in histograms and Q-Q plots and quantitatively with Kolmogorov-Smirnov test. Data are presented with either numbers or percentages, median (IQR), mean (SD), and 95% CI, where relevant. Mann-Whitney U test (for non-parametric data) was used to analyze all comparisons between groups: PVC-High versus PVC-Low, Nurse-Low versus Nurse-High, Forecast-Low versus Forecast-High, and PACU-NRS ≤3 versus PACU-NRS > 3. For the primary outcome we considered a p-value < 0.01, and for other outcomes, a p-value < 0.05, as statistically significant. Bonferroni correction was used to counteract for mass-significance where relevant.

We performed an exploratory multiple linear regression, both adjusted an unadjusted analyses, using a dependent variable, NRS pain at 24 h during rest or mobilization, and adjusting for the following pre-defined covariates: sex, age, patients pain threshold, marital status, education, daily analgesic consumption, PCS, and employment status. To test for the possibility of multicollinearity, Pearson r for parametric data and Spearman rho for non-parametric data was used.

For evaluating and comparing predictive models we calculated Receiver Operating Characteristic curves (ROC). The true positive rate in the model (sensitivity) was plotted against the false positive rate (1 – specificity) for a given cut-off value of the predictive variable, thus aiming to determine the optimal cut-off value. Areas in the interval 0.9–1 represented excellent prediction, 0.8–0.9 good prediction, 0.7–0.8 fair prediction and 0.6–0.7 poor prediction [16, 17]. Statistical analyzes were expressed using IBM SPSS software version 25 for Windows (SPSS Inc. Chicago, IL).

Results

One hundred and fifty patients scheduled for THA were assessed for eligibility. After exclusions, 102 patients were included in the study for evaluation of the primary outcome. For further information see Fig. 1.

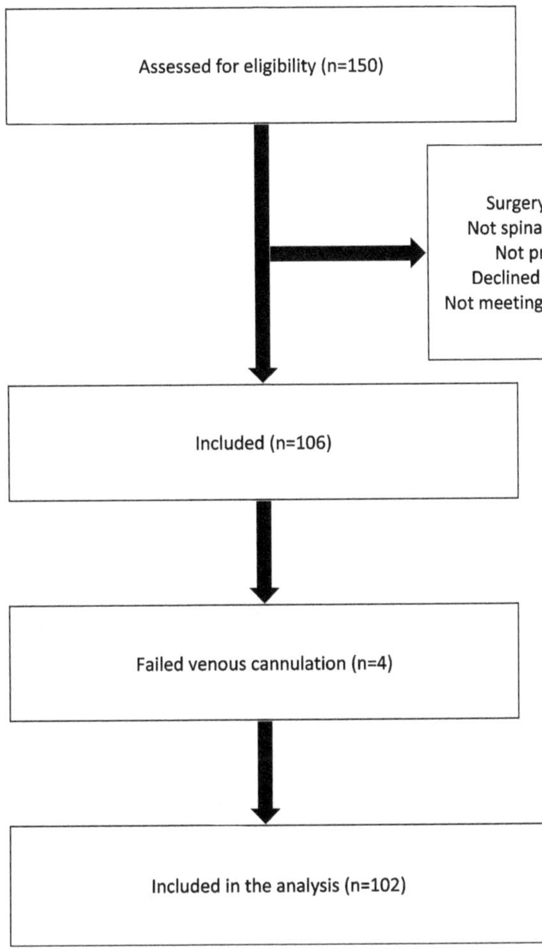

Fig. 1 Patient flow

The study included 35 males and 67 females, mean age was 69 (19) (mean, (SD)) years, the surgery lasted in 53 (46–63) (median, (IQR)) min, and median LOS was 1 (1, 2) day. For further information, see Table 1.

PVC related pain

For the primary outcome, NRS pain during mobilization at 24 h, we found no significant difference between groups PVC-Low 6 (4–8) (median (IQR)) and PVC-High 7 (5–8) (median (IQR)) ($P = 0.10$) (Table 2). For NRS pain at 24 h at rest, we found no significant difference between groups PVC-Low 2 (0–3) (median (IQR) and PVC-High 3 (2–5) (median (IQR), $p = 0.12$. For total 24 h IV morphine eqv. Consumption, we found no significant difference between groups PVC-Low 20 (15–24) (median (IQR)) mg and Group PVC-High 23 (15–28) (median (IQR) mg (median (IQR), $p = 0.20$ (Table 2).

Explorative regression analyses were performed regarding the association between PVC-Low and PVC-High, and postoperative 24 h NRS pain during rest and mobilization, in both unadjusted and adjusted analyses. For 24 h NRS pain during mobilization, the unadjusted analyses demonstrated no significant difference in standardized Beta 0.88 (– 0.18; 1.94) NRS (95% CI) ($p = 0.10$) between groups defined by PVC pain. When adjusted for sex, age, patient's forecast of own pain, marital status, education, daily analgesic consumption, PCS, and employment status, we found a significant difference in standardized Beta NRS (95% CI) 0.24 (0.14; 2.43) ($p = 0.03$) between the groups defined by pain during PVC (Table 3). For NRS pain at rest at 24 h the unadjusted Beta showed a significant difference in NRS (95% CI), 1.13 (0.14; 2.12) (p = 0.03) between groups defined by PVC pain. In the adjusted analyses, however, this difference became non-significant with a standardized Beta NRS (95% CI) 0.18 (– 0.22; 2.06) ($p = 0.11$) (Table 3). We did not find any multicollinearity of parameters in the adjusted analyses.

PACU nurse prediction

We found no significant differences between groups Nurse-Low and Nurse-High for NRS pain during mobilization at 24 h postoperatively Nurse-Low: 5 (4–8)

Table 1 Demographics and baseline data

	Total population n = 102	Missing (n)	PVC-Low (n = 67)	Missing (n)	PVC-High (n = 35)	Missing (n)	PVC-Low vs High p-value
Sex m/f, (n)	35/67	0	26/41	0	9/26	0	0.18
Age, yr, mean (SD)	69 (19)	0	71 (8)	0	66 (10)	0	0.02
Height, cm, mean (SD)	169 (8)	15	168 (8)	11	169 (8)	4	0.58
Weight, kg, median (IQR)	75 (65–85)	15	75 (64–83)	11	75 (66–98)	4	0.41
ASA 1/2/3 (n)	21/62/16	3	15/40/10	2	6/22/6	1	0.57
Education after high school (no/ yes), (n)	24/71	7	16/46	5	8/25	2	0.98
Civil status (married/[a]living alone) (n)	73/ 29	0	48/19	0	25/10	0	0.06
Employed (no/yes), (n)	72/30	0	51/16	0	21/14	0	0.72
Patients forecast (high pain responder/ normal responder) (n)	21/79	2	16/49	2	5/30	0	0.70
Daily use of any analgesics (no/yes), (n)	47/52	3	28/37	2	19/15	1	0.67
PCS (0–52), median (IQR)	14 (7–21)	0	13 (6–18)	0	17 (12–28)	0	0.91
PCS ≤30 / > 30 (n)	87/15	0	58/9	0	29/6	0	
Surgery time (min), median (IQR)	53 (46–63)	0	53 (47–63)	0	52 (44–64)	0	0.91
Length of stay (days), median (IQR)	1 (1–2)	0	1 (1–2)	0	2 (1–2)	0	0.01

PVC Peripheral venous cannulation, *ASA* American Society of Anesthesiologist classification, *PCS* Pain Catastrophizing Scale, [a]Living alone: Divorced, single, widowed, or not in a relationship

and Nurse-high: 6 (4–7) (median (IQR)), $p = 0.78$. No significant differences between groups were found for pain at rest at 24 h postoperatively, and for 24 h morphine consumption. See Table 2 for further details.

Pain at the PACU

For groups based on NRS pain ≤ 3 and NRS pain > 3 at the PACU, we found no significant differences between groups, for pain during mobilization at 24 h postoperatively, PACU-NRS ≤ 3: 5 (4–8) and PACU-NRS > 3: 7 (6–8) (median (IQR)), $p = 0.74$. No significant differences between groups were found for pain at rest. For 24 h morphine consumption, we found a significant difference between group PACU-NRS ≤ 3: 20 (15–25) mg and PACU-NRS > 3: 26 (18–33) mg (median (IQR)), $p = 0.03$, Bonferroni adj. See Table 2 for details.

Patients forecast of pain

We found no significant differences between groups Forecast-Low and Forecast-High regarding NRS pain during mobilization at 24 h postoperatively; Forecast-Low: 6 (4–8) and Forecast-High 6 (4–8) (median (IQR)), $p = 0.79$. No significant differences between groups for NRS pain 24 h during rest and opioid consumption was detected. For further information see Table 2.

Table 2 All patients and comparisons between predictive groups

	All patients (n = 102)	PVC-Low (n = 67)	PVC-High (n = 35)	p-value	Nurse-Low (n = 49)	Nurse-High (n = 32)	p-value	PACU-NRS ≤ 3 (n = 90)	PACU-NRS > 3 (n = 12)	p-value	Forecast-Low (n = 79)	Forecast-High (n = 21)	p-value
Pain (mobilization) 24 h postop.	6 (4–8)	6 (4–8)	7 (5–8)	0.10	5 (4–8)	6 (4–7)	0.78	5 (4–8)	7 (6–8)	0.74	6 (4–8)	6 (4–8)	0.79
Pain (at rest) 24 h postop.	2 (0–4)	2 (0–3)	3 (2–5)	[a]0.12	2 (0–4)	2 (0–4)	0.65	2 (0–4)	3 (2–5)	0.22	2 (1–4)	2 (0–3)	0.19
Morphine consumption (eqv.), IV, mg, (0-24 h)	20 (15–25)	20 (15–24)	23 (15–28)	0.20	19 (15–23)	22 (15–29)	0.16	20 (15–25)	26 (18–33)	[a]0.12	20 (15–28)	20 (15–23)	0.35

[a]Bonferroni correction. *PVC* Peripheral Venous Cannulation. *PACU* Post Anesthesia Care Unit. *NRS* Numerical Rating Scale. Data are median and interquartile range (IQR), pain are numerical rang scale (NRS). Nurse-Low means patients that the PACU nurse evaluates to be an ordinary pain responder and Nurse-High was evaluated to be a high pain responder. Forecast-Low means ordinary pain responder and Forecast-High means high pain responder, according to evaluation by patients themselves before surgery

Table 3 Multiple linear regression model for NRS pain by PVC. Adjusted and unadjusted

Dependent variable	Independent variable	Beta Estimate NRS (95% CI)	*P*-value	R^2
Pain at 24 h (mobilization) Unadjusted	NRS by PVC ≤/> 2	0.88 (− 0.18;1.94)	0.10	0.27
Pain at 24 h (mobilization) Adjusted	NRS by PVC ≤/> 2	0.24[a](0.14;2.43)	0.03	0.20
Pain at 24 h (at rest) Unadjusted	NRS by PVC ≤/> 2	1.13 (0.14;2.12)	0.03	0.05
Pain at 24 h (at rest) Adjusted	NRS by PVC ≤/> 2	0.18[a](−0.22;2.06)	0.11	0.13

Adjusted for; sex, age, patients pain threshold, marital status, education, daily analgesic consumption, PCS and employment
NRS Numerical Rating Scale. *PVC* Peripheral Venous Cannulation. *CI* Confidence Interval [a]Standardized Beta value

ROC curve analyses

We performed ROC curves for groups PVC-Low and PVC-High, and its capability of predicting pain during rest and mobilization 24 h, as well as 24 h opioid consumption. Since all ROC had AUC values less than 0.60, we did not consider these to be reliable predictors (Additional file 2).

Discussion

With this prospective observational cohort study of 102 patients undergoing THA, we investigated four simple and easily available clinical tools to predict patients with higher levels of postoperative pain 24 h after surgery. We did, however, not find any significant difference for postoperative pain during mobilization, at rest, between groups of patients defined by pain by PVC, PACU nurses' prediction, pain levels at the PACU, and patients forecast of pain.

Pain from preoperative peripheral venous cannulation was previously investigated (3) for prediction of postoperative pain in a study with 180 patients undergoing laparoscopic cholecystectomy. Here, Persson and colleagues (3) reported that patients with NRS pain > 2 by PVC reported higher pain scores at rest and received more opioids within the first 90 min at the PACU, compared to those with NRS ≤ 2. Furthermore, in a newer and larger study, Persson and co-workers [18] repeated these findings, but this time in a population of 600 patients undergoing different surgical procedures, receiving different types of anesthesia, and using different places for venous cannulation. Still, they reported that NRS pain > 2 during PVC was associated with moderate to severe postoperative pain at rest at the PACU. We could not confirm these findings, as we found no significant differences for pain at rest at the PACU between PVC-Low and PVC-High. Our study differed from those of Persson and colleagues' in several ways, including different patient populations, differences in age, and the type of anesthesia. Also, we measured pain both at rest and during mobilization, and not only at the PACU but also 24 h postoperatively. We did not find any association between PACU nurses' prediction and patients' pain levels after 24 h, neither at rest nor during mobilization. Interestingly, in the follow-up on background for their choice, we found that the PACU nurses stated that the forecasts of patients being low or a high pain responder, to be primarily based upon the appearance of the patient and on their intuition. These findings were supported by other studies demonstrating that when nurses assess if patients are in pain or not, they primarily base their decision on patients' appearances and their non-verbal behavior [19, 20]. However, this failed to show applicability in this study.

In a recent study in 563 women having breast cancer surgery, Sipilä and colleagues [21] found that patient's expectations of severe postoperative pain were associated with higher clinical pain intensity and increased initial oxycodone use at the PACU. In contrast, in another and smaller prospective study [10] investigating patients' ability to forecast their disability and pain two weeks after hand surgery, only weak correlations between forecasted and realized pain was discovered [10]. In contrast, we did not find any differences in patients pain scores nor opioid usage for the first 24 h postoperatively, based on patients' forecast on being a high pain responder or not. It is possible that differences in type of surgeries and patient populations between these and the present study influences the differences in outcomes, and further studies are needed to elaborate on this clinically relevant topic.

Strengths and limitations

In this prospective study it was a strength that all patients had spinal anesthesia and underwent the same surgical procedure, which was performed by the same two orthopaedic surgeons, and with all patients receiving a standardized perioperative pain treatment. This minimizes variations and bias. Furthermore, PVC was performed by experienced anesthesia nurses, and all were placed in the patients' dominant hand. Also, data at the ward were collected by a limited group of four investigators, reducing observer bias.

We used a cut-off point of NRS 2, for the division of groups, based on the study by Persson et al. [3]. The ROC curve analyses indicated that a cut-off point of NRS 2.5 could have been more appropriate for dividing patients into groups (Additional file 2). However, the AUC-value of the ROC was low and of limited reliability. Missing data was a limitation, especially the relatively large proportion of missing data on PACU nurses' prediction could have influenced our results. Preoperative pain may serve as a predictor for postoperative pain levels [8]. It could therefore be considered as a limitation, that we did not register patients' preoperative pain, but instead, as a proxy here for, registered preoperative analgesic consumption. Another limitation is the sample size calculation, as such calculations typically are based on an equal number of patients in the investigated groups. This was unfortunately not the case, as number of patients differed between the four investigated groups of predictors. As this was a clinical prospective cohort, and not a randomized trial, it can be argued that sample sizes are of limited value, especially when we did not have influence on the distribution of number of patients in the compared groups. Our study can, however, serve as base for sample size calculations of future studies, preferably including larger numbers of participants.

In perspective, the prediction of postoperative pain levels continues to be an important focus for future research, as individualized pain treatment has the potential to improve patient courses. Such research may well be based on the collection of big data including new types of analyses hereof, biomarkers, neuroimaging, physiological and psychological variables, and clinical data as well. It is possible, that results of studies using simple clinical tools, in the future, might be included in such big data in the guidance of pain treatment. Until then, the focus must be on effective pain treatment, regular assessment of pain with frequently monitoring of patients and their needs.

Conclusions

In this prospective cohort study of 102 THA patients, we did not find that preoperative pain by PVC, when using a cut-off point of NRS ≤ 2, were able to predict postoperative pain at 24 h after THA postoperatively. Neither did PACU nurses' prediction of pain, patients forecast of pain, nor did maximum pain levels at the PACU.

Abbreviations

ASA: American Society of Anesthesiologists physical score; CRF: Case Report Form; Eqv: Equivalents; IQR: Inter Quartile Range; IV: Intravenous; LOS: Length of stay; NRS: Numeric Rating Scale; PACU: Post Anesthesia Care Unit; PCS: Pain Catastrophizing Scale; PVC: Peripheral Venous Cannulation; RCT: Randomized controlled trial; THA: Total Hip Arthroplasty; VAS: Visual Analogue Scale; VRS: Verbal Rating Scale; ZUHK: Zealand University Hospital, Koege

Acknowledgements

Thank you to the staff at the department of orthopaedics at Zealand University Hospital, Køge.

Authors' contributions

The study was designed by: AG, EP, OM. Study conduct: AG, JZ, JL, LK, CVS. Data analysis: AG, MS, OM. Critical revision and final approval of the manuscript: All authors.

Author details

[1]Department of Anesthesiology, Zealand University Hospital, Lykkebækvej 1, 4600 Koege, Denmark. [2]Department of Health Sciences, Faculty of Medicine, Lund University, Lund, Sweden. [3]Department of Orthopaedics, Zealand University Hospital, Koege, Denmark. [4]Department of Clinical Medicine, Faculty of Health Sciences, Copenhagen University, Copenhagen, Denmark.

References

1. Gerbershagen HJ, Aduckathil S, van Wijck AJM, Peelen LM, Kalkman CJ, Meissner W. Pain intensity on the first day after surgery: a prospective cohort study comparing 179 surgical procedures. Anesthesiology. 2013;118(4):934–44.
2. Werner MU, Mjöbo HN, Nielsen PR, Rudin A. Prediction of postoperative pain: a systematic review of predictive experimental pain studies. Anesthesiology. 2010;112(6):1494–502.
3. Persson AK, Pettersson FD, Dyrehag L-E, Åkeson J. Prediction of postoperative pain from assessment of pain induced by venous cannulation and propofol infusion. Acta Anaesthesiol Scand. 2016;60(2):166–76.
4. Kehlet H, Dahl JB. Anaesthesia, surgery, and challenges in postoperative recovery. Lancet. 2003;362(9399):1921–8.
5. Lipson Amy R, Miano Sarah J, Daly Barbara J, Douglas SL. The Accuracy of Nurses' Predictions for Clinical Outcomes in the Chronically Critically IllNo Title. Res Rev J Nurs Heal Sci. 2017;3:35–8.
6. Zachariasse JM, Van Der Lee D, Seiger N, De Vos-Kerkhof E, Oostenbrink R, Moll HA. The role of nurses' clinical impression in the first assessment of children at the emergency department. Arch Dis Child. 2017;102(11):1052–6.
7. Horjales-Araujo E, Dahl JB. Is the experience of thermal pain genetics dependent? Biomed Res Int. 2015;2015:349584.
8. Yun H, Ip V, Abrishami A, Peng PWH, Wong J, Chung F, et al. Predictors of postoperative pain and analgesic consumption a qualitative systematic review. Anesthesiology. 2009;111:657–77.
9. Aubrun F, Salvi N, Coriat P, Riou B. Sex- and age-related differences in morphine requirements for postoperative pain relief. Anesthesiology. 2005;103(1):156–60 Available from: http://www.ncbi.nlm.nih.gov/pubmed/15983468.
10. Alokozai A, Eppler SL, Lu LY, Sheikholeslami N, Kamal RN. Can patients forecast their postoperative disability and pain? Clin Orthop Relat Res. 2019;477(3):635–43.
11. Vranceanu A-M. CORR insights®. Clin Orthop Relat Res. 2019;477(4):905–7.
12. Geisler A, Dahl JB, Thybo KH, Pedersen TH, Jørgensen ML, Hansen D, et al. Pain management after total hip arthroplasty at five different Danish hospitals: A prospective, observational cohort study of 501 patients. Acta Anaesthesiol Scand. 2019; Available from: https://onlinelibrary.wiley.com/doi/abs/10.1111/aas.13349.
13. von Elm E, Altman DG, Egger M, Pocock SJ, Gøtzsche PC, Vandenbroucke JP, et al. The Strengthening the reporting of observational studies in epidemiology (STROBE) statement: guidelines for reporting observational studies. Int J Surg. 2014;12(12):1495–9.
14. Sullivan M, Bishop S, Pivik J. The pain catastrophizing scale: user manual. Psychol Assess. 1995;7(4):524 32 Available from: http://sullivan-painresearch.

mcgill.ca/pdf/pcs/PCSManual_English.pdf%5Cn http://psycnet.apa.org/journals/pas/7/4/524/.
15. Hjermstad MJ, Fayers PM, Haugen DF, Caraceni A, Hanks GW, Loge JH, et al. Studies comparing numerical rating scales, verbal rating scales, and visual analogue scales for assessment of pain intensity in adults: a systematic literature review. J Pain Symptom Manage. 2011;41(6):1073–93. Available from. https://doi.org/10.1016/j.jpainsymman.2010.08.016.
16. Landis JR, Koch GG. Landis_Jr__Koch_Gg_1977_Kappa_and_Observer_Agreement. Biometrics. 1977;33(1):159–74.
17. Pepe MS, Janes H, Longton G, Leisenring W, Newcomb P. Limitations of the odds ratio in gauging the performance of a diagnostic, prognostic, or screening marker. Am J Epidemiol. 2004;159(9):882–90 Available from: http://www.ncbi.nlm.nih.gov/pubmed/15105181.
18. Persson AKM, Åkeson J. Prediction of acute postoperative pain from assessment of pain associated with venous Cannulation. Pain Pract. 2019;19(2):158–67.
19. Drayer RA, Henderson J, Reidenberg M. Barriers to better pain control in hospitalized patients. J Pain Symptom Manag. 1999;17(6):434–40.
20. Schafheutle EI, Cantrill JA, Noyce PR. Why is pain management suboptimal on surgical wards? J Adv Nurs. 2001;33(6):728–37.
21. Sipilä RM, Haasio L, Meretoja TJ, Ripatti S, Estlander AM, Kalso EA. Does expecting more pain make it more intense? Factors associated with the first week pain trajectories after breast cancer surgery. Pain. 2017;158(5):922–30.

The effect of transversus abdominis plane block on the chronic pain after colorectal surgery

Zi-Ye Pan, Zhong-Hua Hu, Fan Zhang, Wen-Xiu Xie, Yong-Zhong Tang* and Qin Liao*

Abstract

Background: Chronic postsurgical pain (CPSP) is common and would reduce the quality of life of patients. Transversus abdominal plane (TAP) block has been widely used in lower abdominal surgery and many researches demonstrated that it could improve acute postsurgical pain. We aim to determine whether TAP block could improve chronic postoperative pain at 3 months and 6 months after colorectal surgery.

Methods: A total of 307 patients received selective colorectal surgery under general anesthesia between January, 2015 and January, 2019 in a single university hospital were included: 128 patients received TAP block combined with patient-controlled intravenous analgesia (PCIA) for postsurgical analgesia (group TP) and 179 only administrated with PCIA (group P). Main outcome was the NRS score of pain at 3 months after colorectal surgery. The data was analyzed by two-way repeated measures anova and the chi-square test.

Results: The NRS score at rest and during movement was decreased significantly at 24 h after surgery (rest NRS 1.07 ± 1.34 vs 1.65 ± 1.67, movement NRS 3.00 ± 1.45 vs 3.65 ± 1.89; all $P = 0.003$) in group TP than those of group P. There was no significant difference of NRS score at 48 h after surgery ($P > 0.05$). At 3 months after surgery, the NRS score during movement was also lower in group TP than that in group P (0.59 ± 1.23 vs 0.92 ± 1.65, $P = 0.045$). There was no significant difference of NRS score at 6 months after surgery ($P > 0.05$).
The prevalence of CPSP was 19.5% (25/128) in group TP and 20.7% (37/179) in group P at 3 months after surgery. 13.2% (17/128) of patients suffered from CPSP in group TP and 13.9% (25/179) in group P at 6 months after surgery. Both at 3 months and 6 months after surgery, there was no statistical difference of the prevalence of CPSP between the two groups (all $P > 0.05$) .

Conclusions: TAP block reduced NRS during movement at 3 months after surgery but did not reduce the incidence of CPSP at 3 months and 6 months after selective colorectal surgery.

Keywords: Chronic postsurgical pain, Colorectal surgery, Transversus abdominal plane block, Analgesia

Background

Chronic postsurgical pain (CPSP) is defined by the International Association for the Study of Pain (IASP) as pain that develops after a surgical procedure and persists for at least 3 months after surgery, where all other causes of pain (e.g. infection, recurring malignancy) or pre-existing pain problems are excluded [1, 2]. Few studies reported the prevalence of CPSP after colorectal surgery [3, 4]. A prospective study showed that 19% of patients underwent colorectal surgery reported CPSP at 6 months, 63% of which taking medication for their pain, 53% of which were using opioids to manage their pain [3]. In another retrospective study, 17% of patients reported CPSP after

* Correspondence: tangyongzhong@csu.edu.cn; xy3yyliaoqin@sina.com
Department of Anesthesiology, The Third Xiangya Hospital of Central South University, Changsha 410013, Hunan, China

laparoscopic colorectal surgery, 37% of which suffering from severe pain (pain score ≥ 7) [4]. CPSP has a negative impact on the quality of life, such as mood, sleep, walking ability, and normal work, so it is important to find out methods to reduce CPSP.

It was found that acute postoperative pain was an important risk factor of CPSP, [4–6] and many researches demonstrated that CPSP could be partly improved by optimizing perioperative pain management, including intravenous analgesia, epidural analgesia, paravertebral blocks and regional analgesia [7–9]. Transversus abdominis plane (TAP) block is an effective regional analgesia technique to reduce perioperative pain intensity, [10] especially combined with ultrasound-guided technique. TAP block is the injection of local anesthetics to neurofascial plane between internal oblique and transversus abdominis muscles aiming at blocking the neural afferents from the anterolateral abdominal wall (T7-L1) [11]. TAP block has been widely used in many abdominal operation, with a satisfactory duration of analgesic action for up to 24 h after surgery [10, 12–14]. Many studies confirmed that TAP block can improve acute postoperative pain, [15, 16] but whether TAP block can reduce chronic pain after colorectal surgery has been reported scarcely.

The main aim of our study was to evaluate whether TAP block could improve CPSP after colorectal surgery. We compared the NRS score of different time point for patients who had TAP block and PCIA with those patients without TAP block.

Methods

Our research was approved by the Ethics Committee of Third Xiangya Hospital, Central South University (No: 2019-S473). We reviewed the medical records of patients undertaking colorectal surgery at the third Xiangya hospital of Central South University from January, 2015 to January 2019. Eligibility criteria included patients who were over 18 years old, American Society of Anesthesiologists (ASA) status I-III, receiving selective colorectal surgery under general anesthesia and PCIA for postsurgical analgesia. Exclusion criteria were patients unable to communicate, wound infection after surgery, receiving a second operation.

Study protocol

On entering the surgery room, patients' vital signs were monitored by electrocardiogram, invasive arterial blood pressure, pulse oximetry and bispectral index. General anesthesia was induced with fentanyl (4–6 μg/kg) or sufentanil (0.4–0.6 μg/kg), propofol (1.5–2 mg/kg), midazolam (2–3 mg), rocuronium (1 mg/kg) or cisatracurium besylate (0.15–0.2 mg/kg). Anesthesia was maintained both with intravenous infusion propofol 4 to 7 mg/kg/h, remifentanil 6 to 10 μg/kg/h, and inhalation of 1 to 2% sevoflurane. Fentanyl or sufentanil was used when signs of inadequate analgesia were evident intraoperatively such as increased heart rate or blood pressure. 0.05 mg/kg of cisatracurium was administered at 30–40 min intervals. All patients received 0.25 mg palonosetron hydrochloride intravenously before suture.

For those patients who received TAP block, bilateral TAP block was performed by ultrasound (SonoSite EdgeII, American) before anesthesia induction. 40 ml of 0.5% ropivacaine (AstraZneca AB, Sweden, 20 ml each side) was injected into the transversus abdominis plane under real-time ultrasound guidance.

Postoperatively, electronic analgesic pump with wireless analgesic system was used for 48 h of PCIA (Renxian Medtech, Jiangsu). The PCIA pump was filled with sufentanil 150 μg, azasetron 10 mg, diluted to 150 ml with 0.9% normal saline. It was programmed to give 1.5–2 ml/h background infusion with a 1.5–2 μg bolus of sufentanil solution, with a 5 min lockout time. Patients were routinely informed that they could control the pain by pressing a self-controlled button to only slight pain. Pain was assessed twice a day at rest and during movement with an 11-point Numeric Rating Scale (NRS) (0 = no pain; 10 = pain 'as bad as you can imagine') by the same nurse of acute pain service group within 48 h after operation.

After discharged from hospital, postoperative follow-up team contacted patients via telephone at 3 months and 6 months after operation to complete pain evaluation (NRS score and painful place).

The data extraction

Patients' data including patients' ASA status, sex, age at the time of operation, body mass index was extracted from medical records. Patients' information about surgical and anesthetic management such as anesthesia duration, surgery duration, perioperative opioid dose and pain scores was extracted from Anesthesia records. All patients were allocated to two groups: group TP were those patients who received TAP block and PCIA; and group P were those patients who only received PCIA.

Statistical analysis

In order to facilitate comparison, fentanyl 0.1 mg was equivalent to sufentanil 0.01 mg. Considering that remifentanil is an ultra-short-acting opioid, we analyzed it separately. Opioid usage was analyzed with the unpaired t-test between two groups. Two-way repeated measures anova was used for NRS scores of 24 h, 48 h, 3 months and 6 months after surgery. The chi-square test was used for comparisons of categorical data. Quantitative data were expressed as mean ± SD and categorical variables as percentages. Data were analyzed with the SPSS

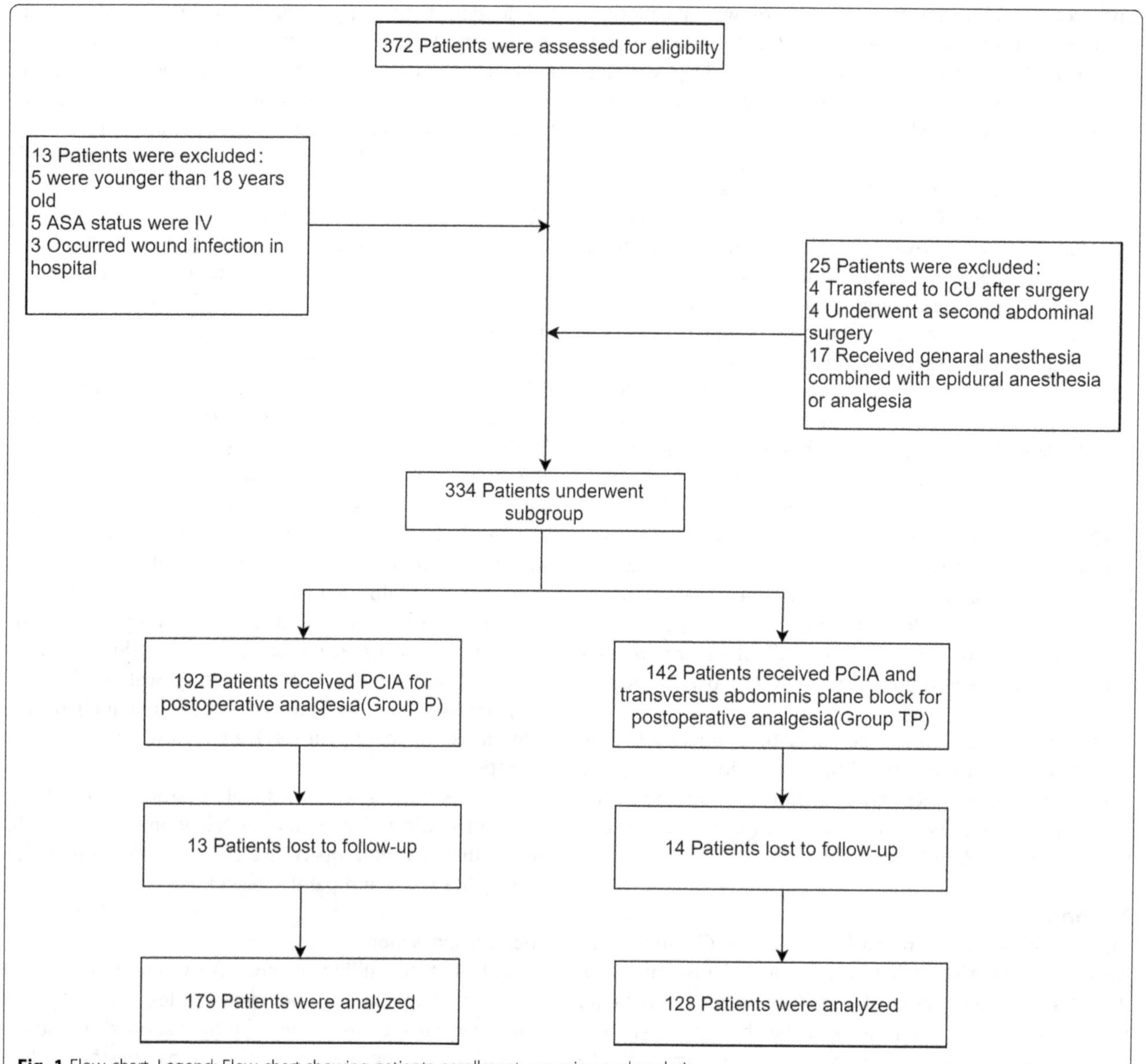

Fig. 1 Flow chart. Legend: Flow chart showing patients enrollment, grouping and analysis

software version 22.0 (SPSS Inc., Chicago, IL). Significance was determined at P<0.05.

Patient and public involvement

Patients and the public were not involved in planning, design, or interpretation of the study. The study involved examination of existing claims data and no participants were recruited for this analysis. This research was done without patient involvement. Patients were not invited to comment on the study design and were not consulted to develop patient relevant outcomes or interpret the results. Patients were not invited to contribute to the writing or editing of this document for readability or accuracy.

Results

Three hundred-seventy-two patients were included in this study between January 2015 and January 2019. Thirty eight patients were excluded (5 patients were younger than 18 years, 5 patients' ASA status was IV, 3 patients occurred wound infection in hospital, 4 patients were transferred to ICU after surgery, 4 patients underwent a second abdominal operation, 17 patients received general anesthesia combined with epidural anesthesia or analgesia). Three hundred-thirty-four patients meeting the selection criteria were reviewed (group $P = 192$; group TP =142). There were 13 patients lost to follow-up in group P and 14 patients in group TP. Finally, 307 patients were enrolled for analysis. The participant flow chart of this study was presented in Fig. 1.

Patients' demographics, ASA status, duration of surgery and anesthesia, and operative method were similar between the two groups (Table 1).

Compared with group P, there was a significant reduction in intraoperative sufentanil usage in group TP (51.3 ± 12.6 vs 64.8 ± 18.8, $P = 0.000$), while there was no significant difference in remifentanil usage between two groups ($P > 0.05$). But the postoperative requirement for sufentanil showed no significant difference at 24 h and 48 h between group TP and group P ($P = 0.255$, $P = 0.300$, respectively) (Table 2).

The NRS score at rest and during movement was decreased significantly at 24 h after surgery (rest NRS 1.07 ± 1.34 vs 1.65 ± 1.67, movement NRS 3.00 ± 1.45 vs 3.65 ± 1.89; all $p = 0.003$) in group TP than those of group P. but there was no significant difference of NRS score at rest and during movement at 48 h ($p > 0.05$). At 3 months after surgery, the NRS score during movement was also lower in group TP than that in group P (0.59 ± 1.23 vs 0.92 ± 1.65, $p = 0.045$). There was no significant difference of NRS score at 6 months after surgery (all $P > 0.05$) (Fig. 2).

In time comparison, both in group TP and group P, the effect of time on pain was statistically significant (all $P < 0.001$) and the degree of pain decreased with time (Fig. 2).

The prevalence of CPSP at 3 months and 6 months after surgery were summarized in Fig. 3. Among 307 patients, CPSP occurred in 62 patients (20.2%) at 3 months after surgery and 42 patients (13.7%) at 6 months after surgery in our patients. The prevalence of CPSP was 19.5% (25/128) in group TP and 20.7%(37/179) in group P at 3 months after surgery; 13.2% (17/128) patients suffered from CPSP in group TP and 13.9% (25/179) at 6 months after surgery. Both at 3 months and 6 months after surgery, there was no statistical difference of the prevalence of CPSP between the two groups (3 months, $P = 0.806$, 6 months, $P = 0.863$, respectively) .

Table 1 Patients' demographics and clinical characteristics

	Group P ($n = 179$)	Group TP ($n = 128$)	Total ($n = 307$)	P
Gender				
Male	79(44.1%)	74(57.8%)	153(49.8%)	0.734
Female	100(55.9%)	54(42.2%)	154(50.2%)	
Age (years)	57.8 ± 11.8	59.6 ± 12.2	58.6 ± 12.0	0.190
BMI (kg/m^2)	22.7 ± 3.2	22.3 ± 2.8	22.5 ± 3.0	0.284
ASA status				
I	1(0.6%)	1(0.8%)	2(0.7%)	0.405
II	102(57.0%)	73(57.0%)	175(57.0%)	
III	76(42.4%)	54(42.2%)	130(42.3%)	
Surgery duration (hours)	3.8 ± 1.4	3.9 ± 1.0	3.8 ± 1.3	0.671
Anesthesia duration (hours)	5.5 ± 1.4	5.6 ± 1.0	5.5 ± 1.3	0.593
Operative Method				
Open	36(20.1%)	16(12.5%)	52(16.9%)	0.080
Laparoscope	143(79.9%)	112(87.5%)	255(83.1%)	

Measurement data is presented as Mean ± SD or number (%). Group P=PCIA only, Group TP = PCIA and TAP block

Table 2 Opioid usage during perioperative period

Opioid usage	Group P ($n = 179$)	Group TP ($n = 128$)	t	P
Intraoperative				
Sufentanil (ug)	64.8 ± 18.8	51.3 ± 12.6	−7.071	0.000*
Remifentanil (mg)	1.4 ± 0.6	1.3 ± 0.5	−1.831	0.068
Postoperative				
Sufentanil usage at 24 h (ug)	45.1 ± 30.2	49.3 ± 34.0	1.141	0.255
Sufentanil usage at 48 h (ug)	84.7 ± 49.1	90.6 ± 50.3	1.038	0.300

Data are presented as Mean ± SD, compared with Group P, *$P<0.05$. Group P= PCIA only, Group TP = PCIA and TAP block

Discussion

Our research assumptions were partially supported. TAP block not only significantly decreased the intraoperative opioids, but also lessen pain intensity at 24 h and 3 months after colorectal surgery; however, such an effect did not occur at other time point.

In group TP, patients received bilateral TAP block before surgery, the NRS score both at rest and during movement at 24 h after surgery was significantly lower than that in group P. This result was similar to some studies, which showed that TAP block with levobupivacaine could reduce postoperative visual analogue pain scores in the first 24 h after major abdominal surgery, [17] and TAP block provided superior analgesia with lower pain scores at rest and movement in the first 24 h after colorectal surgery, when compared to PCA alone [18]. In our study, TAP block significantly decreased intraoperative sufentanil use, but there was no significant difference of sufentanil consumption at 24 h and 48 h after surgery and NRS score at 48 h after surgery between the two groups. Bhattacharjee et al. [19] also found that preincisional TAP block decreased intraoperative fentanyl requirements, and median time to request first postoperative analgesic was 290 min. According to McDonnell et al. [10] and our experience, the duration of TAP was approximately 8-16 h, with complete resolution at 24 h. Maybe this was the cause of the same

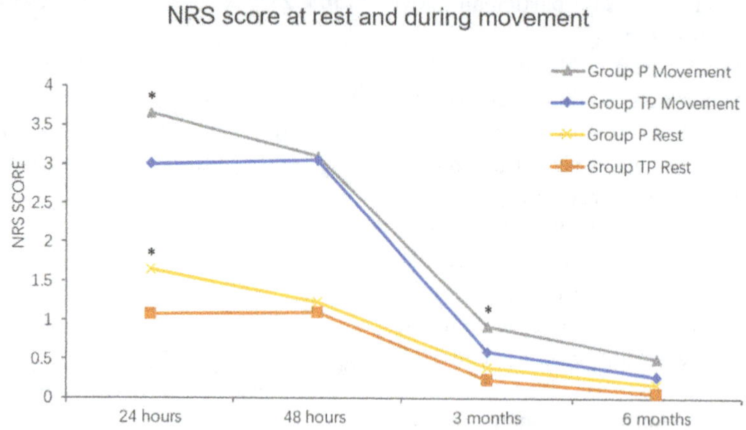

Fig. 2 NRS score at rest and during movement. Legend: The NRS score of patients at rest and during movement at different time points. Data is presented as mean ± SD. Compared with group P, the NRS score (at rest and during movement) was decreased significantly at 24 h in group TP ($P<0.05$), but there was no significant difference at 48 h between two groups ($P > 0.05$). In group TP, the NRS score during movement was significantly lower than that in group P at 3 months after surgery ($P<0.05$). There were no significant difference of NRS score at 6 months after surgery between two groups ($P > 0.05$). NRS = numerical rating scale. Group P=PCIA only, Group TP = PCIA and TAP block. * $P<0.05$

opioid consumptions at 24 h and 48 h after surgery between the two groups. All suggested that TAP block could improve acute postoperative pain and the effect lasted at most 24 h.

In our study, the overall incidence of chronic pain was 20.2% at postoperative 3 months and 13.7% at postoperative 6 months. A prospective research documented that the prevalence of CPSP was 19% at 6 months after colorectal surgery [3]. A retrospective analysis confirmed that the prevalence of CPSP in patients with colorectal cancer was 17% at 38 months after laparoscopic colorectal surgery, [4] which was a little higher than ours at postoperative 6 months. These maybe have something to do with the difference of race and analgesia method.

However, there was no literature on how TAP block affects the incidence of CPSP in colorectal surgery. In our study, at 3 months after surgery, the prevalence of CPSP was 19.5% in group TP and 20.7% in group P; and at 6 months after surgery, the prevalence of CPSP was 13.2% in group TP and 13.9% in group P. There was no significant difference about the prevalence of CPSP between the two groups after elective colorectal surgery. Similarly, a prospective cohort follow-up study indicated TAP block did not influence the prevalence of CPSP at 6 months and 12 months after breast reconstruction [20]. A randomized controlled trial also demonstrated that TAP block did not decrease the incidence of CPSP at 6 months after cesarean delivery [21]. These told us

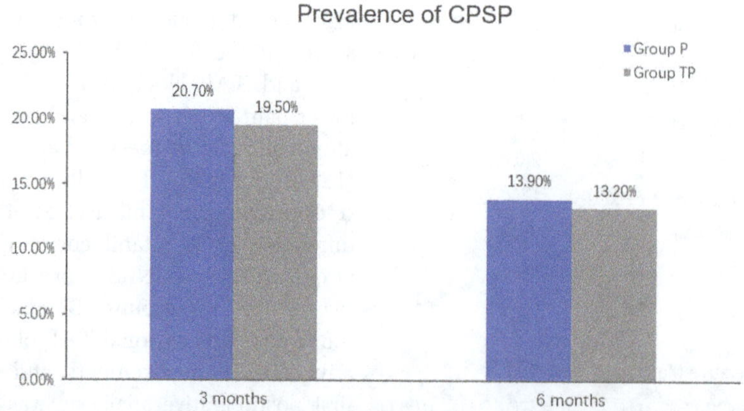

Fig. 3 Prevalence of CPSP. Legend: The prevalence of CPSP at 3 months and 6 months after surgery. Data is presented as percentage. The prevalence of CPSP in group TP showed no significant difference compared with group P at 3 months and 6 months after surgery (all $P > 0.05$). CPSP = chronic postsurgical pain. Group P=PCIA only, Group TP = PCIA and TAP block

that TAP block could not decrease the incidence of CPSP.

Although TAP block did not improve the incidence of chronic pain after colorectal surgery, pain scores at 3 months was lower in group TP than that in group P, which means TAP block has positive effect on CPSP. A randomized controlled trial [14] showed that TAP block could not reduce the incidence of chronic pain after inguinal hernia repair similar to ours but they differed in reduction of the pain scores in rest and movement at 6 months.

Our study has some limitations. The design of the retrospective study made it difficult for us to strictly exclude the use of postoperative non-opioid analgesics, which may also influence postoperative pain scores. In addition, most patients in this study had been operated by the laparoscopic approach and the incidence of chronic pain was not high after intervention, which might be the cause of negative long-term results.

Conclusions

In conclusion, TAP block could relieve pain movement score at 3 months after surgery, but could not reduce the incidence of CPSP at 3 months and 6 months after selective colorectal surgery. Prospective study is required to assess the effect of TAP block on CPSP for prolonged period.

Abbreviations

TAP: Transversus abdominal plane; CPSP: Chronic postsurgical pain; PCIA: Patient controlled intravenous analgesia; NRS: Numerical rating scale

Acknowledgements

This work was supported by grant from National Key R&D Program of China (2018YFC2001800) and by the New Xiangya talent projects of the third Xiangya hospital of Central South University. This study was also supported in part by the Research and Innovation Funds from Xiangya Big data Foundation of Central South University.

Authors' contributions

ZYP reviewed and analyzed the data and wrote the manuscript. ZHH guided the research and revised the manuscript. FZ contributed to the conception and design of the study. WXX aided the research, QL and YZT conceived and designed the study, and revised the manuscript for important intellectual content. All authors read and approved the final manuscript.

References

1. Treede RD, Rief W, Barke A, Aziz Q, Bennett MI, Benoliel R, Cohen M, Evers S, Finnerup NB, First MB, et al. Chronic pain as a symptom or a disease: the IASP classification of chronic pain for the international classification of diseases (ICD-11). Pain. 2019;160(1):19–27.
2. Werner MU, Kongsgaard UE. Defining persistent post-surgical pain: is an update required? Br J Anaesth. 2014;113(1):1–4.
3. Deiss T, Chen LL, Sarin A, Naidu RK. Patient-reported outcomes 6 months after enhanced recovery after colorectal surgery. Perioper Med (Lond). 2018;7:19.
4. Joris JL, Georges MJ, Medjahed K, Ledoux D, Damilot G, Ramquet CC, Coimbra CI, Kohnen LP, Brichant JF. Prevalence, characteristics and risk factors of chronic postsurgical pain after laparoscopic colorectal surgery: retrospective analysis. Eur J Anaesthesiol. 2015;32(10):712–7.
5. Kehlet H, Jensen TS, Woolf CJ. Persistent postsurgical pain: risk factors and prevention. Lancet. 2006;367(9522):1618–25.
6. Glare P, Aubrey KR, Myles PS. Transition from acute to chronic pain after surgery. Lancet. 2019;393(10180):1537–46.
7. Carroll I, Hah J, Mackey S, Ottestad E, Kong JT, Lahidji S, Tawfik V, Younger J, Curtin C. Perioperative interventions to reduce chronic postsurgical pain. J Reconstr Microsurg. 2013;29(4):213–22.
8. Andreae MH, Andreae DA. Regional anaesthesia to prevent chronic pain after surgery: a Cochrane systematic review and meta-analysis. Br J Anaesth. 2013;111(5):711–20.
9. Bouman EA, Theunissen M, Bons SA, van Mook WN, Gramke HF, van Kleef M, Marcus MA. Reduced incidence of chronic postsurgical pain after epidural analgesia for abdominal surgery. Pain Pract. 2014;14(2):E76–84.
10. McDonnell JG, O'Donnell B, Curley G, Heffernan A, Power C, Laffey JG. The analgesic efficacy of transversus abdominis plane block after abdominal surgery: a prospective randomized controlled trial. Anesth Analg. 2007; 104(1):193–7.
11. McDonnell JG, O'Donnell BD, Farrell T, Gough N, Tuite D, Power C, Laffey JG. Transversus abdominis plane block: a cadaveric and radiological evaluation. Reg Anesth Pain Med. 2007;32(5):399–404.
12. Conaghan P, Maxwell-Armstrong C, Bedforth N, Gornall C, Baxendale B, Hong LL, Carty HM, Acheson AG. Efficacy of transversus abdominis plane blocks in laparoscopic colorectal resections. Surg Endosc. 2010;24(10):2480–4.
13. Siddiqui MR, Sajid MS, Uncles DR, Cheek L, Baig MK. A meta-analysis on the clinical effectiveness of transversus abdominis plane block. J Clin Anesth. 2011;23(1):7–14.
14. Theodoraki K, Papacharalampous P, Tsaroucha A, Vezakis A, Argyra E: The effect of transversus abdominis plane block on acute and chronic pain after inguinal hernia repair. A randomized controlled trial. Int J Surg 2019, 63:63–70.
15. Liu L, Xie YH, Zhang W, Chai XQ. Effect of Transversus Abdominis plane block on postoperative pain after colorectal surgery: a meta-analysis of randomized controlled trials. Med Princ Pract. 2018;27(2):158–65.
16. Kanazi GE, Aouad MT, Abdallah FW, Khatib MI, Adham AM, Harfoush DW, Siddik-Sayyid SM. The analgesic efficacy of subarachnoid morphine in comparison with ultrasound-guided transversus abdominis plane block after cesarean delivery: a randomized controlled trial. Anesth Analg. 2010;111(2): 475–81.
17. Saxena A, Bansal R, Mittal A, Shrivastava U. Sharma P, chand T: evaluation of postoperative analgesic efficacy of transversus abdominis plane block after abdominal surgery: a comparative study. J Nat Sci Biol Med. 2013;4(1):177–80.
18. Bharti N, Kumar P, Bala I, Gupta V. The efficacy of a novel approach to transversus abdominis plane block for postoperative analgesia after colorectal surgery. Anesth Analg. 2011;112(6):1504–8.
19. Bhattacharjee S, Ray M, Ghose T, Maitra S, Layek A. Analgesic efficacy of transversus abdominis plane block in providing effective perioperative analgesia in patients undergoing total abdominal hysterectomy: a randomized controlled trial. J Anaesthesiol Clin Pharmacol. 2014;30(3):391–6.
20. Justin O, M PG, Toni Z, Stuart M, Coimbatore S, C ONA, James K, Joel K, P HSO, Hance C. Chronic postsurgical pain outcomes in breast reconstruction patients receiving perioperative Transversus Abdominis plane catheters at the donor site: a prospective cohort follow-up study. Pain Pract. 2016;17(8): 999–1007.
21. McKeen DM, George RB, Boyd JC, Allen VM, Pink A. Transversus abdominis plane block does not improve early or late pain outcomes after cesarean delivery: a randomized controlled trial. Can J Anaesth. 2014;61(7):631–40.

12

Preemptive oxycodone is superior to equal dose of sufentanil to reduce visceral pain and inflammatory markers after surgery

Yi An[1,2], Lei Zhao[1,2*], Tianlong Wang[1,2], Jiapeng Huang[3], Wei Xiao[1,2], Ping Wang[1,2], Lixia Li[1,2], Zhongjia Li[1,2] and Xiaoxu Chen[1,2]

Abstract

Background: Postoperative visceral pain is common after surgery and previous studies have demonstrated that oxycodone is an effective treatment. In this study, we compared the effects of preemptive oxycodone to equal dose of sufentanil on postoperative pain and serum level of inflammatory factors (TNF-α, IL-6, IL-10) after laparoscopic cholecystectomy.

Methods: Forty patients undergoing laparoscopic cholecystectomy were randomized into preemptive oxycodone group or preemptive sufentanil group.

Patients were given either oxycodone 0.1 mg/kg (oxycodone group, $n = 20$) or sufentanil 0.1 μg/kg (sufentanil group, n = 20) for preemptive analgesia. We evaluated pain/sedation scores at 0 h, 0.5 h, 2 h, 4 h, 6 h, 8 h and 24 h after surgery and measured serum concentrations of TNF-α, IL-6 and IL-10 before surgery and at 0 h, 6 h and 24 h after surgery.

Results: Twenty patients were recruited in each group. Numerical rating scale (NRS) of visceral pain in the oxycodone group at 2 h when resting (0.5(0,2.75) vs 3(2,4), $P = 0.008$) and moving (0.5(0,3) vs 3(2.25,4), $P = 0.015$) and 4 h when moving (2(0,3) vs 3(0,4.75), $P = 0.043$) after surgery were significantly lower than the sufentanil group. Serum concentrations of TNF-α at 6 h (38.68 ± 10.49 vs 73.02 ± 16.27, $P<0.001$) and 24 h (43.12 ± 8.40 vs 74.00 ± 21.30, $P<0.001$) in the oxycodone group were lower than the sufentanil group.

Conclusions: Preemptive oxycodone 0.1 mg/kg administration could effectively suppress visceral pain at 2 h and 4 h after surgery and had lower inflammatory marker, serum TNF-α, level when compared to equal dose of sufentanil.

Keywords: Preemptive analgesia, Oxycodone, Sufentanil, Visceral pain, TNF-α

* Correspondence: zhaoalei@sina.com

[1]Department of Anesthesiology, Xuanwu Hospital, Capital Medical University, 45 Changchun Street, Xicheng District, Beijing 100053, China

[2]National Clinical Research Center for Geriatric Disorders, Beijing, China

Background

Laparoscopic cholecystectomy (LC) carries short operation time, mild surgical trauma and minimal blood loss, which could greatly enhance recovery after surgery (ERAS) [1, 2]. However, acute pain after LC causes severe physical discomfort, prolong the recovery duration and delay discharge [3, 4]. LC postoperative pain consists of incision pain, visceral pain and referred pain (shoulder pain). Visceral pain is a major part of pain within 24 h after surgery [5] and is difficult to locate and lack targeted treatments. Organ injury and peritoneal inflammation, local acidosis and visceral mucosa ischemia caused by pneumoperitoneum may be causes of visceral pain after LC surgery [2, 6]. Moreover, Morten et al. [7] have shown that patients with higher visceral pain in the first week after LC were associated with chronic pain.

Degree of analgesia intraoperatively is another factor impacting postoperative pain. The nociceptive stimulation during operation will increase pro-inflammatory cytokines such as TNF-α, IL-6 and decrease anti-inflammatory cytokines such as IL-10 [8] and cause systemic inflammatory response, which will influence recovery process and prognosis.

Opioids are the most common medication used by anesthesiologists to treat pain. There are three opioids receptors, μ receptor, κ receptor and δ receptor. Sufentanil is high selective μ receptor agonist with fast onset and strong analgesic effect [9, 10]. However, sufentanil is less effective to relieve visceral pain than oxycodone [11]. Oxycodone not only activate the μ receptor but also occupy the κ receptor and relieve pain of organs composed of smooth muscle [12].

Besides drug types, the timing of drug delivery also impacts perioperative pain. Preemptive analgesia starts administration of analgesic interventions before nociceptive stimulation and is intended to suppress the progress of stress state and central sensitization before they start [13, 14]. Previous studies have shown a reduction in postoperative pain and use with preemptive analgesia [13, 15].

We hypothesized that preemptive oxycodone can reduce the degree of postoperative visceral pain and decrease the incidence of postoperative remedial analgesia and PONV. The primary outcome was to evaluate whether preemptive oxycodone administration is superior to equal dose of sufentail on visceral pain after LC in postoperative time points. Secondary outcomes included the serum level of TNF-α, IL-6 and IL-10, the dose of opioid used intraoperative, the postoperative sedation level and the degree of postoperative nausea and vomiting (PONV) and complications after surgery.

Methods

This double-blinded prospective randomized controlled trial was conducted from March 2018 to September 2018 at the Xuanwu Hospital, Beijing, China, after approval from Xuanwu Hospital Ethics Committee in March 2018. The trial was registered with China Clinical Trial Registry (registration number: ChiCTR-IOR-17013738, principal investigator's name: Lei Zhao, date of registration: 6th December 2017). Forty patients scheduled for LC were included and the written informed consents were obtained from all patients before participation. This manuscript adheres to the applicable CONSORT guidelines.

Inclusion criteria were patients aged 18–65 years, with an American Society of Anesthesiologists (ASA) physical status I-II, body mass index 18-35 kg/m^2 [16]. Patients with severe systematic disease, history of gastrointestinal hemorrhage or peptic ulcer, suffering acute or chronic pain, dependence on alcohol or opioid, using psychological drugs, allergic to agents used in this trial were excluded. Patients who had to be converted to open surgery, used drugs out of initial anesthetic plan (inhalational anesthetic agents, other analgesics, et al.), experienced special complications (stroke, acute coronary syndrome, circulatory instability caused by arrythmia, liver injury, et al.) during surgery were excluded from this trial.

Forty patients were randomly assigned into either oxycodone group (group O, $n = 20$) or sufentanil group (group S, n = 20) using a computer-generated list by anesthesiologist who is not involved in this trial. Allocation was blinded to patients, anesthesiologists and other healthcare providers. Numerical rating scale (NRS) and characteristics of LC postoperative pain were explained to patients during preoperative interview. Incisional pain is defined as a pain restricted to incision site on abdominal wall, visceral pain is defined as a deep, dull and hard to locate pain, while the referred pain is defined as the right shoulder pain in LC. Patients were educated to distinguish these three types of pain from our definitions.

Heart rate (HR), blood pressure (BP), SpO_2 were monitored after entering the operation room and Bispectral index (BIS) electrodes were placed on patients' forehead. After adequate preoxygenation with 100% oxygen, a bolus of 0.1 mg/kg oxycodone was administered as preemptive analgesia [15, 17] in oxycodone group followed by sufentanil 0.2μg/kg, etomidate 0.2 mg/kg and rocuronium 0.6 mg/kg as anesthesia induction. Patients in sufentanil group were administered sufentanil 0.1 μg/kg as preemptive analgesia followed by sufentanil 0.2μg/kg, etomidate 0.2 mg/kg and rocuronium 0.6 mg/kg as anesthesia induction. Tracheal intubation was performed 5 min after preemptive oxycodone/sufentanil administration. Ventilation model was PCV-VG, tidal volume 6-8 ml/kg, FiO_2 50%, I: E = 1:2, and $P_{ET}CO_2$ was monitored and maintained between 35 and 45 mmHg. Anesthesia was maintained with total intravenous anesthesia (TIVA) using propofol and remifentanil by target controlled infusion (TCI) pumps after tracheal intubation was accomplished. Propofol was infused using Marsh model with 1μg/ml as initial concentration and adjusted by ±0.5μg/ml. Remifentanil was infused using Minto model with 4 ng/ml as initial concentration and adjusted by ±1 ng/ml. The target was to maintain BIS between 40 and 60 and have no body movements during the whole process of operation.

BP and HR were stabilized between ± 20% of baseline. Parecoxib 40 mg was given 30 min before the end of surgery in both groups. Ondansetron 4 mg and oxycodone 0.05 mg/kg were administered when pneumoperitoneum was stopped and local anesthesia was administrated with 0.5% ropivacaine.

Extubation was performed after patients met extubation criteria. All participants were immediately (0 h) investigated for degree of incision pain, visceral pain and shoulder pain (NRS) when resting (breathing) or moving (cough and deep breathing). Degree of sedation and PONV were also evaluated. In post anesthesia care unit (PACU), oxycodone 2 mg was administered as remedial anesthesia if NRS ≥ 4 and it could be repeated every 10 min until NRS ≤ 3. Researchers recorded the drug amount and pain assessments in PACU. Follow-up evaluations were conducted at 0.5 h, 2 h, 4 h, 6 h, 8 h and 24 h postoperatively by anesthesiologists blinded to grouping and offered the same questions to patients. Postoperative complications were also recorded.

Blood samples were collected before operation (T0), at the end of operation (T1), 6 h (T2) and 24 h (T3) after operation. Serum samples were stored at − 80 °C refrigerator after centrifugation with 3000 rpm for 15 min and used ELISA to measure serum level of TNF-α, IL-6 and IL-10.

Statistical analysis

The result of our pilot experiment was used as reference standard of the calculation of sample size. Setting an α of 0.05(2-tailed) and a power of 80%, the sample size was 17 in each group calculated by the formula $n = [Z\alpha/2 + Z\beta]2 /(P1\text{-}P2)^2$ and a sample size of 20 patients per group was chosen to allow for potential drop-outs. Data were analyzed by SPSS version 17.0. Continuous data were presented as mean and standard deviation (SD) and non-continuous data in median (quartile). The demographics and intraoperative situations were compared by Student *t* test or χ^2 test. The NRS, degree of sedation and PONV were compared with Mann-Whitney U test. Serum concentration of TNF-α, IL-6 and IL-10 were analyzed by repeated measurement analysis of variance, $P < 0.05$ was considered as a statistical significance.

Results

Seventy one patients were assessed for eligibility based on inclusion and exclusion criteria, with 26 patients excluded for not meeting inclusion criteria due to poor physical status ($n = 10$), emergency surgery ($n = 6$), long term psychotropic drugs use ($n = 4$) and refusing to participation (n = 6). After surgery, 5 patients were excluded for converting to open surgery and failing to follow up as planned. Finally, 40 patients were included in present analysis (group O: group S = 1:1, $n = 20$) (Fig. 1).

Demographics and intraoperative characteristics of all participants are summarized in Table 1 and no statistical significance was found between the groups.

Medication quantities and perioperative complications are shown in Table 2 and no statistical significance was found between the groups. The incidence of nausea and vomiting in the oxycodone group is similar to the sufentanil group without statistical significance. Degree of sedation was evaluated using Ramsey scale and no statistical significance was observed between the groups.

The incision pain, visceral pain and shoulder pain when resting or moving were followed at 0 h, 0.5 h, 2 h, 4 h, 6 h, 8 h, 24 h after surgery. Figure 2 shows the incision pain and shoulder pain when resting or moving and no statistical significance was found.

For visceral pain, we found that oxycodone group has lower pain than sufentanil group at 2 h postoperatively (0.5(0,2.75) vs 3(2,4), $P = 0.008$ Fig. 3). When moving, the NRS was significantly lower in oxycodone group at 2 h (0.5(0,3) *vs* 3(2.25,4), $P = 0.015$) and 4 h (2(0,3) *vs* 3(0,4.75), $P = 0.043$) postoperatively.

One suffered postoperative respiratory depression and two suffered vertigo in the oxycodone group while one

Table 1 Demographic Data and Intraoperative Characteristics

	Group O (*n* = 20)	Group S (*n* = 20)	*P* value
Gender (male/female)	9/11	4/16	0.177
Age (year)	48 ± 13	51 ± 12	0.429
BMI (kg/m2)	25 ± 4	26 ± 4	0.718
ASA(I/II)	5/15	5/15	1.000
Cholecystolithiasis/gallbladder polyps	16/4	19/1	0.339
Pneumoperitoneum time (min)	36 ± 17	29 ± 9	0.201
Operation time (min)	51 ± 20	41 ± 11	0.149
Anesthesia time (min)	78 ± 21	68 ± 15	0.142
Wake-up time (min)	9 ± 3	8 ± 3	0.509
Extubating time (min)	12 ± 3	12 ± 4	0.964
Bile spillover(Y/N)	6/14	3/17	0.449
Blood loss (ml)	Minimal	Minimal	NA
Drainage(Y/N)	5/15	1/19	0.184

Data were expressed as mean ± SD
ASA American Society of Anesthesiologists, *BMI* body mass index, *Group O* oxycodone group, *Group S* sufentanil group, *Y* yes, *N* no

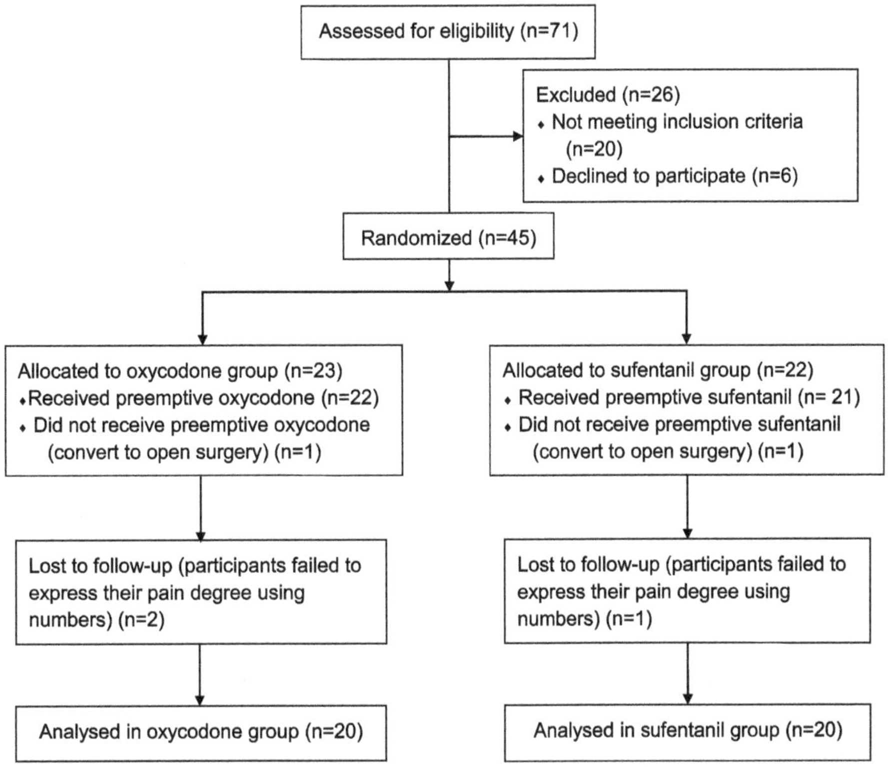

Fig. 1 Flow diagram. ASA, American Society of Anesthesiologist

patient had recurrence of atrial fibrillation in the sufentanil group. Two patients suffered chest tightness in both groups respectively and were relieved after oxygen inhalation.

Serum TNF-α concentration in both groups gradually rose from preoperation to 24 h after surgery (Fig. 4). The comparison between the two groups showed the oxycodone group was statistically lower in TNF- α at 6 h (38.68 ± 10.49 vs 73.02 ± 16.27, *P*<0.001) and 24 h (43.12 ± 8.40 vs 74.00 ± 21.30, *P*<0.001) after surgery. For IL-6 and IL-10, no statistical significance could be found between the groups.

Table 2 Medication Quantities and Complications

	Group O	Group S	*P* value
Propofol (mg/kg/h)	4.84 ± 0.92	5.07 ± 1.46	0.799
Remifentanil (μg/kg/min)	0.26 ± 0.07	0.27 ± 0.06	0.253
Hypertension (Y/N)	3/17	1/19	0.598
Hypotension (Y/N)	16/4	16/4	1.000
Tachycardia (Y/N)	1/19	2/18	1.000
Bradycardia (Y/N)	0/20	1/19	1.000
Myocutaneous antagonist (Y/N))	4/16	8/12	0.301
Remedial analgesia (Y/N)	3/17	5/15	0.693
Exhaust time (h)	15 ± 10	13 ± 7	0.858
PONV (Y/N)	17/3	17/3	1.000

Either nausea or vomiting is recorded as "Y"
Group O oxycodone group, *Group S* sufentanil group, *PONV* postoperative nausea and vomiting, *Y* yes, *N* no

Discussion

Preemptive analgesia is an effective strategy to provide adequate analgesia before patients are exposed to nociceptive stimulus. It decreases the physiologic reaction caused by pain and blocks the peripheral nociceptive stimulus transmition to the spinal cord, which inhibits hyperalgesia in central nervous system [18, 19]. Previous studies have shown that it could achieve better analgesic effect [20, 21]. Our study used equivalent dose of oxycodone and sufentanil as preemptive analgesia. Oxycodone takes effect about 2 min after injection, reaches peak level in serum in 3–5 min [22] and the duration of action is 3–4 h. Sufentanil takes effect in 3 min [9] and lasts for 0.5–1 h.

Previous study of Lenz et al. demonstrated that patients suffer most severe pain between 2 h and 6 h after surgery [23]. In our study, we found that visceral pain at 2 h and 4 h postoperatively were less with preemptive oxycodone. In addition, there was no difference on the incidence of adverse events between both groups. Preemptive oxycodone could be a good choice to reduce the hard to treat visceral pain in LC surgery.

Opioids is commonly used during surgery, but it is complicated by PONV, respiratory depression,

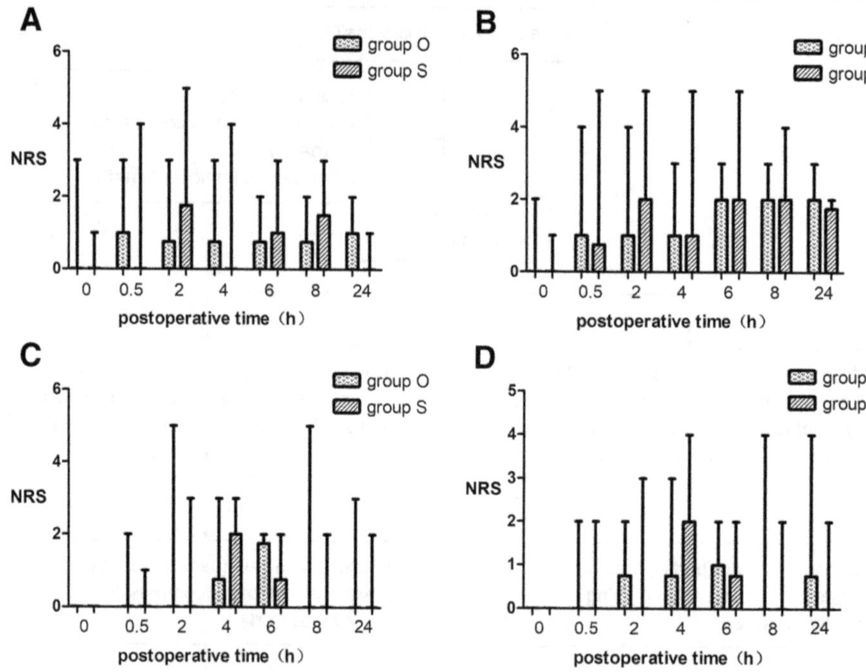

Fig. 2 Incision Pain and Shoulder Pain when resting and moving. The results are represented by box graph. The transverse line in rectangular box is the median, the lower bound means the lower quartile and the upper bound is the upper quartile. The lower/upper bar is the minimum/maximum. **a**. incision pain when resting. **b**. incision pain when moving. **c**. shoulder pain when resting. **d**. shoulder pain when moving. No statistical significance was found. Group O = oxycodone group. Group S = sufentanil group

hyperalgesia, opioid tolerance and anesthetic related mortality postoperatively [24–27]. These side effects are related to the activation of μ receptor by opioids. Sufentanil has strong affinity with μ receptor and it is easy to pass blood brain barrier with its highly fat solublity and achieves central analgesic effect. However, sufentanil is not the best choice in LC. The incision of LC is small and the visceral pain is the main component of intraoperative and postoperative pain. Peripheral κ opioid receptor has been suggested as a possible target for attenuating visceral pain [28]. Oxycodone has κ receptor agonist properties and is more potent in the treatment of visceral pain [29, 30]. It elevates the threshold for visceral pain stimulation [31] so that the pain signal is blocked in the peripheral and the input to central nervous system is then weakened [28]. In addition, the low fat solubility reduces the proportion of oxycodone passing through blood brain barrier so that the incidence of complications related to the μ receptor may be lower.

It is worth noting that there was no statistically significant difference on remifentanil dose between

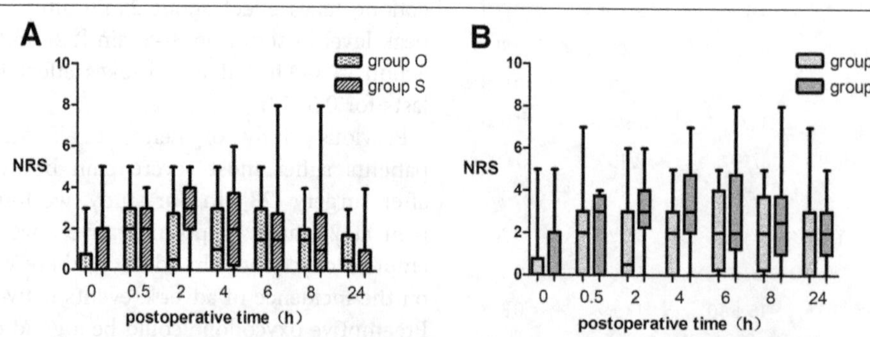

Fig. 3 Visceral Pain when Resting and Moving. The results are represented by box graph. The transverse line in rectangular box is the median, the lower bound means the lower quartile and the upper bound is the upper quartile. The lower/upper bar is the minimum/maximum. **a**. Visceral pain when resting. **b**. Visceral pain when moving. Group O = oxycodone group. Group S = sufentanil group

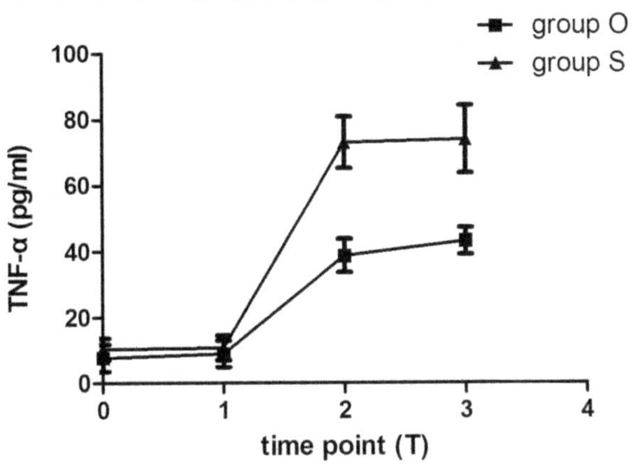

Fig. 4 Serum Concentration of TNF-α. The square and the triangle is the mean and the transverse line is standard deviation. Group O = oxycodone group. Group S = sufentanil group

the two groups. This indicated that preemptive administration of oxycodone did not increase the dose of opioid used intraoperatively than preemptive sufentanil.

Whether analgesia is adequate could be reflected by the level of inflammatory factors during and after surgery. Previous studies suggested that TNF-α was the initial factor in systematic inflammatory reaction. It acts early and motivates the creation of other cytokines [32]. In addition, TNF-α also associates with pain and is involved in the formation and maintenance of hyperalgesia [33]. Song et al. demonstrated that TNF-α activation was critical in inflammatory visceral hyperalgesia [34]. These studies suggest that sufficient analgesia to reduce the TNF-α production is one of the most effective means to alleviate postoperative visceral pain. In our study, analysis of TNF-α showed that the concentrations at 6 h and 24 h after surgery in oxycodone group were significantly lower than the sufentanil group ($P < 0.001$). The results demonstrated that preemptive administration of oxycodone 0.1 mg/kg in LC could effectively suppress the release of TNF-α. According to the role of TNF-α in inflammatory reaction and pain management, we can infer that the systematic inflammatory syndrome in the oxycodone group is less than the sufentanil group. These findings are consistent with our observations of more reduction of visceral pain with preemptive oxycodone.

There are limitations in our study. First, some of the participants failed to follow-up at 24 h postoperatively because they have already been discharged and a serum specimen was not obtained. Second, the current study is not designed to evaluate hyperalgesia and incidence of chronic pain [33, 35]. Finally, duration of LC is short and surgeries with longer duration are needed for further observation on comparison between preemptive oxycodone and sufentanil administration on postoperative pain.

Conclusions

For patients undergoing LC, preemptive oxycodone 0.1 mg/kg administration could effectively suppress visceral pain at 2 h and 4 h after surgery and inhibit the rising of serum TNF-α level at 6 h and 24 h after surgery without increasing postoperative complications. Preemptive oxycodone appears to be an effective strategy in dealing with visceral pain after LC.

Abbreviations

ASA: American Society of Anesthesiologists; BIS: Bispectral index; BP: Blood pressure; ERAS: Enhance recovery after surgery; HR: Heart rate; LC: Laparoscopic cholecystectomy; NRS: Numerical rating scale; PACU: Post anesthesia care unit; PONV: Postoperative nausea and vomiting; TCI: Target controlled infusion; TIVA: Total intravenous anesthesia

Acknowledgements

We would like to thank Dr. Tianlong Wang, Dr. Lei Zhao and Dr. Jiapeng Huang and their team for the assistance with the study.

Authors' contributions

YA designed the study, conducted the study, analyzed the data and wrote the manuscript. LZ designed the study, conducted the study, analyzed the data and wrote the manuscript. TLW helped design the study, analyze the data and revise the manuscript. JPH helped design the study and revise the manuscript. WX conducted the study, analyzed the data and wrote the manuscript. PW helped conduct the study and write the manuscript. LXL helped conduct the study and write the manuscript. ZJL analyzed the data and wrote the manuscript. XXC helped conduct the study and write the manuscript. All authors read and approved the final manuscript.

Author details

[1]Department of Anesthesiology, Xuanwu Hospital, Capital Medical University, 45 Changchun Street, Xicheng District, Beijing 100053, China. [2]National Clinical Research Center for Geriatric Disorders, Beijing, China. [3]Department of Anesthesiology, Jewish Hospital and Department of Anesthesiology & Perioperative Medicine, University of Louisville, Louisville, KY, USA.

References

1. Ljungqvist O, Scott M, Fearon KC. Enhanced recovery after surgery: a review. JAMA Surg. 2017;152:292–8.
2. Mitra S, Khandelwal P, Roberts K, et al. Pain relief in laparoscopic cholecystectomy--a review of the current options. Pain Pract. 2012;12:485–96.
3. American Society of Anesthesiologists Task Force on Acute Pain Management. Practice guidelines for acute pain management in the perioperative setting: an updated report by the American Society of Anesthesiologists Task Force on acute pain management.[J]. Anesthesiology. 2004;100:1573–81.
4. Bisgaard T, Kehlet H, Rosenberg J. Pain and convalescence after laparoscopic cholecystectomy. Eur J Surg. 2001;167:84–96.
5. Joris J, Thiry E, Paris P, et al. Pain after laparoscopic cholecystectomy: characteristics and effect of intraperitoneal bupivacaine. Anesth Analg. 1995;81:379–84.
6. Volz J, Köster S, Weiss M, et al. Pathophysiologic features of a pneumoperitoneum at laparoscopy: a swine model [J]. Am J Obstet Gynecol. 1996;174:132–40.
7. Blichfeldt-Eckhardt MR, Helle O, Claus A, et al. Early visceral pain predicts chronic pain after laparoscopic cholecystectomy[J]. Pain. 2014;155:2400–7.
8. Singh P, Castillo A, Majid DS. Decrease in IL-10 and increase in TNF-α levels in renal tissues during systemic inhibition of nitric oxide in anesthetized mice. Physiol Rep. 2014;2:e00228.

9. Scott JC, Cooke JE, Stanski DR. Electroencephalographic quantitation of opioid effect: comparative pharmacodynamics of fentanyl and sufentanil. Anesthesiology. 1991;74:34–42.
10. Volpe DA, McMahon Tobin GA, Mellon RD, et al. Uniform assessment and ranking of opioid μ receptor binding constants for selected opioid drugs. Regul Toxicol Pharmacol. 2011;59:385–90.
11. Nie JJ, Sun S, Huang SQ. Effect of oxycodone patient-controlled intravenous analgesia after cesarean section: a randomized controlled study. J Pain Res. 2017;10:2649–55.
12. Kokki H, Kokki M, Sjövall S. Oxycodone, for the treatment of postoperative pain. Expert Opin Pharmacother. 2012;13:1045–58.
13. Trabulsi EJ, Patel J, Viscusi ER, et al. Preemptive multimodal pain regimen reduces opioid analgesia for patients undergoing robotic-assisted laparoscopic radical prostatectomy. Urology. 2010;76:1122–4.
14. Rosero EB, Joshi GP. Preemptive, preventive, multimodal analgesia: what do they really mean? Plast Reconstr Surg. 2014;134:85S–93S.
15. Wang J, Ma H, Zhou H, et al. Effect of preoperative intravenous oxycodone administration on sufentanil consumption after retroperitoneal laparoscopic nephrectomy. Anaesthesiol Intensive Ther. 2016;48:300–4.
16. Kokki M, Broms S, Eskelinen M, et al. Analgesic concentrations of oxycodone--a prospective clinical PK/PD study in patients with laparoscopic cholecystectomy. Basic Clin Pharmacol Toxicol. 2012;110:469–75.
17. Wang N, Wang Y, Pang L, et al. Effect of preemptive analgesia with intravenous oxycodone in the patients undergoing laparoscopic resection of ovarian tumor. Pak J Med Sci. 2015;31:300–3.
18. Campiglia L, Cappellini I, Consales G, et al. Premedication with sublingual morphine Sulphate in abdominal surgery [J]. Clin Drug Invest. 2009;29(1): 25–30.
19. Seltzer Z, Cohn S, Ginzburg R, et al. Modulation of neuropathic pain behavior in rats by spinal disinhibition and NMDA receptor blockade of injury discharge [J]. Pain. 1991;45(1):69–75.
20. Fanelli G, Ghisi D, Berti M, et al. Preoperative administration of controlled-release oxycodone as a transition opioid for total intravenous anaesthesia in pain control after laparoscopic cholecystectomy. Surg Endosc. 2008;22: 2220–8.
21. Van Backer JT, Jordan MR, Leahy DT, et al. Preemptive analgesia decreases pain following anorectal surgery: a prospective, randomized, double-blinded, placebo-controlled trial. Dis Colon Rectum. 2018;61:824–9.
22. Olkkola KT, Kontinen VK, Saari TI, et al. Does the pharmacology of oxycodone justify its increasing use as an analgesic? Trends Pharmacol Sci. 2013;34:206–14.
23. Lenz H, Sandvik L, Qvigstad E, et al. A comparison of intravenous oxycodone and intravenous morphine in patient-controlled postoperative analgesia after laparoscopic hysterectomy. Anesth Analg. 2009;109:1279–83.
24. Pasternak GW. Molecular biology of opioid analgesia. J Pain Symptom Manag. 2005;29(5 Suppl):S2–9.
25. Angst MS. Intraoperative use of remifentanil for TIVA: postoperative pain, acute tolerance, and opioid-induced hyperalgesia. J Cardiothorac Vasc Anesth. 2015;29(Suppl 1):S16–22.
26. Weber L, Yeomans DC, Tzabazis A. Opioid-induced hyperalgesia in clinical anesthesia practice: what has remained from theoretical concepts and experimental studies? Curr Opin Anaesthesiol. 2017;30:458–65.
27. Monk TG, Saini V, Weldon BC, et al. Anesthetic management and one-year mortality after noncardiac surgery. Anesth Analg. 2005;100:4–10.
28. Rivière PJ. Peripheral kappa-opioid agonists for visceral pain. Br J Pharmacol. 2004;141:1331–4.
29. Staahl C, Christrup LL, Andersen SD, et al. A comparative study of oxycodone and morphine in a multi-modal, tissue-differentiated experimental pain model. Pain. 2006;123:28–36.
30. Staahl C, Dimcevski G, Andersen SD, et al. Differential effect of opioids in patients with chronic pancreatitis: an experimental pain study. Scand J Gastroenterol. 2007;42:383–90.
31. Arendt-Nielsen L, Olesen AE, Staahl C, et al. Analgesic efficacy of peripheral kappa-opioid receptor agonist CR665 compared to oxycodone in a multi-modal, multi-tissue experimental human pain model: selective effect on visceral pain. Anesthesiology. 2009;111:616–24.
32. Kraft AD, McPherson CA, Harry GJ. Heterogeneity of microglia and TNF signaling as determinants for neuronal death or survival. Neurotoxicology. 2009;30:785–93.
33. Temugin B, Chul-Kyu P, Zhen-Zhong X, et al. Extracellular caspase-6 drives murine inflammatory pain via microglial TNF-α secretion. J Clin Invest. 2014; 124:1173–86.
34. Dan-dan S, Yong L, Dong T, et al. Neuron-glial communication mediated by TNF-α and glial activation in dorsal root ganglia in visceral inflammatory hypersensitivity. Am J Physiol Gastrointest Liver Physiol. 2014;306:G788–95.
35. Fletcher D, Martinez V. Opioid-induced hyperalgesia in patients after surgery: a systematic review and a meta-analysis. Br J Anaesth. 2014;112: 991–1004.

13

A preliminary assessment of vital-signs-integrated patient-assisted intravenous opioid analgesia (VPIA) for postsurgical pain

Ban Leong Sng[1,2*], Daryl Jian'an Tan[2], Chin Wen Tan[1], Nian-Lin Reena Han[3], Rehena Sultana[4] and Alex Tiong Heng Sia[1,2]

Abstract

Background: We developed a Vital-signs-integrated Patient-assisted Intravenous opioid Analgesia (VPIA) analgesic infusion pump, a closed-loop vital signs monitoring and drug delivery system which embodied in a novel algorithm that took into account patients' vital signs (oxygen saturation, heart rate). The system aimed to allow responsive titration of personalized pain relief to optimize pain relief and reduce the risk of respiratory depression. Moreover, the system would be important to enable continuous monitoring of patients during delivery of opioid analgesia.

Methods: Nineteen patients who underwent elective gynecological surgery with postoperative patient controlled analgesia (PCA) with morphine were recruited. The subjects were followed up from their admission to the recovery room/ ward for at least 24 h until assessment of patient satisfaction on the VPIA analgesic infusion pump.

Results: The primary outcome measure of incidence of oxygen desaturation showed all patients had at least one episode of oxygen desaturation (< 95%) during the study period. Only 6 (31.6%) patients had oxygen desaturation that persisted for more than 5 min. The median percentage time spent during treatment that oxygen saturation fell below 95% was 1.9%. Fourteen (73.7%) out of 19 patients encountered safety pause, due to transient oxygen desaturation or bradycardia. The patients' median [IQR] pain scores at rest and at movement after post-op 24 h were 0.0 [2.0] and 3.0 [2.0], respectively. The average morphine consumption in the first 24 h was 12.5 ± 7.1 mg. All patients were satisfied with their experience with the VPIA analgesic infusion pump.

Conclusions: The use of VPIA analgesic infusion pump, when integrated with continuous vital signs monitor and variable lockout algorithm, was able to provide pain relief with good patient satisfaction.

Keywords: Infusion pump, Postoperative pain, Vital sign monitoring, Oxygen desaturation

* Correspondence: sng.ban.leong@singhealth.com.sg
[1]Department of Women's Anaesthesia, KK Women's and Children's Hospital, 100 Bukit Timah Road, Singapore, Singapore
[2]Anaesthesiology and Perioperative Sciences Academic Clinical Program, Duke-NUS Medical School, 8 College Road, Singapore, Singapore

Background

More than 230 million major surgeries are performed annually in the world that could result in moderate to severe post-surgical pain [1]. Patient-controlled analgesia (PCA) with an opioid pump is often the commonly used technique to relief pain. Opioids adverse effects such as nausea, vomiting, sedation and respiratory depression may occur especially in high risk patients. The risk of opioid-induced respiratory depression was significantly increased in the patients with advanced age, respiratory disease and obstructive sleep apnoea [2, 3], leading to the increased length of stay and overall costs [4]. Intermittent monitoring measures were highly labor intensive, yet not reliably recognized opioid-induced respiratory depression in the postoperative period [5]. According to Anaesthesia Patient Safety Foundation, patients having vital signs charted every 4 h were usually left unmonitored > 90% of the time. Since these patients were commonly administered with supplemental oxygen, this might eventually complicate the monitoring by masking hypoventilation, causing the signs of respiratory depression to be recognized only in its later stage [6].

Our overall aim was to develop a Vital-signs-integrated Patient-assisted Intravenous opioid Analgesia (VPIA) analgesic infusion pump with closed-loop vital signs monitoring and drug delivery system which embodied a novel algorithm that accounted for patients' vital signs (oxygen saturation, heart rate). In this preliminary study, our primary aim was to investigate the incidence of oxygen desaturation (defined as oxygen saturation < 95% in a patient for more than 60 s) in postoperative patients using our VPIA analgesic infusion pump. The side effects of opioid administration (nausea, vomiting and sedation), patients' satisfaction and vital signs monitoring data were also evaluated.

Methods

This study was approved by the SingHealth Centralized Institutional Review Board, Singapore (SingHealth CIRB Ref: 2015/3062), and registered on Clinicaltrials.gov (NCT02804022). Written informed consent was obtained from every patient before any study procedure. The study period was between January 2017 and June 2017 and was conducted at KK Women's and Children's Hospital, Singapore.

We recruited female patients aged 21 to 70 years old with American Society of Anesthesiologists (ASA) status I or II, undergoing elective surgery and intending to use postoperative PCA with morphine for postoperative analgesia. The exclusion criteria were the patients with allergies to morphine, history of significant respiratory disease or obstructive sleep apnea, unwilling to wear oxygen saturation monitoring devices throughout the study duration, pregnancy and unable to comprehend the use of PCA. The recruitment was performed either in the pre-operative assessment clinic or on the same day of surgery if they had not attended pre-operative assessment clinic. An information brochure describing the use of VPIA analgesic infusion pump for post-operative analgesia, including potential side effects and complications was provided to the patients.

Setting up of infusion pump

The algorithm and the VPIA analgesic infusion pump ("Intellifuse pump"; Model: Opiva) was designed by Innovfusion Pte Ltd., Singapore (Fig. 1). Intravenous morphine used in the VPIA analgesic infusion pump was administered according to the institutional guidelines: morphine diluted in normal saline to a concentration of 1 mg/ml, with bolus doses of 1 mg morphine delivered as per patient demand. In the VPIA analgesic infusion pump, vital signs monitoring (oxygen saturation, pulse rate) was programmed into the VPIA variable lockout algorithm, in which a temporary pause to the pump was triggered when vital signs safety threshold was breached; and subsequently the lockout interval was increased upon re-starting thereby improving the safety of intravenous morphine administration. That means when the vital signs were within normal range, the system was able to increase or decrease the lockout interval according to the analgesic needs of the patient. This lockout interval was a safety mechanism that limited the

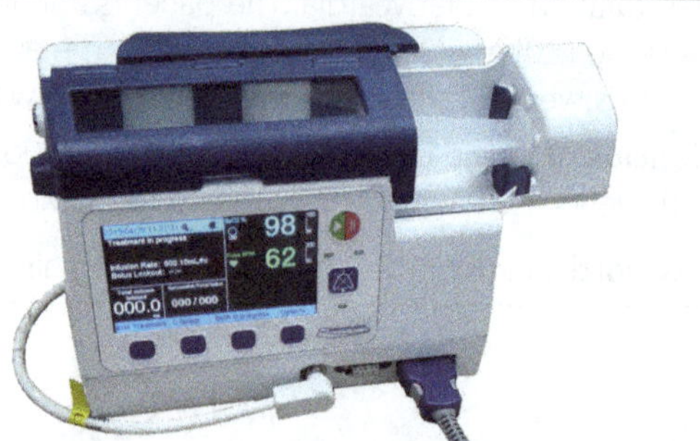

Fig. 1 An illustration of Vital-signs-integrated Patient-assisted Intravenous opioid Analgesia (VPIA) analgesic infusion pump. The algorithm and the VPIA analgesic infusion pump ("Intellifuse pump"; Model: Opiva) was designed by Innovfusion Pte Ltd., Singapore. The written permission has been given for publication by Innovfusion Pte Ltd., Singapore

frequency of demands. By allowing an adequately long interval between each dose, the patients were given sufficient time to achieve the opioid's effects before the next dose. However, if the interval were prolonged, the effectiveness of patient controlled analgesia would be reduced.

The detailed VPIA variable lockout algorithm was illustrated in Fig. 2. The bolus lockout interval was empirically set at 7 min, and was adjusted automatically according to the patient successful demands and the patient safety in the event of abnormal vital signs monitoring. The monitoring data was performed by taking average epochs of 15 s to summarize the vital signs. Missing vital signs were dropped from the analysis. However, if there was no available vital sign for the whole duration of each epoch, a safety pause would be triggered. The VPIA variable lockout algorithm reassessed for the recovery of the patient's' vital signs at the end of the safety lockout period. If the patient's vital signs did not recover to the safe levels, the pump automatically raised the on-board alarm. Conversely, if the patient's vital signs recovered beyond the threshold limits by the end of the safety lockout period, the lockout interval would be prolonged. If at any time, there were critically abnormal vital sign parameters, the system would trigger the "emergency safety stop" function to cease the patient's boluses. The system would be manually restarted by a clinician or a nurse after reviewing the patient.

All patients had established intravenous access before surgery. The patients were instructed on the use of the VPIA analgesic infusion pump prior to the study and educated to press the demand button whenever they needed pain relief. While in the recovery room after surgery, the VPIA analgesic infusion pump was secured with a 50 ml syringe filled with1 mg/ml morphine that was connected to the patient's intravenous line for analgesia. The patient's oxygen saturation and heart rate was continuously monitored by the VPIA analgesic system at least for 24 h after surgery.

Data collection

We collected and analyzed three sets of data: (1) patient demographic, surgical and anesthetic characteristics; (2) VPIA analgesic infusion pump data including opioid consumption, patient demands, successful demands, pattern of demands, oxygen saturation and heart rate; and (3) VPIA analgesic infusion pump user feedback survey that was conducted at the end of the study.

Following the initiation of VPIA analgesic infusion pump, attending nurses who were educated on the usage and side effects of morphine therapy would monitor the patient at regular intervals and document pain scores

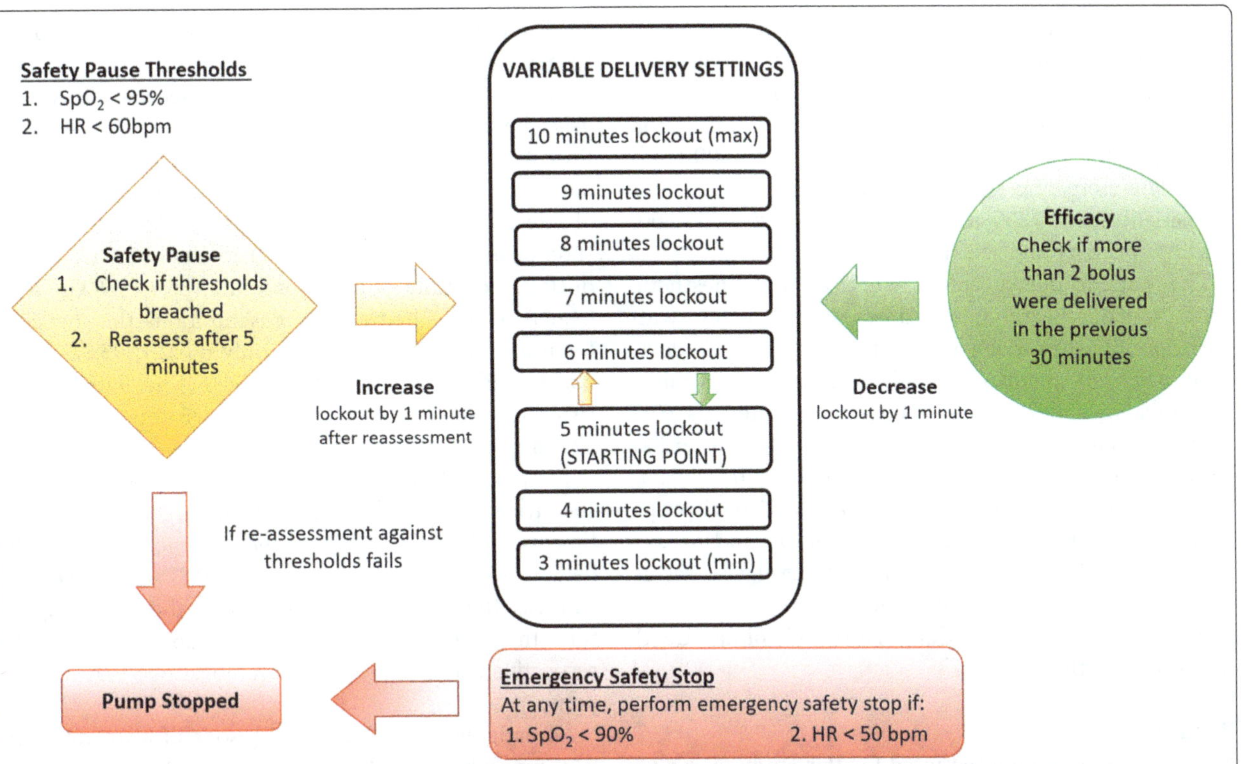

Fig. 2 The proposed Vital-signs-integrated Patient-assisted Intravenous opioid Analgesia (VPIA) analgesic infusion pump and the variable lockout algorithm

(0–10 numeric rating scale), blood pressure, heart rate, oxygen saturation and sedation score (0 for "awake, alert", 1 for "occasionally drowsy, easy to rouse, responds to calling", 2 for "occasionally drowsy, difficult to rouse, responds to shaking only"; 3 for "unresponsive and unarousable-- defined as no response to voice or physical stimulation"; D for "distressed -- defined as awake and in great pain"). Side effects such as nausea and vomiting were also recorded.

An independent observer would assess the patient during the period she was placed on the VPIA analgesic infusion pump. The patient's overall satisfaction (numerical score between 0 and 100%) with the postoperative analgesia provided, the feedback on pain relief effectiveness and any side effect from the therapy were also gathered. Once the indications for PCA opioid for pain management were deemed unnecessary by the patient's primary care team, the VPIA analgesic infusion pump was disconnected.

Table 1 Baseline and demographic characteristics of recruited subjects

Parameters	No. of patients	Mean (SD)/ Percentage
Age; years	19	51.5 (8.8)
Race	19	
Chinese	13	68.4%
Indian	3	15.8%
Malay	2	10.5%
Others	1	5.3%
Weight; kg	19	62.0 (9.9)
BMI; kg/m^2	19	24.7 (4.4)
ASA Status	19	
I	5	26.3%
II	14	73.7%
Intraoperative morphine (mg)	19	8.7 (1.3)
Intraoperative fentanyl (mcg)	19	102.0 (35.3)

SD: Standard deviation

Sample size calculation and statistical analysis

The primary outcome measure of the study was the incidence of oxygen desaturation (defined as oxygen saturation < 95% in a patient for more than 60 s) in the patients using the VPIA analgesic infusion pump. The secondary outcome measures were bradycardia, sedation, nausea/vomiting, pain scores, total consumption of morphine, patient's satisfaction score. Patient's oxygen saturation and heart rate were measured every minute for at least 24 h. Assuming that a patient had < 3% oxygen desaturation, 0.005 width of interval and 95% confidence interval, we would require 18,000 oxygen saturation readings. Each patient would provide at least 1200 readings. Therefore, the study was adequately powered for 18 patients with 1200 readings (= 18 X 1200 ~ 21,600) for both primary and secondary aims.

The patient demographics, surgical and anesthetic characteristics were summarized as frequency with corresponding proportion, as mean ± standard deviation (SD) or median [range], whichever applicable. The incidence rate and 95% confidence intervals (CI) of binary outcomes (such as desaturation, bradycardia) were estimated based on the exact method by Wilson [7], which demonstrated to have good statistical properties even for small number of subjects and/or extreme probabilities [8, 9]. Significance level was set at 0.05 and all tests were two-tailed. SAS version 9.3 software (SAS Institute; Cary, North Carolina, USA) was used for the analysis.

Results

Nineteen patients were recruited for this study over a 6-month period (January 2017 to June 2017), with their baseline and demographic characteristics shown in Table 1. The mean age of patients was 51.5 ± 8.8 years (range 36–66 years), the average body mass index (BMI) was 24.7 ± 4.4 kg/m^2. All patients recruited went through scheduled open surgery, with the majority (n = 15) under total abdominal hysterectomy and bilateral salpingo-oophorectomy (TAHBSO). The rest were open myomectomy (n = 2) and salpingo-oophorectomy (n = 2). Intraoperative morphine and fentanyl was administered with a mean dosage of 8.7 ± 1.3 mg and 102.0 ± 35.3 μg respectively.

The patients were offered pain relief via VPIA analgesic infusion pump once they were transferred to the Post-Anesthesia Care Unit (PACU). The primary outcome measure of incidence of oxygen desaturation (Table 2) showed that all patients had at least one episode of oxygen saturation (SpO_2) below 95% transiently during the study period. Only 13 (68.4, 95%CI 46.0–84.6%) patients had oxygen desaturations that persisted for more than 60 s. However, only 8 (42.1, 95%CI 23.1–63.7%) and 6 (31.6, 95%CI 15.4–54.0%) patients had persisted oxygen desaturation for 3 and 5 min, respectively. The median total time spent and the percentage of time that SpO_2 fell below 95% was 35.3 min and 1.9%, respectively. During the 1st 4 h post-surgery, the median time period and the percentage of time that SpO_2 fell below 95% was 2.08 min and 0.87%, respectively; whereas the median time spent and the percentage of time that SpO_2 fell below 95% was 26.8 min and 1.4%, respectively after 4 h until the removal of VPIA infusion pump.

All patients had at least one episode of heart rate (HR) < 60/min with 3 (15.8, 95%CI 5.5–37.6%) patients experiencing their HR < 60/min for longer than 60 s duration (Table 2). The median time period and the percentage of

Table 2 The characteristics of oxygen saturation and heart rate in recruited subjects

Parameters	No. of patients	
Incidence of oxygen desaturation		**Percentage % (95% CI)**
At least one episode SpO2 < 95%	19	100
SpO2 < 95% persisted for > 60 s	13	68.4 (46.0–84.6)
SpO2 < 95% persisted for > 3 min	8	42.1 (23.1–63.7)
SpO2 < 95% persisted for > 5 min	6	31.6 (15.4–54.0)
		Median [IQR]
Post-surgery 0 h until the removal of pump		
Total time spent of SpO2 < 95%, min		35.3 [6.8–73.8]
The % of time of SpO2 < 95%		1.9 [0.4–4.2]
0–4 h post-surgery		
Total time spent of SpO2 < 95%, min		2.1 [0.2–9.2]
The % of time of SpO2 < 95%		0.87 [0.07–3.8]
> 4 h post-surgery		
Total time spent of SpO2 < 95%, min		26.8 [2.7–68.8]
The % of time of SpO2 < 95%		1.4 [0.3–3.4]
Incidence of bradycardia		**Percentage % (95% CI)**
At least one episode of HR < 60/min	19	100
HR < 60/min persisted for > 60 s	3	15.8 (5.5–37.6)
HR < 60/min persisted for > 3 min	1	5.3 (1.0% - 24.6)
HR < 60/min persisted for > 5 min	1	5.3 (1.0% - 24.6)

time that HR fell below 60/min was 1.2 min and 0.13%, respectively. Only 1 (5.3, 95%CI 1.0–24.6%) patient had HR < 60 for both 3 and 5 min. There was no clinically significant respiratory event of note.

Fourteen out of 19 (73.7%) patients encountered the safety pauses, whereas ten (52.6%) patients had experienced an emergency safety stop during the study period. The median [range] number of safety pause was 5 [1–21]. The reasons for the safety pause included either the occurrence of oxygen desaturation or bradycardia. Eleven (57.9%) patients had the safety pause due to $SpO_2 < 95\%$ but all had HR > 60/min during the episode. Six (31.6%) patients had HR < 60/min but all had $SpO_2 >$ 95% during the episode. There were 2 (10.6%) patients experiencing oxygen desaturation < 90% for more than 1 min. The median number of demands of bolus was 21 per patient. Post-operative side effects included nausea / vomiting (6/19) and pruritus (1/19).

The average morphine consumption during the stay was 3.6 ± 3.0 mg (Table 3), whereas the last pain score before sending to ward was 3 [0–6]. Minimal to moderate sedation was observed in 15 patients, whereas 4 other patients exhibited no sedation, having a median of overall sedation scoring of 1 [0–2]. Only one patient showed nausea or vomiting during this period. At 12 h post-surgery, the pain score at rest and movement in 19 patients was 2 [0–6] and 5 [0–10], respectively (Table 3). At 24 h post-surgery, patients had pain scores of 0 [0–7] and 3 [0–8] at rest and movement, respectively. The average morphine consumption in the first 24 h was 12.5 ± 7.1 mg.

User feedback received on VPIA analgesic infusion pump showed that all patients agreed that the pump was safe and effective to use, although they remained neutral on the mobility of the pole where the pump was mounted onto (Table 4).

Discussion

The results of this preliminary assessment on our novel VPIA analgesic infusion pump suggested that the use of this drug delivery system, when integrated with continuous physiological monitoring and a variable lockout algorithm, was able to provide pain relief with good patient satisfaction in post-operative acute pain management. No significant adverse event was observed in this study.

Several studies evaluated the incidence of oxygen desaturation after different types of analgesia, but few analyzed the oxygen saturation continuously for 24–60 h after surgery [10]. Our results showed that all patients had at least one episode of oxygen desaturation ($SpO_2 <$ 95%) transiently, whereas only 13 (68.4%) patients had persistent oxygen desaturations more than 60 s. Moreover, only 8 (42.1%) and 6 (31.6%) patients had persisted

Table 3 Pain characteristics during Post Anesthesia Care Unit (PACU) and ward stay

Parameters	No. of patients	Mean (SD) / Median [range] / Percentage
During PACU stay	19	
Morphine (mg)	19	3.6 (3.0)
Last pain score before discharge (0–10)	19	3 [0–6]
Last sedation score before discharge (0–3)	19	1 [0–2]
Nausea/vomiting before discharge (0–3)	19	0 [0–1]
During Ward stay		
12 h Post-op	19	
Pain score (at rest) (0–10)	19	2 [0–6]
Pain score (movement) (0–10)	19	5 [0–10]
Sedation score (0–3)	19	0 [0–1]
Nausea/vomiting (0–3)	18	0 [0–3]
24 h Post-op	19	
Pain score (at rest) (0–10)	19	0 [0–7]
Pain score (movement) (0–10)	19	3 [0–8]
Sedation score (0–3)	19	0 [0–1]
Nausea/vomiting (0–3)	19	0 [0–1]
Morphine consumption (24 h; mg)	19	12.5 (7.1)
Side effect		
Nausea / vomiting	6	31.6%
Pruritus	1	5.3%

oxygen desaturation for 3 and 5 min, respectively. It was important to understand the percentage of time spent with oxygen desaturation. Motamed et al. [11] demonstrated that the time spent with $SpO_2 < 95\%$ was about 65 and 40% during 1st and 2nd postoperative night, respectively. This was much higher than our results that showed the median time period and percentage of time spent with $SpO_2 < 95\%$ was 35.3 min and 1.9%, respectively. The reason behind this might due to our novel VPIA analgesic infusion system that integrated with continuous vital signs monitor and a variable lockout algorithm.

Hospital practice of intermittent vital signs monitoring with opioid delivery became an increasing concern. More than 75% of patients with moderate to severe sleep apnea were undiagnosed and conventional risk stratification for heightened post-op monitoring could potentially miss the patients at increased risk of respiratory depression [12]. Respiratory depression was reported in up to 5% patients with the use of PCA opioids [5, 13]. A retrospective study on Chinese patients receiving PCA intravenous morphine showed that the incidence of respiratory depression (as defined by $SpO_2 < 90\%$ for longer than 1 min) was 1.62%. The present study showed a higher incidence due to the difference in the definition of oxygen desaturation and the continuous monitoring system because conventional intermittent routine monitoring could under-diagnose the events of oxygen desaturation [14]. Early recognition and the detection of risk of opioid-induced respiratory depression by continuous monitoring vital signs could mitigate the chance of patients' increased length of stay, the risk of hospital-acquired infections and the increased costs [15].

Table 4 Post-operative feedback (n = 19) on the VPIA analgesic infusion pump

Parameters	Values [range]
Feedback (1–5; 1: Strongly disagree; 5: strongly agree)	
Patient handset button	4 [4–5]
Mobility of pole with mounted pump	3 [3–4]
No interference of vital signs monitoring with treatment	4 [1–5]
Pump safety	4 [3–5]
Pump effectiveness	4 [3–5]

This study concentrated on varying the duration of the lockout interval as a safety mechanism. This safety of margin allowed an interval to be long enough for the drugs to take effect in the patients from the present bolus dose before the next bolus was delivered. There was no recommended optimal lockout interval, hence this would need to be individualized to the patient's pain relief and safety requirements [16]. Our results showed that the morphine consumption was 12.5 mg in 24 h after surgery which was comparable with other groups. Chou et al. found that the average morphine consumption of 40 mg in postoperative 48 h in 80 patients that underwent total abdominal hysterectomy and later [17]. Another study on patients after total knee arthroplasty showed an average morphine consumption of 27 mg in 48 h, indicating the different opioid consumptions across various surgical procedures [18].

We also gathered the patient-centered outcomes through the patients' feedback on the device setup (patient handset, pole stand) and their overall treatment experiences (the interference with treatment, the safety and the effectiveness). The overall feedback was positive but the patients remained neutral on the reduced mobility of the pump due to the integration of the vital signs monitor. Future design of a more portable setup would be desirable.

This preliminary study was an initial assessment of our newly developed VPIA analgesic infusion pump. The limitations of this study would include the small number of subjects conducted in only gynecological surgeries. The larger trials in patients with different demography, medical comorbidities and surgical procedures would need to be investigated. This system could be more refined with higher risk patients in future. The physical design of the pump would be reduced to enable great mobility on the patient transfer. The artefact interference with the algorithms could led to false alerts in the present system. Hence., future study plans will include refining new vital signs sensors, incorporating a respiratory rate monitoring and better integration with the delivery system to ensure better data capture.

Conclusions

In conclusion, this preliminary assessment on the VPIA analgesic infusion pump system has found that this novel pump was able to detect and automatically respond to oxygen desaturation and bradycardia by instituting safety pause, and to provide pain relief with good patient satisfaction in post-operative acute pain management. The larger studies with adequate number of subjects would be needed to evaluate the efficiency of this drug delivery system.

Abbreviations

ASA: American Society of Anesthesiologists; BMI: Body mass index; CI: Confidence intervals; IQR: Interquartile range; PACU: Post-Anesthesia Care Unit; PCA: Patient controlled analgesia; SD: Standard deviation; SpO2: Oxygen saturation; TAHBSO: Total Abdominal Hysterectomy and Bilateral Salpingo-oophorectomy; VAS: Visual analogue scale; VPIA: Vital-signs-integrated Patient-assisted Intravenous opioid Analgesia

Acknowledgments

We would like to thank Miss Agnes Teo (Senior Clinical Research Coordinator) and Miss Denise Anne (Clinical Research Coordinator) for their administrative support in this work. The design and layout of the algorithm was performed by Innovfusion Pte Ltd., Singapore.

Authors' contributions

All authors (BLS, DJT, CWT, NLRH, RS, ATHS) contributed to the study design, data analysis and discussion, drafting and/or revising the manuscript. All authors approved the final version of the manuscript, and agree to be accountable for all aspects of this work.

Author details

[1]Department of Women's Anaesthesia, KK Women's and Children's Hospital, 100 Bukit Timah Road, Singapore, Singapore. [2]Anaesthesiology and Perioperative Sciences Academic Clinical Program, Duke-NUS Medical School, 8 College Road, Singapore, Singapore. [3]Division of Clinical Support Services, KK Women's and Children's Hospital, Singapore, Singapore. [4]Centre for Quantitative Medicine, Duke-NUS Medical School, 8 College Road, Singapore, Singapore.

References

1. Weiser TG, Regenbogen SE, Thompson KD, Haynes AB, Lipsitz SR, Berry WR, et al. An estimation of the global volume of surgery: a modelling strategy based on available data. Lancet. 2008;372(9633):139–44.
2. Maddox RR, Williams CK, Oglesby H, Butler B, Colclasure B. Clinical experience with patient-controlled analgesia using continuous respiratory monitoring and a smart infusion system. Am J Health Syst Pharm. 2006; 63(2):157–64.
3. Schein JR, Hicks RW, Nelson WW, Sikirica V, Doyle DJ. Patient-controlled analgesia-related medication errors in the postoperative period. Drug Saf. 2009;32(7):549–59.
4. Etches RC. Respiratory depression associated with patient-controlled analgesia: a review of eight cases. Can J Anaesth. 1994;41(2):125.
5. Paul JE, Buckley N, McLean RF, Antoni K, Musson D, Kampf M, et al. Hamilton acute pain service safety studyUsing root cause analysis to reduce the incidence of adverse events. Anesthesiology. 2014;120(1):97–109.
6. Weinger MB, Lee LA. No patient shall be harmed by opioid-induced respiratory depression. APsF Newsletter. 2011;26(2):21–8.
7. Wilson EB. Probable inference, the law of succession, and statistical inference. J Am Stat Assoc. 1927;22(158):209–12.
8. Newcombe RG. Interval estimation for the difference between independent proportions: comparison of eleven methods. Stat Med. 1998;17(8):873–90.
9. Brown LD, Cai TT, DasGupta A. Interval estimation for a binomial proportion. Stat Sci. 2001;16(2):101–17.
10. Madej TH, Whetaley RG, Jackson IJB, Hunter D. Hypoxaemia and pain relief after lower abdominal surgery: comparison of extradural and patient controlled analgesia. Br J Anaesth. 1992;69:554–7.
11. Motamed C, Spencer A, Farhat F, Bourgain JL, Lasser P, Jayr C. Postoperative hypoxaemia: continuous extradural infusion of bupivacaine and morphine vs patient-controlled analgesia with intravenous morphine. Br J Anaesth. 1998;80:742–7.
12. Ankichetty S, Chung F. Considerations for patients with obstructive sleep apnea undergoing ambulatory surgery. Curr Opinion Anesthesiol. 2011; 24(6):605–11.
13. Macintyre P, Loadsman J, Scott D. Opioids, ventilation and acute pain management. Anaesth Intensive Care. 2011;39(4):545–58.
14. Tsui S, Tong W, Irwin M, Ng K, Lo J, Chan W. The efficacy, applicability and side-effects of postoperative intravenous patient-controlled morphine analgesia: an audit of 1233 Chinese patients. Anaesth Intensive Care. 1996; 24(6):658–64.
15. Cohen MJ, Schecter WP. Perioperative pain control: a strategy for management. Surgical Clin. 2005;85(6):1243–57.
16. Ginsberg B, Gil KM, Muir M, Sullivan F, Williams DA, Glass PS. The influence of lockout intervals and drug selection on patient-controlled analgesia following gynecological surgery. Pain. 1995;62(1):95–100.
17. Chou W-Y, Wang C-H, Liu P-H, Liu C-C, Tseng C-C, Jawan B. Human opioid receptor A118G polymorphism affects intravenous patient-controlled analgesia morphine consumption after total abdominal hysterectomy. Anesthesiology. 2006;105(2):334–7.
18. Chou WY, Yang LC, Lu HF, Ko JY, Wang CH, Lin SH, et al. Association of μ-opioid receptor gene polymorphism (A118G) with variations in morphine consumption for analgesia after total knee arthroplasty. Acta Anaesthesiol Scand. 2006;50(7):787–92.

14

Efficacy of different dose of dexmedetomidine combined with remifentanil in colonoscopy

Li Jia, Meng Xie, Jing Zhang, Jingyu Guo, Tong Tong and Yuying Xing*

Abstract

Background: Dexmedetomidine has advantages during colonoscopy as it allows the patient to cooperate during the procedure. Few studies examined the dexmedetomidine-remifentanil combination. This study was to evaluate the effects of different doses of the dexmedetomidine-remifentanil combination in colonoscopy.

Methods: This was a prospective trial carried out at the Fourth Hospital of Hebei Medical University between 02/2018 and 10/2018. The patients were randomized: group I (dexmedetomidine 0.2 $\mu g \cdot kg^{-1}$), group II (dexmedetomidine 0.3 $\mu g \cdot kg^{-1}$), and group III (dexmedetomidine 0.4 $\mu g \cdot kg^{-1}$), all combined with remifentanil. The primary outcomes were the patient's body movements during the procedure and adverse events.

Results: Compared with at admission (T_0), the SBP, HR, and RR at immediately after giving DEX (T_1), at the beginning of the examination (T_2), 5 min after the beginning of the examination (T_3), 10 min after the beginning of the examination (T_4), and at the end of the examination (T_5) in the three groups were all reduced (all $P < 0.05$), but all were within the clinically normal range. SpO_2 remained > 98% in all patients during the examination. Compared with T_0, the BIS values of the three groups were decreased at T_1 and T_2 (all $P < 0.05$). There were no significant differences in BIS among the three groups (all $P > 0.05$). The minimum BIS value in group III was lower than in groups I and II ($P < 0.05$). The degree of satisfaction with the anesthesia effect was higher in groups II and III that in group I ($P < 0.05$). No hypotension occurred, seven patients had bradycardia, and four patients had nausea/vomiting.

Conclusions: Dexmedetomidine 0.3 $\mu g \cdot kg^{-1}$ combined with remifentanil was effective for colonoscopy and had few adverse reactions.

Keywords: Colonoscopy, Dexmedetomidine, Piperidines, Analgesia, Conscious sedation

Background

Colonoscopy can be performed for the screening of cancer, adenomas, and polyps, for the assessment of known or possible bleeding, and for the evaluation of possible causes of abdominal pain, gastrointestinal symptoms, and/or changes in bowel habits [1, 2]. The National Colorectal Cancer Roundtable aims to reach 80% screening prevalence in the eligible American population [3, 4], representing 5.1 million colonoscopies each year [5].

Beyond the discomfort and inconveniences associated with bowel preparation [6], colonoscopy is

* Correspondence: 281575038@qq.com
Department of Anesthesiology, Fourth Hospital of Hebei Medical University, No. 12, Jiankang Road, Shijiazhuang 050000, Hebei, China

associated with discomfort and sometimes pain. At present, the commonly used methods are the intravenous injection of propofol, etomidate, ketamine, and other drugs to make the patient's unconscious [7]. The disadvantage is that the patient cannot cooperate during the examination (e.g., for changing position), and medical staff is needed to assist in turning over the patient, if necessary. This may compress the patient's stomach and abdomen, which may cause gastric reflux and aspiration, which may cause pneumonia, with morbidity and even mortality [8, 9].

Dexmedetomidine (DEX) is a new type of highly selective α2 receptor agonist. It has sedative, analgesic, and anxiolytic effects, and is known as a "wake-up sedative". Compared with propofol and fentanyl, it provides sedation without the risk of respiratory depression and can provide cooperative or semi-rousable sedation [10, 11]. It has incomparable advantages during colonoscopy as it allows the patient to cooperate during the procedure [12–15]. Dexmedetomidine can be used with other drugs such as remifentanil to achieve deeper sedation, but few studies examined the dexmedetomidine-remifentanil combination for colonoscopy.

Therefore, this study aimed to evaluate the effects of dexmedetomidine combined with remifentanil at different doses for colonoscopy. The results could provide clues about the most optimal doses and improve the patient experience of colonoscopy.

Methods

Study design and patients

This was a prospective trial that was carried out in patients who were scheduled to undergo colonoscopy at the Fourth Hospital of Hebei Medical University between February 2018 and October 2018. All patients were inpatients. This study was approved by the Medical Ethics Committee of the Fourth Hospital of Hebei Medical University (2017MEC113) and written informed consent was obtained from all subjects participating in the trial. The trial was registered at the Chinese Clinical Trial Registry (ChiCTR2000029105, Principal investigator: Li Jia, Date of registration: 2020-01-13). This study adheres to CONSORT guidelines.

The inclusion criteria were: 1) ASA grade was I-II; 2) 18–75 years of age; 3) weight of 50–80 kg; 4) no obvious abnormalities in preoperative ECG, blood routine, electrolytes, and other tests; 5) no history of allergies to narcotic drugs; 6) no history of sedation, analgesics, or alcohol abuse; and 7) no mental illness. The exclusion criteria were: 1) emergency patients; 2) severe abnormalities in heart, lung, kidney, liver, and other functions; 3) sleep apnea syndrome or difficult airways; 4) bronchial asthma; or 5) recent respiratory infections.

Grouping and intervention

The patients were randomly divided into three groups using the random number table method: group I (DEX 0.2 $\mu g{\cdot}kg^{-1}$), group II (DEX 0.3 $\mu g{\cdot}kg^{-1}$), and group III (DEX 0.4 $\mu g{\cdot}kg^{-1}$) (Fig. 1). Patients, surgeon and postoperative observes were blind to group allocation. The routine preoperative preparation was performed. The patient was placed on the left side with the knees bent after entering the room. The Bene View T5 monitor (Mindray Biomedical Electronics Co., Shenzhen, China) and Aspect 2000 EEG monitor (Aspect Medical Systems, Inc., Newton, MA, USA) were connected to monitor the systolic blood pressure (SBP), diastolic blood pressure (DBP), heart rate (HR), pulse oximetry (SpO_2), respiratory rate (RR), and bispectral index (BIS). Oxygen mask inhalation was given at 5 L/min. An upper limb venous access was opened. For group I, 0.2 $\mu g{\cdot}kg^{-1}$ DEX (batch number: 10122334, Jiangsu Hengrui Pharmaceutical Co., Ltd.) and a loading dose of 1 $\mu g{\cdot}kg^{-1}$ remifentanil (batch number: 6120721 Yichang Renfu Pharmaceutical Co., Ltd.) was injected successively, both within 2 min with an intravenous pump. Then, remifentanil was given at a maintenance dose of 0.1 $\mu g{\cdot}kg^{-1}{\cdot}min^{-1}$. Colonoscopy started after 2 min. The infusion of remifentanil was stopped after the end of colonoscopy. For group II, the patients were injected intravenously with 0.3 $\mu g{\cdot}kg^{-1}$ DEX. The patients in group III were injected intravenously with 0.4 $\mu g{\cdot}kg^{-1}$ DEX. The dose of remifentanil was the same in all three groups. If bradycardia occurred during the examination (HR $<$ 50 beats/min), atropine 0.5 mg was injected intravenously. Ephedrine 5–10 mg was injected intravenously if hypotension (SBP $<$ 90 mmHg) appeared. And after the colonoscopy, patients were monitored in PACU for 30 min and transferred to the ward.

Data collection

The data of patients, including SBP, DBP, HR, SpO_2, and RR at admission (T_0), immediately after giving DEX (T_1), at the beginning of the examination (T_2), 5 min after the beginning of the examination (T_3), 10 min after the beginning of the examination (T_4), and at the end of the examination (T_5), and the BIS value at T_0, T_1, and T_2, and the minimum value of BIS during the examination were recorded. We investigated whether the patient was cooperating quietly and whether there were body movements during the examination; whether the patient could wake up; if the patient was needed to turn and whether the patient could do it on his own to complete the examination; number of patients with slight limb activity who did not need additional medications; number of patients with great limb mobility who were unable to cooperate quietly and complete the examination and required additional medications (intravenous injection of 50 mg propofol); number of patients

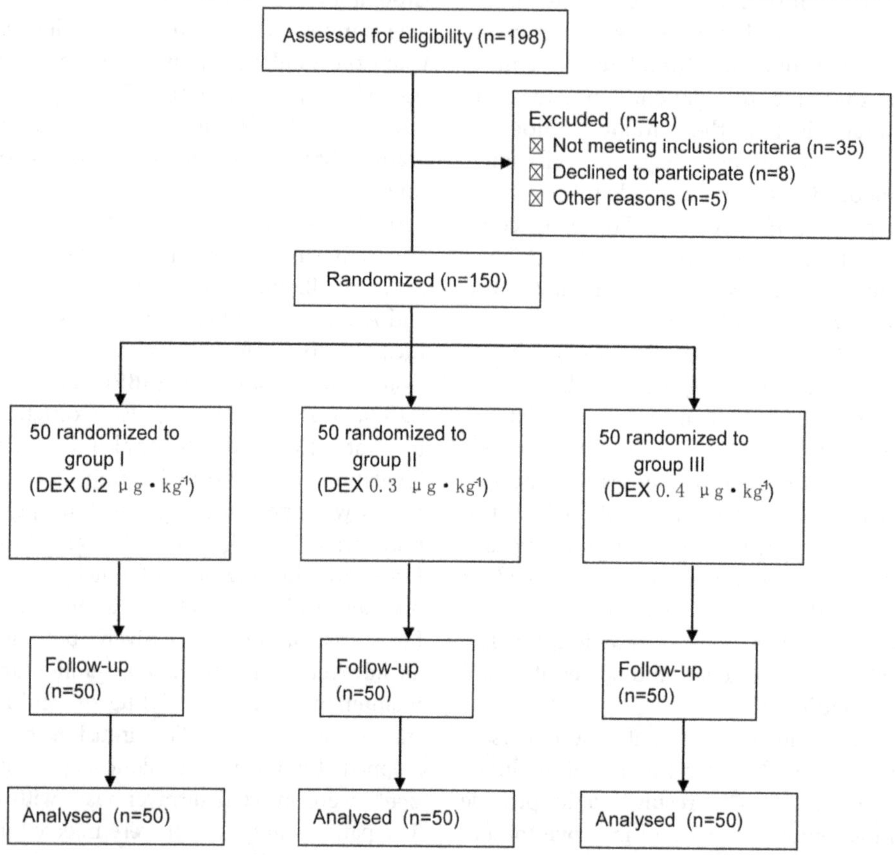

Fig. 1 Flow Diagram

who could wake up; and number of patients who could turn over the body on their own and cooperate to the examinations were recorded. Adverse reactions such as bradycardia, hypotension, and nausea and vomiting were recorded. The examination duration was also recorded. At the end of the examination, the satisfaction degree of the surgeon on the anesthesia effect, which was divided into three grades of excellent, good, and poor, were investigated. Excellent: the patient was quiet during the examination, had no limb movement, was able to wake up during the operation, and was able to turn over the body to cooperate with the examination. Good: the patient had only slight limb movement, which did not affect the examination, was able to wake up during the operation and was able to turn over the body to cooperate with the examination. Poor: the patient had a large degree of limb activity, and it was difficult to complete the examination quietly or cooperatively, or the patient had no limb activity, but could not wake up, or could wake up but could not turn over the body to cooperate with the examination. All examinations were performed by a senior doctor in the endoscopy department of our hospital.

Outcomes

The primary outcomes of this study were the patient's body movements during the procedure and adverse events such as bradycardia, hypotension, nausea, and vomiting. The secondary outcomes were the duration of colonoscopy and the satisfaction of the surgeon to the anesthesia effect.

Statistical analysis

The sample size was calculated based on the patient's movements during the examination. Our preliminary study found that the incidence of patient movements in 11 patients with remifentanil for analgesia was 55%. A reduction of 25% after combined with dexmedetomidine was considered clinically significant. Therefore, a minimum sample size of 46 patients for each group would be required with a significance level of 5% to achieve a power of 80%. Taking into consideration a potential dropout rate of 10%, we recruited 50 patients per group. Normally distributed continuous variables were presented as mean ± standard deviation and were analysed using Student's t test. Mann-Whitney U test was used for non-normally distributed continuous variables, which were presented as median (interquartile range) [M(Q)]. Categorical variables were expressed as frequency (percentage) and were analysed using the Pearson chi-square test. Wilcoxon rank sum test was used for comparison of rank variables. $p < 0.05$ was statistically significant.

Results

Characteristics of the participants

There were no significant differences in general data (age, sex, weight, and examination duration) among the three groups (all $P > 0.05$) (Table 1). There were no significant differences in SBP, DBP, HR, and RR at T_0 among the three groups (all $P > 0.05$) (Table 2).

Changes in circulation and breathing parameters

Compared with T_0, the SBP, HR, and RR at T_{1-5} in the three groups were all reduced (all $P < 0.05$), but all were within the clinically normal range (Table 2, Fig. 2). SpO_2 remained > 98% in all patients during the examination.

Adverse reactions

During the examination, 13, six, and three patients in groups I, II, and III, respectively, had slight body movements that did not interfere with the operation or required propofol injection (all $P < 0.05$). Two patients in group I had body movements that interfered with the operation and needed additional propofol. All patients in each group can be waked up during the examination. For patients who needed to turn over, except for one patient in group III who needed assistance, all patients could turn over on their own. There were 0, one, and six participants of bradycardia in groups I, II, and III, respectively (all $P < 0.05$). No hypotension occurred in the three groups. Nausea and vomiting occurred in one participant in group I, one in group II, and two in group III (Table 3).

Bispectral index

Compared with T_0, the BIS values of the three groups were decreased at T_1 and T_2 (all $P < 0.05$). There were no significant differences in BIS among the three groups (all $P > 0.05$). The minimum BIS value in group III was lower than in groups I and II ($P < 0.05$) (Table 4).

Surgeon's satisfaction

Thirty-five participants in group I were excellent, 13 were good, and two were poor; those numbers were 44, six, and 0, respectively, in group II; and 47, three, and 0, respectively, in group III. The degree of satisfaction with the anesthesia effect was higher in groups II and III that in group I ($P < 0.05$) (Table 5).

Discussion

Dexmedetomidine has advantages during colonoscopy as it allows the patient to cooperate during the procedure [12, 13]. Few studies examined the dexmedetomidine-remifentanil combination. Therefore, this study aimed to evaluate the effects of different doses of the dexmedetomidine-remifentanil combination in colonoscopy. The results strongly suggest that dexmedetomidine 0.3 $\mu g{\cdot}kg^{-1}$ combined with remifentanil was effective for colonoscopy and had few adverse reactions.

Dexmedetomidine is a new type of highly selective $\alpha 2$ receptor agonist and has eight times the affinity to $\alpha 2$ receptors as clonidine [10, 11, 16]. Compared with clonidine, dexmedetomidine has stronger sedative, analgesic, and anxiolytic effects [10, 11, 16]. Its sedative and hypnotic characteristics are that the patients can be awakened and cooperate, and the sleep state is similar to that of natural sleep [10, 11, 16]. It is also the only sedative that allows patients to be easily awakened to cooperate without breathing depression [10, 11, 16]. Bekker et al. [17] reported for the first time the use of dexmedetomidine for craniotomy and left temporal tumor resection, during which it could be used to locate the language area and awaken intraoperatively during surgery. Ramsay et al. [18] used dexmedetomidine as the only intravenous anesthetic in the laser ablation for severe subglottic stenosis and artificial upper trachea replacement. The patients' blood oxygen saturation was above 90% without oxygen inhalation, and hemodynamics were relatively stable. The results of this study showed that the hemodynamic parameters and respiratory parameters of the three groups of participants were within the clinically normal range, and SpO_2 was above 98% in all participants, which was consistent with the results of the above studies.

Cortinez et al. [19] showed that dexmedetomidine had mild-to-moderate analgesic effects on cold compression tests, but had limited effects on acute pain such as electricity and thermal pain. Its analgesic mechanism is different from opioids, which can have a synergistic effect and reduce the amount of opioids [20]. Therefore, the combination of dexmedetomidine and opioids can achieve the purpose of analgesia and

Table 1 Comparison of demographics and clinical characteristics of the three groups

Group	Cases	Age (years)	Weight (kg)	ASA (I / II)	Sex (male/female)	procedure time, min
I	50	53.4 ± 3.3	67.5 ± 2.6	20/30	27/23	20.3 ± 1.4
II	50	51.6 ± 2.5	63.3 ± 1.8	22/28	26/24	21.2 ± 1.0
III	50	55.8 ± 2.8	63.9 ± 2.6	19/31	24/26	20.7 ± 1.2

Table 2 Hemodynamic and respiratory changes in the three groups

Group	Items (mmHg/bpm)	T_0	T_1	T_2	T_3	T_4	T_5
I	SBP	125 ± 23	111 ± 22[a]	114 ± 22[a]	112 ± 23[a]	114 ± 22[a]	116 ± 24[a]
	DBP	69 ± 11	62 ± 12[a]	63 ± 12[a]	63 ± 12[a]	66 ± 12	69 ± 16
	HR	80 ± 14	74 ± 14[a]	75 ± 13[a]	73 ± 12[a]	74 ± 12[a]	76 ± 12[a]
	RR	18 ± 2	16 ± 3[a]	16 ± 3[a]	16 ± 4[a]	16 ± 4[a]	16 ± 4[a]
II	SBP	124 ± 20	111 ± 19[a]	110 ± 19[a]	112 ± 20[a]	115 ± 20[a]	117 ± 22[a]
	DBP	70 ± 11	64 ± 11[a]	64 ± 11[a]	65 ± 12[a]	68 ± 13	70 ± 14
	HR	73 ± 14	67 ± 12[a]	69 ± 15[a]	72 ± 16[a]	72 ± 16[a]	73 ± 16[a]
	RR	18 ± 2	16 ± 3[a]	15 ± 3[a]	15 ± 3[a]	15 ± 2[a]	15 ± 2[a]
III	SBP	123 ± 16	117 ± 21[a]	107 ± 18[a]	99 ± 18[a]	105 ± 19[a]	106 ± 18[a]
	DBP	72 ± 12	70 ± 14	75 ± 13[a]	73 ± 12[a]	74 ± 12[a]	76 ± 12[a]
	HR	81 ± 15	72 ± 13[a]	73 ± 13[a]	75 ± 13[a]	74 ± 13[a]	75 ± 13[a]
	RR	18 ± 3	16 ± 3[a]	15 ± 3[a]	15 ± 3[a]	15 ± 3[a]	15 ± 3[a]

[a]$P < 0.05$ vs. T_0; all $P > 0.05$ among the three groups for all parameters at all time points. n = 50/group

sedation. Remifentanil is a new type of short-acting μ opioid receptor agonist. Wilhelm et al. [21] reported that after remifentanil anesthesia, the patients could be waked up faster, and the orientation was recovered faster. Neurocognitive tests showed that it was better than fentanyl, which was more suitable for short outpatient surgery. Therefore, in this study, dexmedetomidine and remifentanil were used for painless colonoscopy. This combination has been reported before for colonoscopy [13], but the exact dose of dexmedetomidine has not been examined within the same trial.

The recommended dose of dexmedetomidine for general anesthesia is a loading dose not exceeding 1 $\mu g \cdot kg^{-1}$. Due to the synergistic effect with remifentanil, the present study examined three doses (0.2, 0.3, and 0.4 $\mu g \cdot kg^{-1}$) combined with remifentanil 1–2 $\mu g \cdot kg^{-1}$ and 0.1 $\mu g \cdot kg^{-1} \cdot min^{-1}$ maintenance dose [22]. Remifentanil at a rate of 0.1 ± 0.05 $\mu g \cdot kg^{-1} \cdot min^{-1}$ did not affect ventilation and wakefulness [23]. Therefore, in this study, the loading dose of remifentanil was 1 $\mu g \cdot kg^{-1}$, and the maintenance dose was 0.1 $\mu g \cdot kg^{-1} \cdot min^{-1}$. After remifentanil was given at a loading dose, the time to peak efficacy was 1.6 min [24]. Therefore, colonoscopy

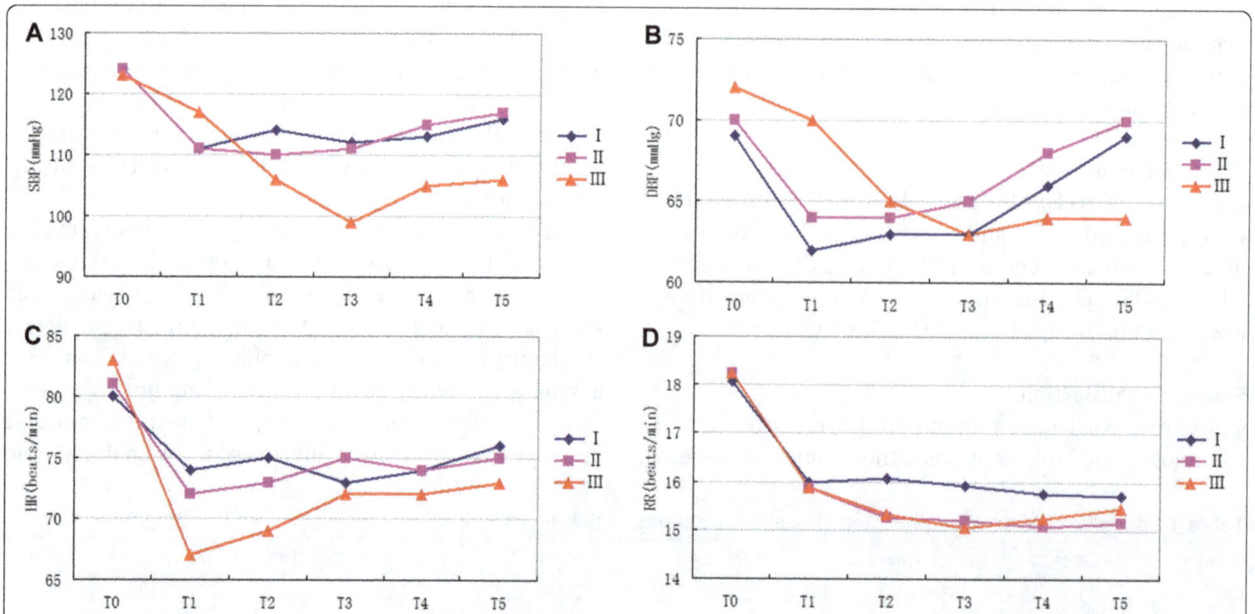

Fig. 2 A: Changes of SBP of three groups of patients. **B:** Fig. 2 Changes of DBP of three groups of patients. **C:** Fig. 3 Changes of HR of three groups of patients. **D:** Fig. 4 Changes of RR of three groups of patients

Table 3 Comparison of the analgesic effect and occurrence of adverse events in the three groups

Items	Group I	Group II	Group III
Slight body movement	13	6^{a}	3^{ab}
Severe body movement	2	0	0
Could be awaked up	50	50	50
Could change position independently (patients need change position)	8 (8)	11 (11)	8 (9)
Bradycardia	0	1^{a}	6^{ab}
Hypotension	0	0	0
Nausea and vomiting	1	1	2

$^{a}P < 0.05$ vs. group I; $^{b}P < 0.05$ vs. group II
n = 50/group

started 2 min after the administration of remifentanil, and dexmedetomidine also began to have effect at this time since, after dexmedetomidine infusion, the rapid distribution-related half-life is about 6 min [25].

The results of the present study showed that only two patients in group I had body movements that interfered with the examination, but the examination could be completed after the addition of propofol. Both groups II and III achieved satisfactory analgesic effects, and the patients were quiet, with no or only mild body movements, which showed that dexmedetomidine combined with remifentanil was effective for analgesia during colonoscopy. The SBP, HR, and RR of the participants during the examination in the three groups were lower than before surgery. During the examinations, the minimum BIS value in the three groups was about 73, and all patients could wake up at any time. Except for one patient in group III who needed assistance for turning over, they could turn over on their own and cooperate to change the position. At the end of the examination, the rate of excellent and good anesthesia for groups II and III reached 100%. This showed that dexmedetomidine combined with remifentanil was suitable for colonoscopy.

During the examination and after the operation, no hypotension occurred in the three groups, and the occurrence of nausea and vomiting was low, but the occurrence rate of bradycardia in group III was higher than that in groups I and II. Dexmedetomidine is a highly

Table 4 Comparison of the BIS values at different time points among the three groups

Group	T_0	T_1	T_2	Minimum value
I	95.1 ± 5.3	91.5 ± 8.2^{a}	93.4 ± 7.2^{a}	86.7 ± 7.5^{a}
II	96.4 ± 2.2	92.4 ± 7.3^{a}	92.5 ± 6.7^{a}	84.4 ± 8.1^{a}
III	97.2 ± 2.4	92.2 ± 8.5^{a}	88.3 ± 9.2^{a}	74.5 ± 8.3^{abc}

$^{a}P < 0.05$ vs. T_0; $^{b}P < 0.05$ vs. group I; $^{c}P < 0.05$ vs. group II
n = 50/group

Table 5 Comparison of the satisfaction degree to the anesthesia effect of the surgeon among the three groups ($n = 50$)

Group	Excellent	Good	Poor
I	35	13	2
II	44^{a}	6^{a}	0^{a}
III	47^{a}	3^{a}	0^{a}

$^{a}P < 0.05$ vs. group I
n = 50/group

selective α2 receptor agonist, which activates postsynaptic α2 receptors in the central nervous system and simultaneously inhibits sympathetic nerve activity, causing lower blood pressure and heart rate.

During the examination, the minimum BIS value in groups I and II were decreased to about 86, and the minimum BIS value in group III was about 73. When all patients were waked up or talked to, the BIS value could return to more than 90. Except for one participant in group III who needed assistance, all the other patients were able to cooperate with the examiner to turn over the body on their own, and most patients did not experience any discomfort. It indicated that dexmedetomidine 0.2–0.4 $\mu g \cdot kg^{-1}$ could produce good sedation, which was consistent with the results of Souter et al. [26]. Nevertheless, the minimum BIS value in group III was lower than those in the other two groups, suggesting that 0.4 $\mu g \cdot kg^{-1}$ dexmedetomidine combined with remifentanil had a risk of deeper sedation when used for colonoscopy.

This trial has limitations. It was performed at a single center. There was no control group. Only three doses of dexmedetomidine were tested, without changes in the dose of remifentanil. Finally, besides BIS, no objective score was used.

Conclusions

In conclusion, 0.3 $\mu g \cdot kg^{-1}$ dexmedetomidine combined with remifentanil (loading dose of 1 $\mu g \cdot kg^{-1}$, maintenance dose of 0.1 $\mu g \cdot kg^{-1} \cdot min^{-1}$) had a good effect, and few adverse reactions for colonoscopy.

Abbreviations
DEX: Dexmedetomidine; SBP: Systolic blood pressure; DBP: Diastolic blood pressure; HR: Heart rate; SpO2: Pulse oximetry; RR: Respiratory rate; BIS: Bispectral index

Acknowledgments
Not applicable.

Authors' contributions
JL helped with study concept and design, acquisition of subjects and data, analysis and interpretation of data, and preparation of manuscript. XM helped with acquisition of subjects and data, analysis and preparation of manuscript. ZJ helped with acquisition of subjects and data and preparation of manuscript. GJ helped with study concept and design and preparation of manuscript. TT helped with acquisition of subjects and preparation of manuscript. XY helped with study concept and design, and interpretation of

data, and preparation of manuscript. The authors read and approved the final manuscript.

References

1. Rex DK, Boland CR, Dominitz JA, Giardiello FM, Johnson DA, Kaltenbach T, et al. Colorectal cancer screening: recommendations for physicians and patients from the U.S. multi-society task force on colorectal cancer. Gastroenterology. 2017;153(1):307–23. https://doi.org/10.1053/j.gastro.2017.05.013.
2. Wolf AMD, Fontham ETH, Church TR, Flowers CR, Guerra CE, LaMonte SJ, et al. Colorectal cancer screening for average-risk adults: 2018 guideline update from the american cancer society. CA Cancer J Clin. 2018;68(4):250–81. https://doi.org/10.3322/caac.21457.
3. Meester RG, Doubeni CA, Zauber AG, Goede SL, Levin TR, Corley DA, et al. Public health impact of achieving 80% colorectal cancer screening rates in the United States by 2018. Cancer. 2015;121(13):2281–5. https://doi.org/10.1002/cncr.29336.
4. Fedewa SA, Ma J, Sauer AG, Siegel RL, Smith RA, Wender RC, et al. How many individuals will need to be screened to increase colorectal cancer screening prevalence to 80% by 2018? Cancer. 2015;121(23):4258–65. https://doi.org/10.1002/cncr.29659.
5. Joseph DA, Meester RG, Zauber AG, Manninen DL, Winges L, Dong FB, et al. Colorectal cancer screening: estimated future colonoscopy need and current volume and capacity. Cancer. 2016;122(16):2479–86. https://doi.org/10.1002/cncr.30070.
6. Johnson DA, Barkun AN, Cohen LB, Dominitz JA, Kaltenbach T, Martel M, et al. Optimizing adequacy of bowel cleansing for colonoscopy: recommendations from the us multi-society task force on colorectal cancer. Gastroenterology. 2014;147(4):903–24. https://doi.org/10.1053/j.gastro.2014.07.002.
7. Triantafillidis JK, Merikas E, Nikolakis D, Papalois AE. Sedation in gastrointestinal endoscopy: current issues. World J Gastroenterol. 2013;19(4):463–81. https://doi.org/10.3748/wjg.v19.i4.463.
8. Green SM, Mason KP, Krauss BS. Pulmonary aspiration during procedural sedation: a comprehensive systematic review. Br J Anaesth. 2017;118(3):344–54. https://doi.org/10.1093/bja/aex004.
9. Agrawal D, Marull J, Tian C, Rockey DC. Contrasting perspectives of anesthesiologists and gastroenterologists on the optimal time interval between bowel preparation and endoscopic sedation. Gastroenterol Res Pract. 2015;2015:497176. https://doi.org/10.1155/2015/497176.
10. Cormack JR, Orme RM, Costello TG. The role of alpha2-agonists in neurosurgery. J Clin Neurosci. 2005;12(4):375–8. https://doi.org/10.1016/j.jocn.2004.06.008.
11. Pasin L, Greco T, Feltracco P, Vittorio A, Neto CN, Cabrini L, et al. Dexmedetomidine as a sedative agent in critically ill patients: a meta-analysis of randomized controlled trials. PLoS One. 2013;8(12):e82913. https://doi.org/10.1371/journal.pone.0082913.
12. Dere K, Sucullu I, Budak ET, Yeyen S, Filiz AI, Ozkan S, et al. A comparison of dexmedetomidine versus midazolam for sedation, pain and hemodynamic control, during colonoscopy under conscious sedation. Eur J Anaesthesiol. 2010;27(7):648–52. https://doi.org/10.1097/EJA.0b013e3283347bfe.
13. Nishizawa T, Suzuki H, Hosoe N, Ogata H, Kanai T, Yahagi N. Dexmedetomidine vs propofol for gastrointestinal endoscopy: a meta-analysis. United European Gastroenterol J. 2017;5(7):1037–45. https://doi.org/10.1177/2050640616688140.
14. Amri P, Nahrini S, Hajian-Tilaki K, Hamidian M, Alipour SF, Hamidi SH, et al. Analgesic effect and hemodynamic changes due to dexmedetomidine versus fentanyl during elective colonoscopy: a double-blind randomized clinical trial. Anesth Pain Med. 2018;8(6):e81077. https://doi.org/10.5812/aapm.81077.
15. Edokpolo LU, Mastriano DJ, Serafin J, Weedon JC, Siddiqui MT, Dimaculangan DP. Discharge readiness after propofol with or without dexmedetomidine for colonoscopy: a randomized controlled trial. Anesthesiology. 2019;131(2):279–86. https://doi.org/10.1097/ALN.0000000000002809.
16. Yildiz M, Tavlan A, Tuncer S, Reisli R, Yosunkaya A, Otelcioglu S. Effect of dexmedetomidine on haemodynamic responses to laryngoscopy and intubation : perioperative haemodynamics and anaesthetic requirements. Drugs R D. 2006;7(1):43–52. https://doi.org/10.2165/00126839-200607010-00004.
17. Bekker AY, Basile J, Gold M, Riles T, Adelman M, Cuff G, et al. Dexmedetomidine for awake carotid endarterectomy: efficacy, hemodynamic profile, and side effects. J Neurosurg Anesthesiol. 2004;16(2):126–35. https://doi.org/10.1097/00008506-200404000-00004.
18. Ramsay MA, Luterman DL. Dexmedetomidine as a total intravenous anesthetic agent. Anesthesiology. 2004;101(3):787–90. https://doi.org/10.1097/00000542-200409000-00028.
19. Cortinez LI, Hsu YW, Sum-Ping ST, Young C, Keifer JC, Macleod D, et al. Dexmedetomidine pharmacodynamics: part ii: crossover comparison of the analgesic effect of dexmedetomidine and remifentanil in healthy volunteers. Anesthesiology. 2004;101(5):1077–83. https://doi.org/10.1097/00000542-200411000-00006.
20. Liu Y, Liang F, Liu X, Shao X, Jiang N, Gan X. Dexmedetomidine reduces perioperative opioid consumption and postoperative pain intensity in neurosurgery: a meta-analysis. J Neurosurg Anesthesiol. 2018;30(2):146–55. https://doi.org/10.1097/ANA.0000000000000403.
21. Wilhelm W, Schlaich N, Harrer J, Kleinschmidt S, Muller M, Larsen R. Recovery and neurological examination after remifentanil-desflurane or fentanyl-desflurane anaesthesia for carotid artery surgery. Br J Anaesth. 2001;86(1):44–9. https://doi.org/10.1093/bja/86.1.44.
22. Bailey PL, Egan TD, Stanley TH. Intravenous opioid anesthetics. In: Miller RD, editor. Anesthesia. 5th ed. Philadelphia: Churchill Livingstone; 2001.
23. Zhao G, Yin X, Li Y, Shao J. Continuous postoperative infusion of remifentanil inhibits the stress responses to tracheal extubation of patients under general anesthesia. J Pain Res. 2017;10:933–9. https://doi.org/10.2147/JPR.S123423.
24. Glass PS, Hardman D, Kamiyama Y, Quill TJ, Marton G, Donn KH, et al. Preliminary pharmacokinetics and pharmacodynamics of an ultra-short-acting opioid: Remifentanil (gi87084b). Anesth Analg. 1993;77(5):1031–40. https://doi.org/10.1213/00000539-199311000-00028.
25. Ebert TJ, Hall JE, Barney JA, Uhrich TD, Colinco MD. The effects of increasing plasma concentrations of dexmedetomidine in humans. Anesthesiology. 2000;93(2):382–94. https://doi.org/10.1097/00000542-200008000-00016.
26. Souter MJ, Rozet I, Ojemann JG, Souter KJ, Holmes MD, Lee L, et al. Dexmedetomidine sedation during awake craniotomy for seizure resection: effects on electrocorticography. J Neurosurg Anesthesiol. 2007;19(1):38–44. https://doi.org/10.1097/01.ana.0000211027.26550.24.

15

Comparative evaluation of epidural bupivacaine alone and bupivacaine combined with magnesium sulfate in providing postoperative analgesia

Li-Qin Li[1], Mei-Dan Fang[2], Cong Wang[3], Hong-Liu Lu[2], Li-Xue Wang[2], Hong-Yu Xu[2] and Hou-Zhong Zhang[2*]

Abstract

Background: The comparative efficacy of epidural bupivacaine alone and bupivacaine combined with magnesium sulfate in providing postoperative analgesia remains controversial.

Methods: We searched Mediline (OvidSP), EMBASE (OvidSP) and Cochrane Central Register of Controlled Trials (CENTRAL) to identify trials that compared epidural bupivacaine and magnesium sulfate combination (intervention) with bupivacaine alone (control). Grading of Recommendations, Assessment, Development and Evaluations (GRADE) framework was used to assess the quality of evidence.

Results: Eleven studies fulfilled our inclusion criteria after screening. We found that epidural bupivacaine combined with magnesium sulfate could prolong the time for first rescue analgesics (SMD 4.96; 95% CI [2.75, 7.17], $P <$ 0.00001, $I^2 = 98\%$), reduce the number of patients who need rescue analgesics (RR 0.38; 95% CI [0.20, 0.74], $P =$ 0.004, $I^2 = 75\%$) and requirement for rescue analgesics (SMD -2.65; 95% CI [− 4.23, − 1.06], $P = 0.001$, $I^2 = 96\%$).

Conclusions: Magnesium suifate as an adjuvant of epidural bupivacaine improved postoperative analgesia. However, we rated the quality of evidence to be very low because of high heterogeneity, imprecise of results and small sample sizes. Furthermore, further large high-quality trials are still needed to confirm the effects of magnesium sulfate on postoperative analgesia.

Keywords: Magnesium sulfate, Postoperative analgesia, Epidural anesthesia, Bupivacaine

Background

Alleviation of postoperative pain is an important objective for the anesthesiologists. Inadequaten postoperative pain control is associated with deep vein thrombosis and pulmonary embolism, quality-of-life impairment, delayed recovery time and higher health-care costs [1, 2]. Epidural anaesthesia is an effective technique, with the advantage of safety, efficiency and prolonged postoperative pain relief [3]. A number of adjuvants have been used with bupivacaine via epidural route over the years with the purpose of prolonging the duration of postoperative analgesia and minimising the side effects. Nevertheless researchers continue to find the optimum adjuvants, as the currently researched adjuvants (e.g. opioids, tramadol, dexmedetomidine) still have some adverse effects such as nausea and vomiting, pruritus, bradycardia, and hypotension [4–6].

Magnesium is the fourth most plentiful cation in the body and possess certain analgesic property in both animal and human models of pain [7, 8]. Magnesium ion ($Mg2+$) is a non-competitive N-methyl-D-aspartate (NMDA) receptor antagonist that blocks inward current flow through ion channels linked to NMDA receptors in a voltage-dependent fashion, has the potential to prevent central sensitization induced by peripheral nociceptive

* Correspondence: 2994266687@qq.com
[2]Department of Anesthesiology, Jilin University Second Hospital, No. 218 Ziqiang street, Changchun, Jilin 130021, People's Republic of China

stimulation. For these reasons, it seems plausible that magnesium as an adjuvant of epidural bupivacaine can prolong postoperative analgesia and reduce side effects. Therefore we conducted this meta-analysis to test our hypothesis.

Materials and methods

For this meta-analysis, we followed the recommendation with Preferred Reporting Items for Systematic Reviews and Meta-Analyses (PRISMA) guidelines [9], and the quality of the evidence was assessed using the GRADE approach and recommendations from the Cochrane Collaboration [10].

Eligibility and exclusion criteria

The purpose of this meta-analysis was to evaluate the safety and efficacy of magnesium sulfate as an adjuvant of epidural bupivacaine. Studies will be included if they meet the following criteria: (1) randomized controlled trials (RCTs); (2) adults (≥18 years old); (3) comparing the analgesic efficacy of epidural bupivacaine and magnesium sulfate combination (intervention), with bupivacaine alone (control) for anesthesia or postoperative pain management; (4) study provided data at least on one of the outcomes (time to the first rescue analgesia, number of patients required rescue analgesia, requirement for rescue analgesia, duration of motor block, and side effects); (5) full text published in English. We excluded studies in which another drug (eg.fentanyl, morphine) was added in the intervention or control group, and magnesium sulfate was administered by another route (e.g. intrathecal, intravenous or intramuscular).

Endpoints

Primary outcomes: (1) the time to the first request for rescue analgesics; (2) the number of patients required postoperative rescue analgesics; (3) requirement for rescue analgesics. Secondary outcomes: (1) duration of motor block; (2) adverse events related to postoperative analgesia protocols (the incidence of hypotension, bradycardia, nausea and vomiting, pruritus, shivering).

Search strategy and study selection

We searched Mediline (OvidSP), EMBASE (OvidSP) and Cochrane Central Register of Controlled Trials (CENTRAL) on october 24, 2019 in order to identify trials that compared epidural bupivacaine and magnesium sulfate combination (intervention) with bupivacaine alone (control). The exact search strategies are shown in Appendix 1. After importing the search results into EndNote X9, duplicated studies were excluded. Two investigators (Li and Wang) independently determined eligibility on the basis of the title, abstract and full text according to the inclusion and exclusion criteria, with disagreements resolved by discussion and consensus with a third agent (Fang).

Data extraction and quality assessment

Two review authors (Li and Wang), independently extracted data using a predesigned form and verified for consensus before entry into Review Manager 5.0. Li and Wang independently assessed the risk of bias for each included study using the criteria outlined in the Cochrane Handbook for Systematic Reviews of Interventions [11]. We rated the overall risk of bias of a study as low if ≦1 domain were 'high risk' or 'unclear', high if two or more of the domains were identified as 'high risk' or 'unclear'. Resolving any disagreements by discussion and consensus with a third reviewer (Fang).

Statistical analysis

We used the software Review Manager 5.0 for statistical analysis. Only primary and secondary outcomes defined previously were included in our analysis. For continuous data (e.g. the time to the first request for rescue analgesics, requirement for rescue analgesics and duration of motor block), considering the different modes of postoperative pain management and species of rescue analgesics, we calculated standardized mean differences (SMDs) with corresponding 95% confidence intervals (95% CI). We rated the effect size of SMDs as small effect (0.2–0.5), medium effect (0.5–0.8) and large effect (≥0.8). For those studies that did not report a mean and standard deviation (SD), we did not hand and transformate the date, because we did not know if it was normally distributed. We calculated risk ratios (RR) with corresponding 95% CI for dichotomous outcomes (e.g. the number of patients required postoperative rescue analgesics, adverse events related to postoperative analgesia protocols).

Assessment of heterogeneity and subgroup analysis

We assessed statistical heterogeneity using the I^2 statistic, as described in the Cochrane Handbook for Systematic Reviews of Interventions [11], and an I^2 value > 50% is considered to indicate substantial heterogeneity. To explore the sources of clinical heterogeneity, we planned to perform subgroup analyses of bolus injection versus bolus followed a continuous injection according to the administration of magnesium sulfate. We used a randomized-effect model if there was significant heterogeneity among studies ($I^2 > 50\%$), otherwise the fixed effects model was used. A P-value < 0.05 and the 95% CI did not cross the equivalent line were considered statistically significant differences from control.

Sensitivity analysis and assessment of publication bias

We decided to perform sensitivity analyses for the primary outcomes by removing studies with high risk of of bias or using two different models (the randomized effect model and the fixed effect model). If sufficient studies (10 or more) were included for the primary or second outcomes, we had intended to use a funnel plot to explore the possibility of publication bias.

Results

Study selection and characteristics of included studies

The literature search identified 4392 studies totally and 112 references from CENTRAL, 2481 references from MEDLINE (OvidSP), and 1799 studies from Embase (Ovidsp). Eleven studies fulfilled our inclusion criteria after screening [12–22]. The details of retrieval was shown in Fig. 1. The various characteristics of the included studies were shown in Table 1. Seven trials applied magnesium sulfate as a bolus followed by a continuous infusion [12–18], while the remaining four trials applied a bolus injection [19–22]. In eight studies enrolled participants undergoing Lower abdominal or lower limb surgeries [12, 13, 15, 17–20, 22], with participants administered epidural anesthesia. Participants in Mohammad 2015 and Radwan 2017 underwent unilateral thoracic surgery and spine surgery respectively with general plus epidural anesthesia. Two studies enrolled participants undergoing cesarean section, with participants in Sun 2012 administered combines spinal epidural anesthesia, and participants in Elsharkawy 2018 administered epidural anesthesia. Total enrollment ranged from 40 to 100 participants, with the number of participants in each study epidural bupivacaine and magnesium sulfate combination ranging from 20 to 50, control 20 to 50.

Risk of Bias of the included trials

Fig. 2 and Fig. 3 presents the risk of bias of the included studies. We assessed 3 of these trials as low risk of bias [12, 13, 16], while the remaining 8 trials as high risk of bias according to our pre-specified criteria [14, 15, 17–22].

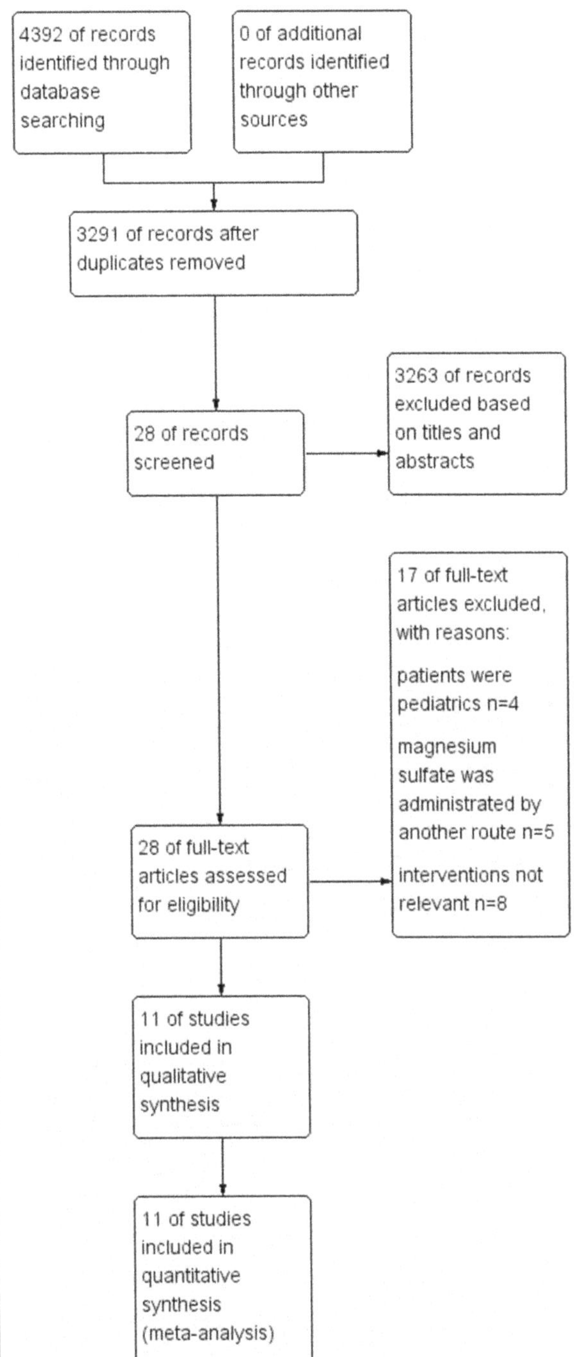

Fig. 1 The details of retrieval

Primary outcome: the time to the first request for rescue analgesics

Nine studies reported the time to the first request for rescue analgesics, in which the data of six studies were reported as mean ± standard deviation (SD) [12–15, 17, 20], while the remaining two studies reported the data in fig [16, 19, 22].. As a result, only six studies involving 400 patients were included for analysis [12–15, 17, 20]. The meta-analysis showed that the time to the first request for rescue analgesics was prolonged significantly in the magnesium sulfate group compared with the control group (SMD 4.96; 95% CI [2.75, 7.17], $P < 0.00001$, $I^2 = 98\%$; Fig. 4). We deemed the quality of the evidence to be very low because: (1) four studies had 'high' risk of bias; (2) the

Table 1 Characteristics of included trials

Study	Patients (MgSO4/ control)	Surgery	Anesth-esia strateg-y	Intervention	Control	Postoperative analgesia
Aly 2011	30/30	Orthoped-ic surgeries	EA	bupivacaine 0.5% + 50 mg magnesium sulphate (MgSO4) in 10 ml as an initial bolus dose followed by infusion of 10 mg/ h (2 ml/h) during the surgery.	N/S in same volume	When surgery was completed, all patients received PCEA using a PCEA device containing fentanyl 2 µg/ml and bupivacaine 0.03% (0.3 mg/ml). The PCEA was programmed to deliver 2.5 ml/h infusion with a bolus dose of 1.5 ml on demand. The lockout interval between boluses was 6 min. If patients had inadequate analgesia, supplementary rescue analgesia with intramuscular pethidine 50 mg was available.
Daabiss 2013	40/40	Total knee replacem-ent surgery	EA	Bupivacaine 0.5% + 50 mg magnesium sulphate (MgSO4) in 10 ml as an initial bolus dose followed by infusion of 10 mg/h (diluted in 10 ml saline) during the surgery.	N/S in same volume	When surgery was complete, all patients received PCEA using a PCEA device containing fentanyl 2 µg/ml and bupivacaine 0.08%. The PCEA was programmed to administer a demand bolus dose of fentanyl 5 ml with no background infusion and lockout interval 20 min. If patients had inadequate analgesia, supplementary rescue analgesia with intramuscular pethidine 50 mg was available.
Elshark-awy 2018	30/30	Cesarean section	EA	Epidural 20 ml levobupivacaine hydrochloride 0.5% followed by 5 ml of 10% preservative-free MgSO4(500 mg) prepared in two separate syringes	N/S in same volume	If the recorded VAS was ≥3, the patient was given diclofenac potassium 75 mg oral tablets as the first rescue analgesia every 12 h. If the VAS was still > 3 within 30 min, patients were given incremental dose of 0.5 µg/kg fentanyl.
Ghatak 2010	30/30	Lower abdomina-l and lower limb surgeries	EA	Bupivacaine 0.5% (19 ml) + magnesium sulphate 50 mg (in 1 ml 0.9% saline)	N/S in same volume	In the event of pain, (VAS ≥40), both intraoperatively as well as postoperatively, a bolus of epidural bupivacaine 0.25% (8 ml) was administered by the anaesthesiologist inside the operation theatre and the nursing staff in the recovery room
Gupta 2013	30/30	Total abdomina-l hysterectomies	EA	1 ml of 50 mg/ml magnesium sulphate in 10 ml epidural anaesthetic solution (9 ml 0.125% bupivacaine)	N/S in same volume	If patients had inadequate analgesia (VAS > 3), epidural fentanyl 1mcg/kg in 10 ml normal saline was administered as supplementary rescue analgesic.
Moham-mad 2015	20/20	Unilatera-l thoracic surgery	GA + EA	Toward the end of the surgery, approximately 20 min prior to anticipated extubation. Bupivacaine 0.25% 8 ml + magnesium sulfate 50 mg in 1 ml 0.9% saline.	N/S in same volume	Epidural infusion with 5 ml/h of 0.1% bupivacaine was started 15 min after the bolus dose, and it was continued during the postoperative period via epidural catheter using an infusion pump. Patients complaining of pain in the postoperative period with VAS score ≥ 4, received tramadol 50 mg IV as rescue analgesia and time to the first request for analgesia was noted.
Omar 2018	50/50	Infraumb-ilical abdomina-l and pelvic surgeries	EA	15 ml mixture of 14 ml levobupivacaine 0.5% + 0.5 ml MgSO410% (50 mg) + 0.5 ml of 0.9 NaCl in epidural catheter at induction then continuous epidural infusion of this mixture by 5 ml/h till the end of the surgery	N/S in same volume	If patients had inadequate analgesia (i.e.,: if VAS ≥4 when measured each hour or if patient expressed intolerable pain in between VAS measurements periods) supplementary rescue analgesic was used, pethidine 1 mg/kg i/m/and paracetamol (Perfalgan®) 1 g i.v. drip.
Radwan 2017	22/22	Spine surgeries	GA + EA	14 ml levobupivacaine 0.5% + 50 mg magnesium sulphate in 1 ml saline. Subsequently continuous epidural infusion of levobupivacaine 0.125% + 2 mg/ml magnesium sulphate. Drugs were prepared in 20 cc syringe and the rate of infusion in each group was 5 ml/h.	N/S in same volume	One gram of iv paracetamol was given to the patients when VAS > 3 and every 8 h thereafter. A second rescue analgesic in the form of 50 mg iv meperidine was given to patients if VAS remained > 3 one hour after iv paracetamol.

Table 1 Characteristics of included trials *(Continued)*

Study	Patients (MgSO4/ control)	Surgery	Anesth-esia strateg-y	Intervention	Control	Postoperative analgesia
Shruthi 2016	20/20	Infraumb-ilical surgery	EA	15 ml of bupivacaine 0.5% + 50 mg of magnesium sulphate (MgSO4) made up to 1 ml.	N/S in same volume	Postoperative analgesia was managed with epidural bolus of bupivacaine 0.125% 8 ml boluses and/or Paracetamol 1 g infusion as per discretion of treating consultants.
Shahi 2014	40/40	Lower limb surgery	EA	Bupivacaine 0.5% (14 ml) + magnesium sulfate 50 mg (in 1 ml 0.9% saline)	N/S in same volume	In the event of pain, (VAS ≥40), both intraoperatively as well as postoperatively, a bolus of epidural bupivacaine 0.125% (12 ml) was administered by the anesthesiologist inside the operation theatre and the nursing staff in the recovery room.
Sun 2012	50/50	Cesarean section	CSEA	After delivery of the fetus, received 0.1% bupivacaine 10 mL and Mg 500 mg.	Nothing added	Postoperatively, oral diclofenac 12.5 mg was given for rescue analgesia whenever the VAS pain score was > 3 cm

***CSEA* Combines spinal epidural anesthesia, *EA* Epidural anesthesia, *GA* General anesthesia, *N/S* Normal saline, *VAS* Visual analogue scale**

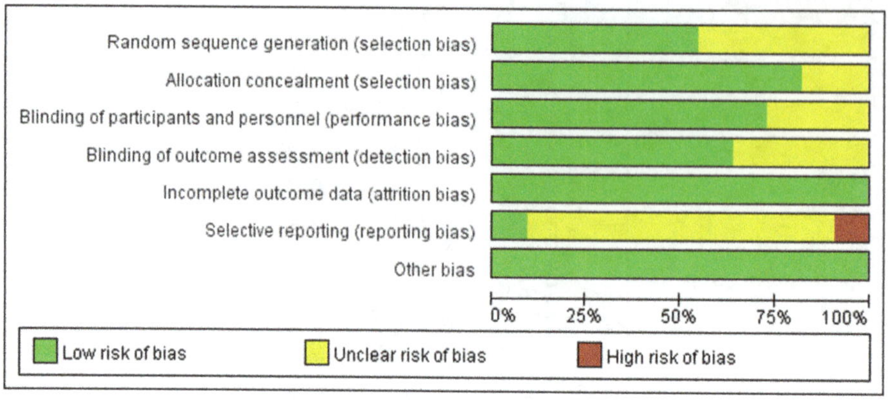

Fig. 2 Risk of bias graph. Review authors' judgements about each risk of bias item presented as percentages across all included studies

result was imprecise (wide confidence interval); and (3) there was significant heterogeneity among studies.

Subgroup analysis was conducted according to the administration of magnesium sulfate. Five studies administrated magnesium sulfate by bolus injection [12–15, 17], and only one study by bolus followed a continuous injection [20]. We noted the time to the first request for rescue analgesics was also prolonged significantly in the magnesium sulfate group compared with the control group when the study by bolus followed a continuous injection was excluded (SMD 3.67; 95% CI [1.75, 5.58], $P = 0.0002$, $I^2 = 97\%$). We also found significant difference between the subgroups ($P < 0.0001$) and the bolus followed a continuous injection subgroup had a greater effect on the time to the first rescue analgesics.

Primary outcome: the number of patients required postoperative rescue analgesics

Five studies including 304 patients reported the number of patients required rescue analgesics [12, 16, 18, 19, 21]. The merged effect analysis showed that it was significantly less in magnesium group compared with control group (RR 0.38; 95% CI [0.20, 0.74], $P = 0.004$, $I^2 = 75\%$, Fig. 5). We judged, the quality of the evidence to be very low based on the GRADE framework: (1) three studies had a 'high' risk of bias; (2) there was significant heterogeneity among studies.

Subgroup analysis was conducted according to the administration of magnesium sulfate. Patients required postoperative rescue analgesics was significantly less in magnesium group when magnesium sulfate was administrated by bolus injection (RR 0.49; 95% CI [0.24, 0.97], $P = 0.04$, $I^2 = 70\%$). No significant difference was shown between the two groups when magnesium sulfate was administrated by bolus followed a continuous injection (RR 0.17; 95% CI [0.01, 1.97], $P = 0.16$, $I^2 = 84\%$).

Primary outcome: requirement for rescue analgesics

The requirement for rescue analgesia was reported in five studies involving 300 participants [12, 14, 17, 19, 22]. The meta-analysis showed that the magnesium sulfate group had significantly lower consumption of rescue analgesics than the control group (SMD -2.65; 95% CI [− 4.23, − 1.06], $P = 0.001$, $I^2 = 96\%$; Fig. 6). We rated the quality of the evidence to be very low: (1) four studies had 'high' risk of bias; (2) the result was imprecise; and (3) there was significant heterogeneity among studies.

Subgroup analysis was conducted according to the administration of magnesium sulfate. A significant reduction was shown in the magnesium group when magnesium sulfate was administrated by bolus injection (SMD -2.92; 95% CI [− 5.43, − 0.42], $P = 0.02$, $I^2 = 97\%$). No significant difference was shown between two groups when magnesium sulfate was administrated by bolus followed a continuous injection (SMD -2.31; 95% CI [− 5.26, 0.65], $P = 0.13$, $I^2 = 98\%$).

Secondary outcome: duration of motor block

Two studies reported duration of motor block [12, 15]. The result showed that the duration of motor block in magnesium sulfate group was significantly longer than contol group (SMD 6.29; 95% CI [0.33, 12.24], $P = 0.04$, $I^2 = 97\%$; Fig. 7). We rated the quality of the evidence to be very low: (1) the result was imprecise; (2) there was significant heterogeneity among studies; and (3) limited availability of evidence.

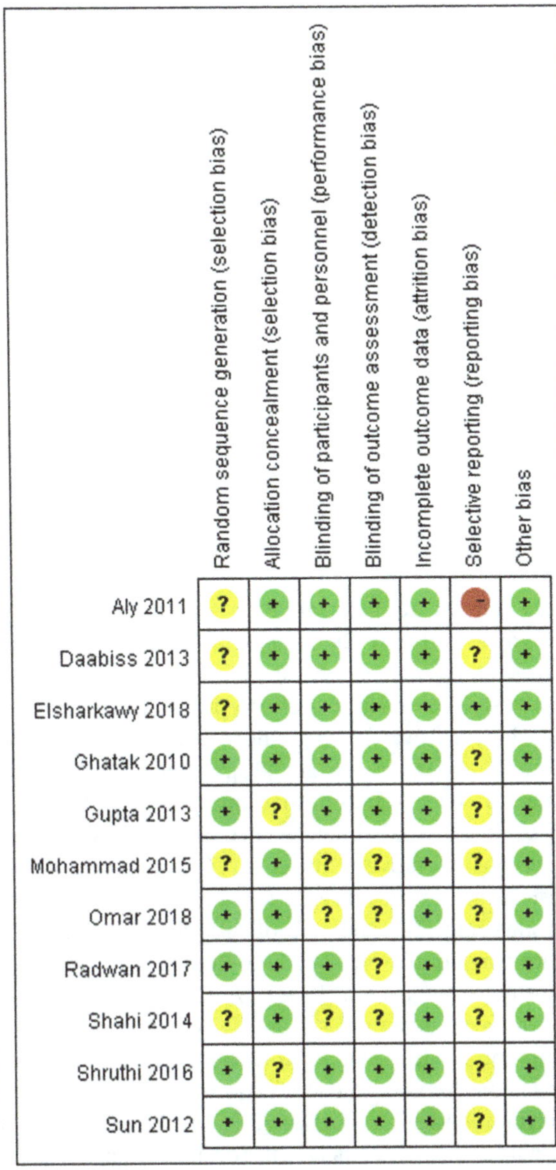

Fig. 3 Risk of bias summary: review authors' judgements about each risk of bias item for each included study

Secondary outcome: adverse events related to postoperative analgesia protocols

A meta-analysis of adverse events was shown in Fig. 8, such as hypotension (RR 0.80; 95% CI [0.64,1.00], $P=0.05$, $I^2=0\%$), bradycardia (RR 0.80; 95% CI [0.47, 1.36], $P=0.41$, $I^2=0\%$), nausea and vomiting (RR 0.57; 95% CI [0.31, 1.06], $P=0.08$, $I^2=0\%$) and pruritus (RR 0.67; 95% CI [0.11, 3.91], $P=0.65$, $I^2=0\%$) showed no statistically significant differences, except that the incidence of shivering in magnesium sulfate group was significantly lower than control group (RR 0.31; 95% CI [0.18, 0.53], $P<0.0001$, $I^2=24\%$). We rated the evidence for adverse events to be moderate quality.

Sensitivity analysis and assessment of publication bias

Based on the prior definition, there were only three studies with a low risk of bias [12, 13, 16], so we did not conduct the sensitivity analysis based on the risk of bias. Sensitivity analyses of primary outcomes using the fixed effect model yielded stable overall results. Consider that each outcome included fewer than 10 studies, there were insufficient data for any publication bias analysis.

Discussion

This meta-analysis aimed to assess the efficacy and safety of magnesium sulfate as an adjuvant in epidural bupivacaine in providing postoperative analgesia. We found that epidural bupivacaine combined with magnesium sulfate could prolong the time for first rescue analgesics. Furthermore, the addition of magnesium sulfate could reduce the number of patients who need rescue analgesics and requirement for rescue analgesics without adverse events. In addition, our meta-analysis showed that the incidence of shivering was lower with bupivacaine-magnesium sulfate than bupivacaine alone. Nevertheless, duration of motor blockade was significantly prolonged in group magnesium sulfate.

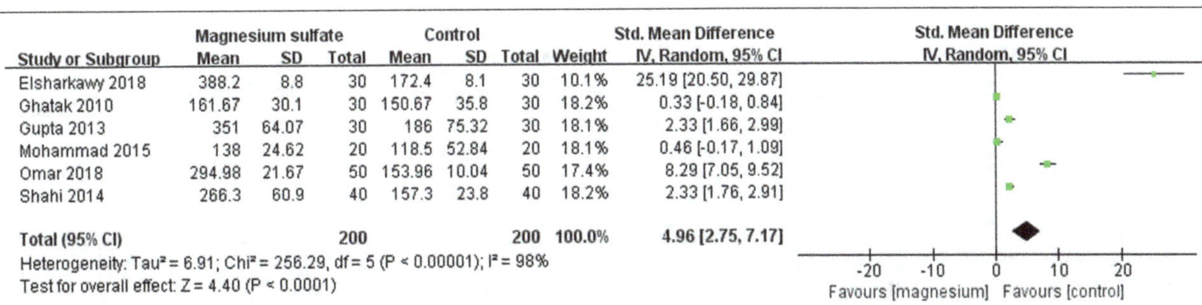

Fig. 4 Forest plot of comparison: Magnesium sulfate vs Control, Outcome: the time to the first request for rescue analgesics

Study or Subgroup	Magnesium sulfate Events	Magnesium sulfate Total	Control Events	Control Total	Weight	Risk Ratio M-H, Random, 95% CI
Aly 2011	9	30	21	30	24.1%	0.43 [0.24, 0.78]
Elsharkawy 2018	4	30	12	30	17.5%	0.33 [0.12, 0.92]
Radwan 2017	1	22	20	22	8.4%	0.05 [0.01, 0.34]
Shruthi 2016	6	20	18	20	22.6%	0.33 [0.17, 0.66]
Sun 2012	24	50	30	50	27.4%	0.80 [0.55, 1.15]
Total (95% CI)		**152**		**152**	**100.0%**	**0.38 [0.20, 0.74]**
Total events	44		101			

Heterogeneity: Tau² = 0.37; Chi² = 16.30, df = 4 (P = 0.003); I² = 75%
Test for overall effect: Z = 2.86 (P = 0.004)

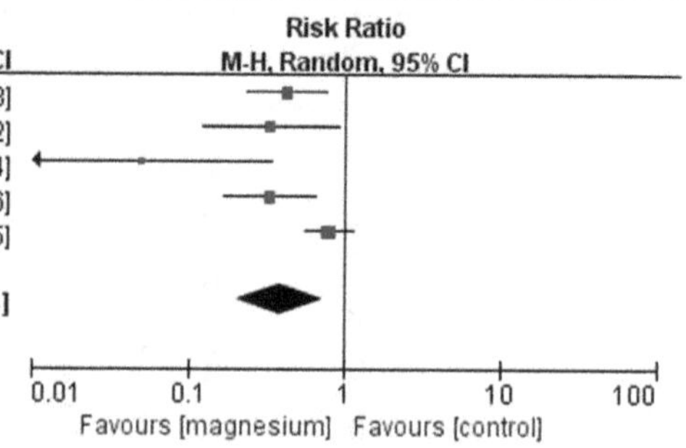

Fig. 5 Forest plot of comparison: Magnesium sulfate vs Control, Outcome: the number of patients required rescue analgesics

We found that many studies did not adequately report randomization methods. Five studies did not describe the generation of random sequences in detail [12, 14, 15, 19, 22], two studies did not describe the methods of allocation concealment [17, 18], three studies did not describe whether the anaesthetists were blind for this study design [14, 15, 20] and four studies did not report in detail their blind assessment of the outcomes [14, 15, 20, 21]. Only one studies reported clinical trials registration [12] and we were not clear about the risk of selective outcome reporting bias. We judged evidence for the time to the first request for rescue analgesics, the number of patients required rescue analgesics, requirement for rescue analgesia and duration of motor block to be very low certainty, and evidence for adverse events to be moderate quality. The low quality of evidence for primary outcomes was largely due to significant heterogeneity among studies and imprecision of the result. The significant heterogeneity might be explained by the differences in the types of surgery performed, the doses and manners of magnesium sulfate administered, and the postoperative pain management models. However, results of subgroup analyses on manners of magnesium administered did not appear to explain heterogeneity and we found that high levels of statistical heterogeneity still remained in both subgroups in each analysis. The surgery types varied between studies to include: cesarean section, unilateral thoracic, spinal, abdominal, orthopaedic. These differences may contribute to inconsistency and reduce the overall applicability of the evidence.

Whether the administrative route is intravenous, epidural, or intrathecal, the actual site of action of magnesium sulfate is probably at the spinal cord NMDA receptors. The analgesic effect primarily depends on Mg2+ blocks inward current flow through ion channels linked to NMDA receptors [23]. Although a previous systematic review found that intravenous administration of magnesium sulfate in orthopedic surgery could reduce postoperative requirement for postoperative analgesics and adverse events such as vomiting, nausea, and shivering [24], the role of intravenous magnesium sulfate was controversial. Some studies had found that intravenous magnesium failed to improve postoperative pain in gastrointestinal surgery [25] and in a pediatric population undergoing tonsillectomy [26]. The reason may be the limited ability of magnesium ions to penetrate the blood-brain barrier [27], so it seems plausible that epidural or intrathecia magnesium might be more effective. An earlier meta-analysis focused on cesarean section revealed that the additional neuraxial magnesium sulfate exerted significant effects on prolonging the duration of neuraxial anesthesia, reducing

Study or Subgroup	Magnesium sulfate Mean	Magnesium sulfate SD	Magnesium sulfate Total	Control Mean	Control SD	Control Total	Weight	Std. Mean Difference IV, Random, 95% CI
Aly 2011	15	26.75	30	36.67	26.04	30	20.6%	-0.81 [-1.34, -0.28]
Daabiss 2013	52.56	9.67	40	92.38	10.91	40	20.1%	-3.83 [-4.57, -3.08]
Elsharkawy 2018	42.55	5.3	30	94.4	9.9	30	18.5%	-6.45 [-7.74, -5.15]
Gupta 2013	119.2	56.24	30	267.2	92.14	30	20.4%	-1.91 [-2.53, -1.30]
Mohammad 2015	100	46.3	20	133.3	55.6	20	20.4%	-0.64 [-1.27, -0.00]
Total (95% CI)			**150**			**150**	**100.0%**	**-2.65 [-4.23, -1.06]**

Heterogeneity: Tau² = 3.10; Chi² = 103.82, df = 4 (P < 0.00001); I² = 96%
Test for overall effect: Z = 3.28 (P = 0.001)

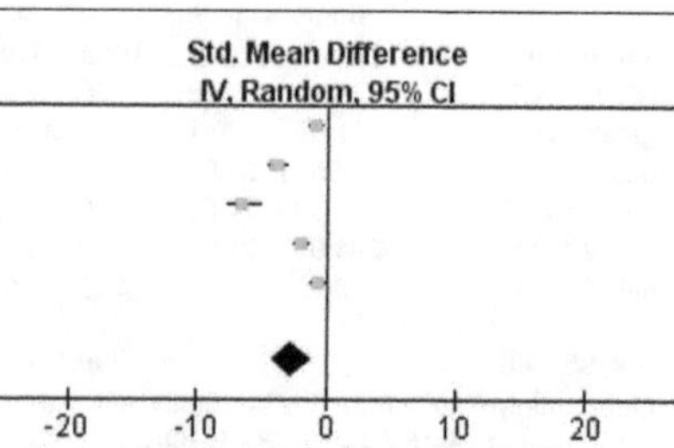

Fig. 6 Forest plot of comparison: Magnesium sulfate vs Control, Outcome: the requirement for rescue analgesia

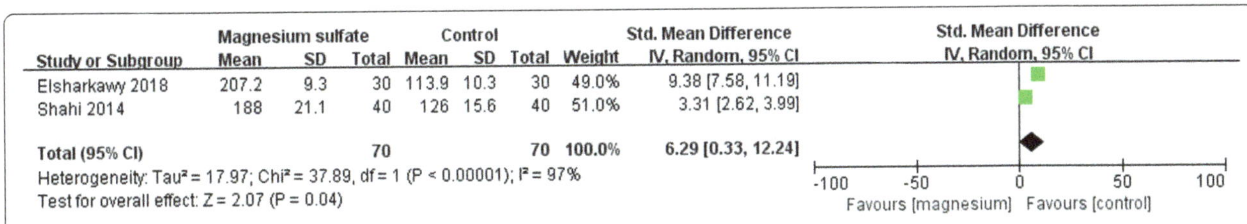

Fig. 7 Forest plot of comparison: Magnesium sulfate vs Control, Outcome: the duration of motor block

postoperative pain scores and decreasing requirement for postoperative analgesics, and was therefore in broad similar to our findings [28]. Furthermore, our findings are similar with the findings in a recent published meta-analysis, where the authors reported a reduction of the need for postoperative rescue analgesics in pediatric when magnesium was added to local anesthetics for caudal anesthesia [29].

In addition, magnesium sulfate has been compared with other epidural adjunct analgesic drugs. One study that evaluated the effects of epidural magnesium sulfate versus dexmedetomidine, and found that the time from epidural medication to first rescue analgesics was longer in dexmedetomidine group, duration of sensory and motor blockade was significantly prolonged in group dexmedetomidine, but risk of sedation increased and there was fall in the mean pulse rate in group dexmedetomidine [15]. Radwan et al. compared magnesium sulfate with fentanyl [21] and Mohammad et al. compared magnesium sulfate with clonidine [14] found the effect of magnesium sulfate on postoperative pain to be comparable to that of the other drugs.

In this meta-analysis, the addition of magnesium sulfate significantly prolonged the duration of motor block. The mechanism might be that magnesium inhibits the motor endplate release of acetylcholine due to inhibition of calcium-dependent channels [30, 31]. As for adverse effects, our meta-analysis showed that the incidence of shivering was lower in magnesium sulfate group. The reason might be that perioperative magnesium supplementation prevented the postoperative hypomagnesaemia and decreased the incidence of postoperative shivering [32].

There are some limitations to this study. Firstly, our meta-analysis demonstrates efficacy of epidural bupivacaine combined with magnesium sulfate when compared with bupivacaine alone in providing postoperative analgesia. Even if It is possible that our findings cannot be interpreted as truly positive because of the small sample sizes and the low quality of evidence assessed by GRADE framework; Secondly, We found that many studies did not adequately report randomization methods; Third, we didn't assess publication bias due to the limited number of studies; Fourth, our findings showed high heterogeneity among studies, especially the existing clinical heterogeneity, such as types of surgery performed, the doses and manners of magnesium sulfate administered, and the postoperative pain management models.

Conclusion

In conclusion, This meta-analysis revealed that magnesium suifate as an adjuvant of epidural bupivacaine improves postoperative analgesia. However, we rated the quality of evidence to be very low because of high heterogeneity, imprecise of results and small sample sizes. Furthermore, further large high-quality trials are still needed to confirm the effects of magnesium sulfate on postoperative analgesia.

Appendix

Search strategy

Cochrane Central Register of Controlled Trials

#1 MeSH descriptor: [Analgesia, Epidural] explode all trees.

#2 MeSH descriptor: [Anesthesia, Epidural] explode all trees.

#3 (epidural* or peridural* or subarachnoid* or extradural* or neuraxial*).

#4 (#1 or #2 or #3).

#5 magnesium OR MgSO4 OR Mg OR MS OR magnesium sulfate or magnesium sulphate.

#6((randomized controlled trial or controlled clinical trial).pt. or randomized.ab. or placebo.ab. or clinical trials as topic.sh. or randomly.ab. or trial.ti.) not (animals not (humans and animals)).sh.

#7 #4 and #5 and #6.

MEDLINE (OvidSP)

1. (Epidural* or peridural* or extradural* or subarachnoid* or neuraxial* or (Anesthesia, Epidural or Analgesia, Epidural)).af.
2. magnesium OR MgSO4 OR Mg OR MS OR magnesium sulfate or magnesium sulphate
3. ((randomized controlled trial or controlled clinical trial).pt. or randomized.ab. or placebo.ab. or clinical

Study or Subgroup	Magnesium sulfate Events	Magnesium sulfate Total	Control Events	Control Total	Weight	Risk Ratio M-H, Fixed, 95% CI
1.5.1 Hypotension						
Aly 2011	4	30	5	30	2.9%	0.80 [0.24, 2.69]
Elsharkawy 2018	8	30	4	30	2.3%	2.00 [0.67, 5.94]
Ghatak 2010	19	30	24	30	13.7%	0.79 [0.57, 1.10]
Shahi 2014	24	40	32	40	18.3%	0.75 [0.56, 1.01]
Shruthi 2016	4	20	8	20	4.6%	0.50 [0.18, 1.40]
Sun 2012	1	50	2	50	1.1%	0.50 [0.05, 5.34]
Subtotal (95% CI)		**200**		**200**	**42.9%**	**0.80 [0.64, 1.00]**
Total events	60		75			
Heterogeneity: Chi² = 3.86, df = 5 (P = 0.57); I² = 0%						
Test for overall effect: Z = 1.94 (P = 0.05)						
1.5.2 Bradycardia						
Aly 2011	2	30	2	30	1.1%	1.00 [0.15, 6.64]
Daabiss 2013	0	40	1	40	0.9%	0.33 [0.01, 7.95]
Ghatak 2010	4	30	6	30	3.4%	0.67 [0.21, 2.13]
Shahi 2014	6	40	8	40	4.6%	0.75 [0.29, 1.97]
Shruthi 2016	6	20	7	20	4.0%	0.86 [0.35, 2.10]
Sun 2012	1	50	0	50	0.3%	3.00 [0.13, 71.92]
Subtotal (95% CI)		**210**		**210**	**14.3%**	**0.80 [0.47, 1.36]**
Total events	19		24			
Heterogeneity: Chi² = 1.15, df = 5 (P = 0.95); I² = 0%						
Test for overall effect: Z = 0.83 (P = 0.41)						
1.5.3 Nausea or vomiting						
Daabiss 2013	1	40	3	40	1.7%	0.33 [0.04, 3.07]
Elsharkawy 2018	1	30	5	30	2.9%	0.20 [0.02, 1.61]
Ghatak 2010	2	30	2	30	1.1%	1.00 [0.15, 6.64]
Omar 2018	3	50	5	50	2.9%	0.60 [0.15, 2.38]
Radwan 2017	0	22	2	22	1.4%	0.20 [0.01, 3.94]
Shahi 2014	3	40	4	40	2.3%	0.75 [0.18, 3.14]
Sun 2012	4	50	4	50	2.3%	1.00 [0.26, 3.78]
Subtotal (95% CI)		**262**		**262**	**14.6%**	**0.57 [0.31, 1.06]**
Total events	14		25			
Heterogeneity: Chi² = 2.84, df = 6 (P = 0.83); I² = 0%						
Test for overall effect: Z = 1.78 (P = 0.08)						
1.5.4 Pruritis						
Elsharkawy 2018	0	30	2	30	1.4%	0.20 [0.01, 4.00]
Radwan 2017	0	22	0	22		Not estimable
Sun 2012	1	50	0	50	0.3%	3.00 [0.13, 71.92]
Subtotal (95% CI)		**102**		**102**	**1.7%**	**0.67 [0.11, 3.91]**
Total events	1		2			
Heterogeneity: Chi² = 1.48, df = 1 (P = 0.22); I² = 33%						
Test for overall effect: Z = 0.45 (P = 0.65)						
1.5.5 Shivering						
Elsharkawy 2018	8	30	17	30	9.7%	0.47 [0.24, 0.92]
Ghatak 2010	0	30	4	30	2.6%	0.11 [0.01, 1.98]
Mohammad 2015	0	20	8	20	4.9%	0.06 [0.00, 0.96]
Shahi 2014	4	40	5	40	2.9%	0.80 [0.23, 2.76]
Shruthi 2016	0	20	5	20	3.1%	0.09 [0.01, 1.54]
Sun 2012	1	50	6	50	3.4%	0.17 [0.02, 1.33]
Subtotal (95% CI)		**190**		**190**	**26.6%**	**0.31 [0.18, 0.53]**
Total events	13		45			
Heterogeneity: Chi² = 6.61, df = 5 (P = 0.25); I² = 24%						
Test for overall effect: Z = 4.28 (P < 0.0001)						
Total (95% CI)		**964**		**964**	**100.0%**	**0.63 [0.52, 0.77]**
Total events	107		171			
Heterogeneity: Chi² = 22.31, df = 26 (P = 0.67); I² = 0%						
Test for overall effect: Z = 4.63 (P < 0.00001)						
Test for subgroup differences: Chi² = 10.85, df = 4 (P = 0.03), I² = 63.1%						

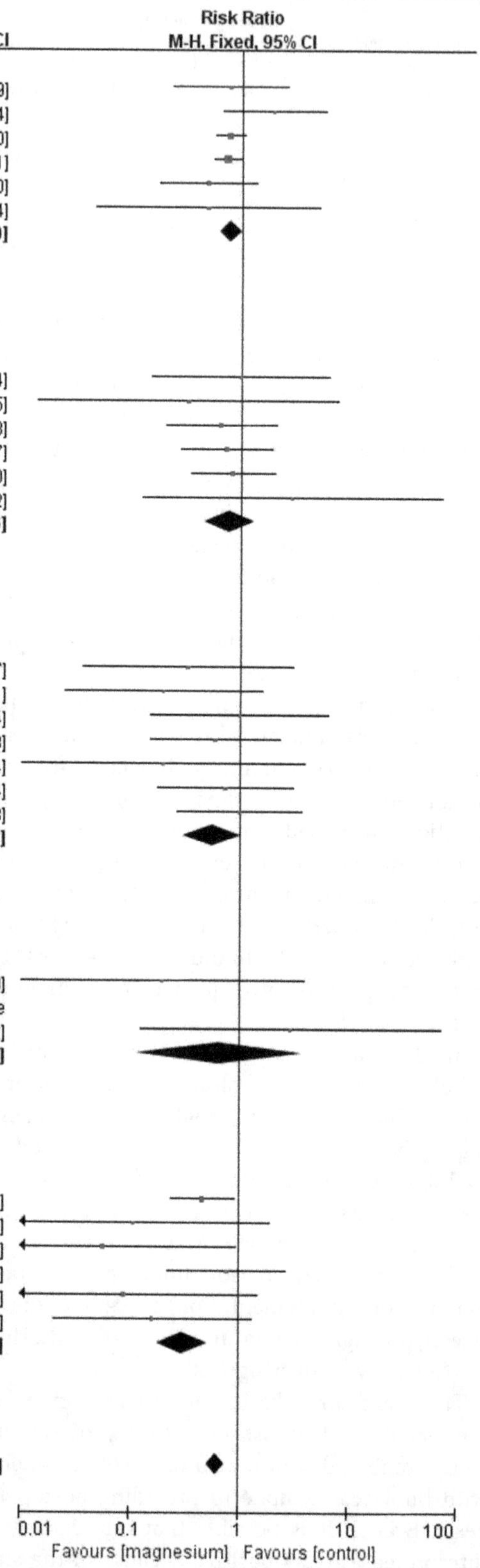

Fig. 8 Forest plot of comparison: Magnesium sulfate vs Control, Outcome:the adverse events

trials as topic.sh. or randomly.ab. or trial.ti.) not (animals not (humans and animals)).sh.
4. 1 and 2 and 3

Embase (OvidSP)

1. (epidural or peridural or extradural or subarachnoid or neuraxial) and (an?esth or analg) or (epidural anesthesia or epidural analgesia)
2. magnesium OR MgSO4 OR Mg OR MS OR magnesium sulfate or magnesium sulphate
3. (placebo.sh. or controlled study.ab. or random*.ti,ab. or trial*.ti,ab. or ((singl* or doubl* or trebl* or tripl*) adj3 (blind* or mask*)).ti,ab.) not (animal not (human and animal)).sh.
4. 1 and 2 and 3

Abbreviations
CI: Confidence intervals; NMDA: N-methyl-D-aspartate; PRISMA: Preferred reporting items for systematic reviews and meta-analyses; RCTs: Randomized controlled trials; RR: Relative risk; SD: Standard deviation; SMDs: Standardized mean differences

Acknowledgements
Not applicable.

Authors' contributions
LLQ participated in the design, collected the data, performed the quality assessment. ZHZ participated in the design and draft the manuscript. WC and FMD collected the data, performed the quality assessment, and helped to draft the manuscript. XHY, LHL, WLX helped to perform statistical analyses and search strategy. All authors read and approved the final manuscript.

Author details
[1]Department of Anesthesiology, Guizhou Provincial People's Hospital, Guiyang, Guizhou, People's Republic of China. [2]Department of Anesthesiology, Jilin University Second Hospital, No. 218 Ziqiang street, Changchun, Jilin 130021, People's Republic of China. [3]Department of Anesthesiology, First Affiliated Hospital to Changchun University of Chinese Medicine, Changchun, Jilin, People's Republic of China.

References
1. Gan TJ. Poorly controlled postoperative pain: prevalence, consequences, and prevention. J Pain Res. 2017;10:2287–98.
2. Joshi GP, Ogunnaike BO. Consequences of inadequate postoperative pain relief and chronic persistent postoperative pain. Anesthesiol Clin North Am. 2005;23(1):21–36.
3. Ng A, Swanevelder J. Pain relief after thoracotomy: is epidural analgesia the optimal technique? Br J Anaesth. 2007;98(2):159–62.
4. Tan X, Shen L, Wang L, et al. Incidence and risk factors for epidural morphine induced pruritus in parturients receiving cesarean section: a prospective multicenter observational study. Medicine (Baltimore). 2019;98(40):e17366.
5. Turkoglu Z, Karacaer F, Biricik E, et al. Comparison of the effects of epidural Levobupivacaine with tramadol or morphine addition on postoperative analgesia following major abdominal surgery. Turk J Anaesthesiol Reanim. 2019;47(4):287–94.
6. Sekhar DP, Kumar L, Kesavan R, et al. Comparison of the analgesic efficacy of a single dose of epidural Dexmedetomidine versus fentanyl as an adjuvant to bupivacaine in abdominal surgery. Anesth Essays Res. 2019;13(3):465–70.
7. Begon S, Pickering G, Eschalier A, et al. Magnesium increases morphine analgesic effect in different experimental models of pain. Anesthesiol. 2002; 96(3):627–32.
8. Kogler J . The analgesic effect of magnesium sulfate in patients undergoing thoracotomy. Acta Clin Croat 2009; 48(1):19–26.
9. Liberati A, Altman DG, Tetzlaff J, et al. The PRISMA statement for reporting systematic reviews and meta-analyses of studies that evaluate healthcare interventions: explanation and elaboration. BMJ. 2009;339:b2700.
10. Guyatt GH, Oxman AD, Vist GE, et al. GRADE: an emerging consensus on rating quality of evidence and strength of recommendations. BMJ. 2008; 336(7650):924–6.
11. Higgins JPT, Green S (editors). Cochrane Handbook for Systematic Reviews of Interventions Version 5.1.0 [updated March 2011]. The Cochrane Collaboration 2011. Available from http://www.cochrane-handbook.org.
12. Elsharkawy RA, Farahat TE, Abdelhafez MS. Analgesic effect of adding magnesium sulfate to epidural levobupivacaine in patients with pre-eclampsia undergoing elective cesarean section. J Anaesthesiol Clin Pharmacol. 2018;34(3):328–34.
13. Ghatak T, Chandra G, Malik A, et al. Evaluation of the effect of magnesium sulphate vs. clonidine as adjunct to epidural bupivacaine. Indian J Anaesth. 2010;54(4):308–13.
14. Mohammad W, Mir SA, Mohammad K, et al. A randomized double-blind study to evaluate efficacy and safety of epidural magnesium sulfate and clonidine as adjuvants to bupivacaine for postthoracotomy pain relief. Anesth Essays Res. 2015;9(1):15–20.
15. Shahi V, Verma AK, Agarwal A, et al. A comparative study of magnesium sulfate vs dexmedetomidine as an adjunct to epidural bupivacaine. J Anaesthesiol Clin Pharmacol. 2014;30(4):538–42.
16. Sun J, Wu X, Xu X, et al. A comparison of epidural magnesium and/or morphine with bupivacaine for postoperative analgesia after cesarean section. Int J Obstet Anesth. 2012;21(4):310–6.
17. Gupta A, Goyal VK, Gupta N, et al. A randomized controlled trial to evaluate the effect of addition of a single dose of epidural magnesium sulphate on the duration of postoperative analgesia in patients undergoing lower abdominal surgeries under epidural anaesthesia. Sri Lankan J Anaesthesiol. 2013;21(1):27–31.
18. Shruthi AH, Sudheesh K, Nethra SS, et al. The effect of a single dose of magnesium Sulphate as an adjuvant to epidural bupivacaine for Infraumbilical surgeries: a prospective double-blind, randomized control trial. Middle East J Anesthesiol. 2016;23(4):449–55.
19. Aly Kandil AH, Hammad RAEA, Shafei MAE, et al. Preemptive use of epidural magnesium sulphate to reduce narcotic requirements in orthopedic surgery. Egypt J Anaesth. 2011;28(1):17–22.
20. Omar H. Magnesium sulfate as a preemptive adjuvant to Levobupivacaine for postoperative analgesia in lower abdominal and pelvic surgeries under epidural anesthesia (randomized controlled trial). Anesth Essays Res. 2018; 12(1):256–61.
21. Radwan T, Awad M, Fahmy R, et al. Evaluation of analgesia by epidural magnesium sulphate versus fentanyl as adjuvant to levobupivacaine in geriatric spine surgeries. Randomized controlled study. Egypt J Anaesth. 2017;33(4):357–63.
22. Daabiss MA, Kandil A. Evaluation of the effect of magnesium vs. midazolam as adjunct to epidural bupivacaine in patients undergoing total knee replacement. Br J Med Pract. 2013;6(2):a610.
23. Mayer ML, Westbrook GL, Guthrie PB. Voltage-dependent block by Mg2+ of NMDA responses in spinal cord neurones. Nat. 1984;309(5965):261–3.
24. Peng YN, Sung FC, Huang ML, et al. The use of intravenous magnesium sulfate on postoperative analgesia in orthopedic surgery: a systematic review of randomized controlled trials. Med (Baltimore). 2018;97(50):e13583.
25. Guo BL, Lin Y, Hu W, et al. Effects of systemic magnesium on post-operative analgesia: is the current evidence strong enough? Pain Physician. 2015;18(5):405–18.
26. Xie M, Li XK, Peng Y. Magnesium sulfate for postoperative complications in children undergoing tonsillectomies: a systematic review and meta-analysis. J Evid Based Med. 2017;10(1):16–25.
27. Ko SH, Lim HR, Kim DC, et al. Magnesium sulfate does not reduce postoperative analgesic requirements. Anesthesiol. 2001;95(3):640–6.
28. Wang SC, Pan PT, Chiu HY, et al. Neuraxial magnesium sulfate improves postoperative analgesia in cesarean section delivery women: a meta-analysis of randomized controlled trials. Asian J Anesthesiol. 2017;55(3):56–67.
29. Kawakami H, Mihara T, Nakamura N, et al. Effect of magnesium added to local anesthetics for caudal anesthesia on postoperative pain in pediatric surgical patients: a systematic review and meta-analysis with trial sequential analysis. PLoS One. 2018;13(1):e0190354.
30. Ghoneim MM, Long JP. The interaction between magnesium and other neuromuscular blocking agents. Anesthesiol. 1970;32(1):23–7.
31. Kim MH, Oh AY, Jeon YT, et al. A randomised controlled trial comparing rocuronium priming, magnesium pre-treatment and a combination of the two methods. Anaesth. 2012;67(7):748–54.
32. Lysakowski C, Dumont L, Czarnetzki C, et al. Magnesium as an adjuvant to postoperative analgesia: a systematic review of randomized trials. Anesth Analg. 2007;104(6):1532–9.

16

Infraclavicular nerve block reduces postoperative pain after distal radial fracture fixation

Stanley S. Wong[1*], Wing S. Chan[1], Christian Fang[2], Chi W. Chan[3], Tak W. Lau[4], Frankie Leung[2] and Chi W. Cheung[1]

Abstract

Background: It is unclear whether regional anesthesia with infraclavicular nerve block or general anesthesia provides better postoperative analgesia after distal radial fracture fixation, especially when combined with regular postoperative analgesic medications. The aim of this study was to compare the postoperative analgesic effects of regional versus general anesthesia.

Methods: In this prospective, observer blinded, randomized controlled trial, 52 patients undergoing distal radial fracture fixation received either general anesthesia ($n = 26$) or regional anesthesia (infraclavicular nerve block, n = 26). Numerical rating scale pain scores, analgesic consumption, patient satisfaction, adverse effects, upper limb functional scores (Patient-Rated Wrist Evaluation, QuickDASH), health related quality of life (SF12v2), and psychological status were evaluated after surgery.

Result: Regional anesthesia was associated with significantly lower pain scores both at rest and with movement on arrival to the post-anesthetic care unit; and at 1, 2, 24 and 48 h after surgery ($p \leq 0.001$ at rest and with movement). Morphine consumption in the post-anesthetic care unit was significantly lower in the regional anesthesia group (p< 0.001). There were no differences in oral analgesic consumption. Regional anesthesia was associated with lower incidences of nausea ($p = 0.004$), and vomiting ($p = 0.050$). Patient satisfaction was higher in the regional anesthesia group ($p = 0.003$). There were no long-term differences in pain scores and other patient outcomes.

Conclusion: Regional anesthesia with ultrasound guided infraclavicular nerve block was associated with better acute pain relief after distal radial fracture fixation, and may be preferred over general anesthesia.

Keywords: General anesthesia, Regional anesthesia, Distal radial fracture fixation, Postoperative pain, Infraclavicular nerve block

* Correspondence: wongstan@hku.hk
[1]Laboratory and Clinical Research Institute for Pain, Department of Anaesthesiology, Li Ka Shing Faculty of Medicine, The University of Hong Kong, Queen Mary Hospital, Room 424, Block K, 102, Pokfulam Road, Hong Kong SAR, China

Background

Distal radial fracture fixation is a commonly performed orthopedic surgery. It is usually associated with moderate pain, but can sometimes also result in severe postoperative pain. Poor postoperative pain control would interfere with rehabilitation, delay recovery, and adversely affect outcomes [1, 2]. Distal radial fracture fixation is performed either under general anesthesia (GA) or regional anesthesia (RA) using a brachial plexus block. The choice of anesthetic technique may affect postoperative pain control.

Regional anesthetic nerve blocks have been shown to reduce acute postoperative pain, opioid consumption, improve patient satisfaction, and shorten postoperative stay [3–6]. However, 2 randomized controlled trials found no overall difference between RA and GA for analgesia after distal radial fracture fixation [7, 8]. Instead, RA was associated with rebound pain and worse pain scores compared with GA at 24 h after surgery. However, standardized regular postoperative analgesics were not given to prevent rebound pain in these clinical trials. Regular analgesic medication is recommended for optimal postoperative pain control and prevention of rebound pain [1, 2, 9–11]. The use of regular postoperative analgesic medication could positively affect the analgesic effect of RA and reduce rebound pain after distal radial fracture fixation. To the best of our knowledge, this has not been studied.

We performed a randomized controlled trial to compare the acute postoperative analgesic effect of RA with ultrasound guided infraclavicular nerve block versus GA plus local anesthetic would infiltration for distal radial fracture fixation. This was conducted with the use of regular postoperative analgesic medication. We also looked at longer-term secondary outcomes including chronic pain, upper limb functional scores, health related quality of life, and psychological well-being at 3 and 6 months after surgery. We hypothesized that RA together with regular postoperative analgesic medication would improve acute postoperative pain control after distal radial fracture fixation.

Methods

This study was conducted in a tertiary university hospital in Hong Kong, China. It was approved by the local university's Institutional Review Board (UW 16–005), and registered at clinicaltrial.gov prior to patient recruitment on 9th February 2017 (NCT03048214). Written consent was obtained from all patients participating in the trial.

This was a prospective, observer blinded, randomized controlled trial. Patients aged between 18 and 80 years old with an American Society of Anesthesiologist (ASA) physical status of I-III scheduled for distal radial fracture fixation (open reduction and internal fixation) were eligible. Exclusion criteria included surgery involving more than fixation of one affected arm; allergy to analgesic drugs including opioids, non-steroidal anti-inflammatory drugs (NSAIDs), local anesthetic drugs, and paracetamol; presence of chronic pain condition; chronic opioid user; alcohol or substance abuse; impaired renal function (defined as serum creatinine level over 120 µmol/L; impaired liver function (defined as plasma bilirubin over 34 µmol/L, international normalized ratio (INR) ≥1.7, alanine aminotransferase (ALT) and aspartate aminotransferase (AST) over 100 U/L; pre-existing neurological or muscular disorders; psychiatric illness; impaired mental state; non-ambulatory; pregnancy; local infection; coagulopathy or on anticoagulants (not including aspirin); or patient refusal.

Eligible patients were randomly assigned to receive either GA plus local anesthetic wound infiltration (GA group) or RA with infraclavicular nerve block (RA group). Patients were randomized using a computer-generated random sequence. A statistician unaware of the nature of the clinical study prepared the sequence. Allocation was concealed in opaque envelopes and opened at the time of intervention by the attending anesthetist. Patients were aware of the type of anesthesia they were receiving. An investigator who was blinded from patient allocation collected the data from the patients. Patients were informed upon enrollment into the study not to tell the investigator collecting data which group they belonged to. The anesthetist who performed the anesthetic was aware of patient allocation, but was not involved in data collection.

Sedative premedication was not prescribed. On arrival to the operating theatre, a 20- or 22-gauge intravenous cannula was inserted. Standard monitoring with pulse oximeter, non-invasive blood pressure, and three lead electrocardiogram (ECG) were applied before induction. Non-invasive blood pressure was measured at least every 5 min throughout the operation. Distal radial fracture fixation was performed in the hospital trauma list, which operated from 8.30 am to 16:30 pm on every weekday.

General anesthesia group (GA)

Patients in the GA group were induced with intravenous propofol 1.5-3 mg/kg, fentanyl 0.25-2mcg/kg and atracurium 0.5 mg/kg. Patients were either intubated with an endotracheal tube or given a laryngeal mask airway as determined by the attending anesthetist. Additional doses of muscle relaxants were given as needed. GA was maintained with sevoflurane, air and oxygen (oxygen and air titrated to give a fraction of inspired oxygen (FiO_2) of between 35 and 50%). Sevoflurane was titrated to 0.7–1.5 minimum alveolar concentration (MAC), and nitrous oxide was not used.

Intravenous morphine sulphate at a dose of 0.05–0.1 mg/kg was given immediately prior to surgical incision. Additional boluses of morphine sulphate at 0.025–0.05 mg/kg could be given at the discretion of the attending anesthetist. Around thirty minutes before end of surgery, intravenous paracetamol at a dose of 1000 mg (15 mg/kg for patients under 50 kg) was given. Ondansetron 4 mg was given intravenously 30 min before the end of surgery. Sevoflurane was switched off after the inner layers of wound were closed. Local wound infiltration with 2 mg/kg of 0.5% levobupivacaine was given by the surgeon during wound closure. Reversal of muscle relaxation was achieved with neostigmine 50mcg/kg and atropine 20mcg/kg given intravenously. Subsequently, the patient was transferred to the post-anesthetic care unit (PACU) for 30 min to 1 h.

Regional anesthesia group (RA)

Infraclavicular nerve blocks were performed under ultrasound guidance using a 22-gauge 50 mm or 100 mm Pajunk® needle for patients in the RA group. The decision whether to use a nerve stimulator was left to the attending anesthetist. Local anesthetic solution was made up of 10 ml of 2% lignocaine with 1:200,000 adrenaline plus 10 ml of 0.75% ropivacaine, made up to a total of 20 ml of local anesthetic solution. Fifteen to twenty milliliters of local anesthetic solution were deposited around the lateral, posterior, and medial cord of the brachial plexus under ultrasound guidance. All regional blocks were performed by a skilled specialist anesthetist or resident fellow under the direct supervision of a specialist anesthetist competent in performing ultrasound guided infraclavicular nerve blocks. Any immediate complications including paresthesia and vascular puncture were noted.

Patients were sedated with propofol infusion during surgery by using the Marsh effect site model to keep the effect site concentration between 0.5–1.5mcg/ml. Propofol level was titrated to put the patients under light sleep where they could be easily aroused with verbal stimulation. Other sedative drugs or opioids were not used in this group. Intravenous paracetamol 1000 mg (15 mg/kg for patients under 50 kg) was given 30 min before the end of surgery. Anesthesia was considered inadequate if there was pain on pinching the surgical site using an artery forcep just prior to surgical incision. Patients with inadequate anesthesia were switched to GA according to protocol.

Postoperative care and assessment

Two milli-grams of intravenous morphine sulphate was given every 5 min until the numerical rating scale (NRS) pain score was less than 4/10 in the PACU. In the general ward, oral analgesics were given once oral fluid was allowed. Regular oral paracetamol 500 mg was given every 6 h for 3 days or until discharge. Oral dihydrocodeine 30 mg as needed every 6 h was prescribed for 3 days or until discharge. Patients were told that they could request dihydrocodeine if their NRS pain score was over 3/10.

Oral fluid diet was allowed on postoperative day (POD) 0. The surgical team assessed for occurrences of postoperative surgical complications every morning and decided on patient suitability for discharge. Patients were assessed for possible complications related to the infraclavicular nerve block on POD 1, and they were reviewed again on POD 2 if complications could not be ruled out on the first assessment. Symptoms assessed included persistent paresthesia, tingling, abnormal sensation, and weakness. These assessments were made in the morning.

NRS pain scores (0–10), where 0 represented no pain, and 10 represented the worse possible pain, was assessed at rest and on movement of the operated upper limb (attempted wrist flexion). These were performed on arrival to the PACU, and at 1, 2, 24, and 48 h after surgery. Frequency and dose of rescue morphine used in the PACU and oral dihydrocodeine used in the ward were recorded daily in the morning. Occurrences of adverse effects including nausea, vomiting, pruritus and dizziness were also recorded every day. The Aonos four-point scale (AFPS) for postoperative emergence agitation was recorded 30 min after arrival at PACU. Patient satisfaction with anesthesia (0–10), where 0 was the least satisfaction, and 10 was the most satisfaction possible, was assessed on POD 1.

An investigator blinded to patient allocation conducted interviews at 3 and 6 months after surgery to collect the following information: NRS pain scores at rest and with movement (wrist flexion); patient satisfaction; health related quality of life measured using the Chinese version of SF12-v2 health survey [12]; psychological status as measured by the Hospital Anxiety and Depression Scale (HADS); and functional outcomes measured using the Disabilities of the Arm, Shoulder and Hand (QuickDASH) questionnaire and Patient Rated Wrist Evaluation (PRWE). Validated Chinese versions of QuickDASH and PRWE were used for Chinese patients [13, 14].

Statistical analysis

The primary outcome was postoperative NRS pain score (0–10) with movement at 24 h after surgery. No suitable references for postoperative NRS pain scores at 24 h that could be used for sample size calculation was found. Based on a previous study on RA versus GA for hand surgery, the standard deviation estimate of the postoperative pain score from brachial plexus block was 2.86

[15]. To detect a difference in NRS pain score of 2.4/10 at a significance level of 0.05 and a power of 0.80, the minimum number of patients required per group was 23. A difference of 2.4 in NRS pain score was chosen because this has been shown to correspond to 'much improvement' in pain relief, which is clinically significant [16]. To take into account for possible dropouts, 26 patients were recruited into each group.

Secondary outcomes included postoperative NRS pain scores at other time points (apart from 24 h postop), postoperative analgesic consumption, patient satisfaction, adverse effects, upper limb functional scores (Patient-Rated Wrist Evaluation, QuickDASH), health related quality of life (SF12v2), and psychological status (HADS score). Patient demographic and operative data were analyzed using Student's t-test and Chi-square test. Postoperative NRS pain scores between the two groups were expressed as median (interquartile range) and compared using the Mann-Whitney U test, as the distribution of the pain scores was non-normal. To adjust for multiple statistical comparisons, post-hoc Bonferroni correction was also applied for comparison of median postoperative NRS pain scores between the two groups for all observed time points. Pain scores between 0 and 48 h and between 3 and 6 months after surgery were also expressed as area under curve (AUC) weighted by the corresponding time interval. The weighted AUC is equivalent to a time weighted average of the pain scores for the specified time interval and is of the same scale as the NRS (0–10). The difference in weighted AUC between the GA and RA groups was compared by the Mann-Whitney U test. Analgesic consumption, functional outcomes (PRWE and QuickDASH), patient satisfaction, health related quality of life and psychological status were analyzed using the Student's t-test. Incidence of adverse effects was compared using the Chi-square test or Fisher's exact test as appropriate. The critical value for statistical significance was $P = 0.05$. Intention to treat analysis was done. The statistical software used was IBM SPSS Statistics for Windows, Version 25.0 (IBM Corp. USA).

Results

Fifty-two patients in total (26 in each group) completed the study, which was conducted from May 2017 to January 2019. Fifty-five patients were assessed for eligibility, and 3 were excluded. Two patients declined to participate and 1 patient did not meet the inclusion criteria. All recruited patients completed the study for primary outcome measure and the results were used for analysis (Fig. 1).

Conversion to GA was required due to inadequate regional anesthetic block in 1 patient in the RA group. Intention to treat analysis was done. One patient from each group was lost to follow up at 6 months and were not included in the analysis for that time point. There were no significant differences between the two groups in patient demographics, duration of anesthesia, duration of surgery, and length of hospital stay (Table 1). Length of stay in the PACU was significantly longer in the GA group compared to the RA group ($p = 0.023$).

Postoperative median NRS pain scores at different time points are shown in Table 2 and Fig. 2. Patients in the RA group had significantly lower NRS pain scores than those in the GA group both at rest and during movement (attempted wrist flexion) on arrival to the PACU ($p<0.001$ for pain at rest and with movement), 1 h ($p<0.001$ at rest and with movement), 2 h ($p<0.001$ at rest and with movement), 24 h ($p = 0.001$ at rest and with movement) and 48 h ($p<0.001$ at rest and with movement) after surgery (Table 2). All of the above differences in NRS pain scores remained statistically significant with adjusted $p < 0.05$ after post-hoc application of Bonferroni multiple comparison correction. There were no significant differences between the two groups in NRS pain scores at rest and with movement (wrist flexion) at 3 and 6 months after surgery (Table 2). Postoperative NRS pain scores were also expressed as weighted AUC. The weighted AUC pain scores from 0 to 48 h after surgery was significantly lower in the RA group ($p < 0.001$ at rest and with movement). There were no differences in weighted AUC pain scores between the two groups from 3 to 6 months after surgery (Table 2).

Consumption of rescue morphine in the PACU was significantly higher in the GA group ($p < 0.001$) (Table 3). Oral paracetamol was given regularly to both groups of patients and there were no significant differences between the two groups (data not shown). There were no significant differences between groups in the consumption of rescue oral dihydrocodeine in the ward (Table 3).

There were no significant differences in the mean Aono's score for emergence agitation in the PACU between the two groups (Table 3). Patients in the GA group were significantly more likely to experience nausea ($p = 0.004$) and vomiting ($p = 0.050$) after surgery (Table 3). There were no significant differences in the incidence of other adverse effects (Table 3). No immediate complications were reported. There were no significant differences in the incidence of paresthesia, tingling, and abnormal sensation over the operated limb (Table 3). Significantly more patients in the GA group experienced weakness in the acute postoperative period ($p = 0.035$) (Table 3). Patient satisfaction with anesthesia was significantly higher in the RA group on POD 1 (8.8 vs 7.3, $p = 0.003$) and at 3 months (8.4 vs 7.1, $p = 0.007$) after surgery, but

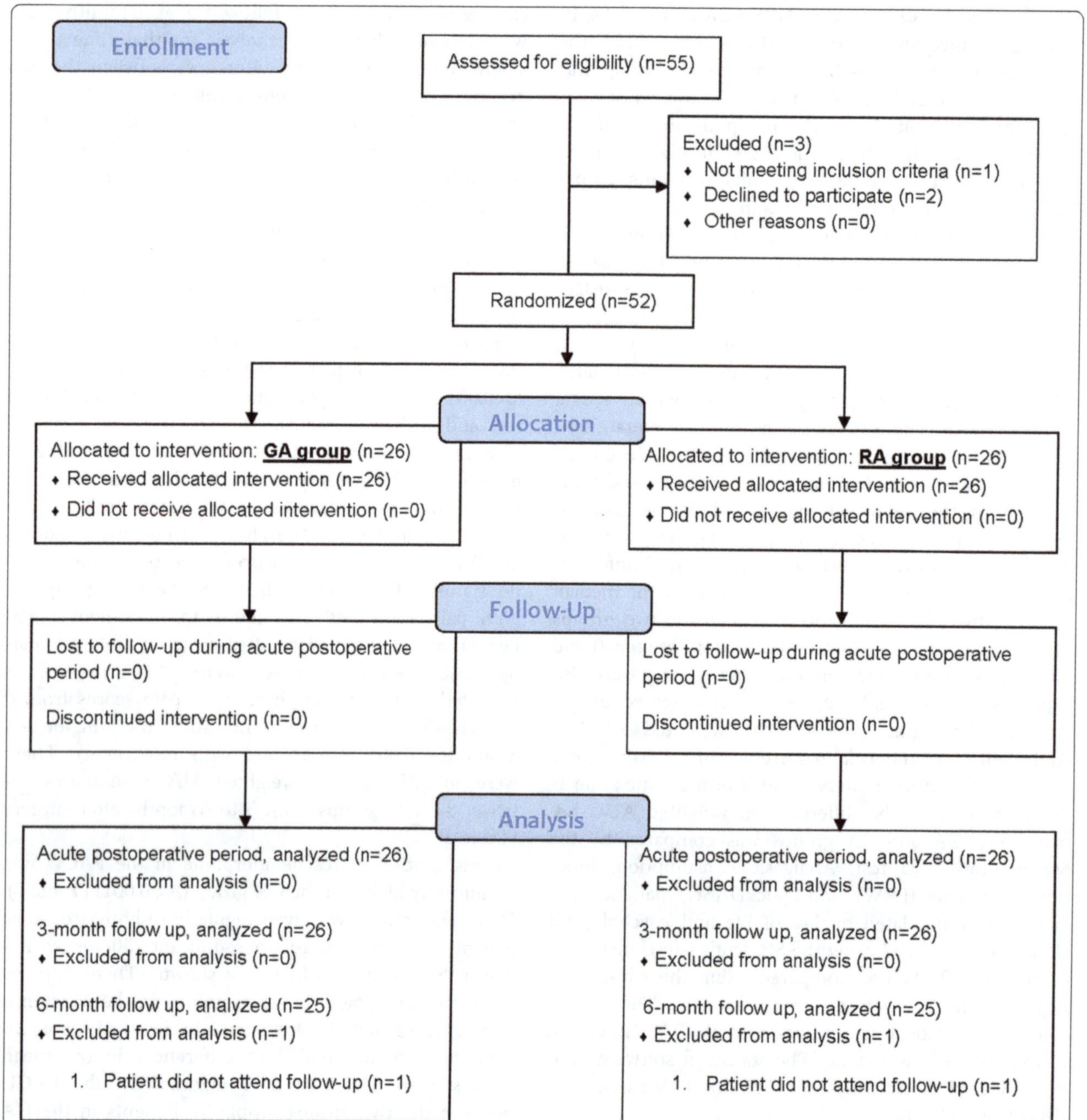

Fig. 1 Flow diagram of patients enrolled in the study

there were no differences at 6 months. There were no differences in the proportion of patients willing to repeat the same anesthetic technique (data not shown).

There were no differences in functional scores as measured by PRWE and QuickDash (Disability/symptom score) at 3 and 6 months after surgery (Table 4). There were also no differences between the two groups in SF12-v2 and HADS at 3 and 6 months after surgery (data not shown).

Discussion

RA with infraclavicular nerve block was associated with reduced NRS pain scores at rest and with movement compared to GA plus local anesthetic wound infiltration on arrival to the PACU, at 1, 2, 24 and 48 h after surgery. Patients in the RA group used significantly less morphine in the PACU, but oral dihydrocodeine consumption was similar between the two groups. There were no differences in pain scores, upper limb functional

Table 1 Patient characteristics and operative data

Patient characteristics and operative data	GA (*n* = 26)	RA (n = 26)	*P* values
Sex (Female)	73.1% (19)	69.2% (18)	0.760
Age (year)	58.9 ± 12.8	59.2 ± 8.5	0.919
Body weight (kg)	60.1 ± 14.5	58.8 ± 9.5	0.518
ASA, I:II	30.8: 69.2% (8: 18)	53.8: 46.2% (14: 12)	0.092
Right: left distal radius fracture	42.3: 57.7% (11: 15)	42.3: 57.7% (11: 15)	1.000
Duration of anesthesia (min)	87.7 ± 21.8	97.6 ± 38.9	0.261
Duration of surgery (min)	56.1 ± 20.1	65.0 ± 37.3	0.288
Duration in PACU (min)	62.0 ± 23.7	48.8 ± 15.5	0.023*
Length of hospital stay (Days)	1.5 ± 0.81	1.5 ± 1.2	0.895

Values in mean ± SD or % (n)
Kg indicates kilograms; *ASA* American Society of Anesthesiologists physical status; *min* minutes; *PACU* post-anesthetic care unit; *SD* standard deviation
* significantly different at $P \leq 0.05$

scores (PRWE and QuickDASH), psychological status (HADS) or health related quality of life (SF12v2) at 3 and 6 months after surgery.

Our results showed that RA was associated with better acute postoperative pain control compared to GA up to 48 h after distal radial fracture fixation. This is in contrast to the results from two previous randomized controlled trials conducted by Galos et al. and Rundgren et al. that compared RA versus GA for distal radial fracture fixation. In those 2 clinical trials, RA was not associated with overall analgesic benefit [7, 8]. Patients with RA had lower initial pain scores 2 h after surgery, but experienced rebound pain with worse pain scores 24 h after surgery [7, 8]. However, no significant rebound pain was observed in our study. A number of randomized controlled trials comparing RA versus GA for other

Table 2 Postoperative NRS pain scores at rest and with movement

NRS pain scores	GA (*n* = 26)	RA (*n* = 26)	*P* values
At rest			
On arrival to PACU	5.5 [2–8]	0 [0–0]	< 0.001*
Postoperative 1 h	5 [5–8]	0 [0–0]	< 0.001*
Postoperative 2 h	5 [3.75–8]	0 [0–0]	< 0.001*
Postoperative 24 h	4.5 [2–6]	1.5 [0–3]	0.001*
Postoperative 48 h	4.5 [3–6]	1 [0–2]	< 0.001*
Postoperative 3 months	2 [0–3.25]	2 [1–3]	0.737
Postoperative 6 months	1 [0–2.5]	2 [0–3]	0.991
Weighted AUC 0–48 h	5.1 [2.8–5.8]	1.1 [0–2.1]	< 0.001*
Weighted AUC 3–6 months	1.5 [0.5–2.5]	1.5 [0.5–3.0]	0.992
On movement of the operated limb	(*n* = 26)	(*n* = 26)	
On arrival to PACU	7.5 [2.75–8.25]	0 [0–0]	< 0.001*
Postoperative 1 h	6 [5–8]	0 [0–0]	< 0.001*
Postoperative 2 h	6.5 [4–8.25]	0 [0–0]	< 0.001*
Postoperative 24 h	6 [4–7.25]	2 [2–4.25]	0.001*
Postoperative 48 h	5 [4–7]	2 [1.75–3]	< 0.001*
Postoperative 3 months	4 [2–7]	3 [1.75–5]	0.332
Postoperative 6 months	3 [0.5–5]	3 [0–3.25]	0.254
Weighted AUC 0–48 h	6.0 [4.5–6.9]	1.5 [1.4–3.2]	< 0.001*
Weighted AUC 3–6 months	3.5 [2.3–5.5]	3.3 [0.9–4.1]	0.254

Weighted AUC indicates weighted area under curve; *h* hours; *NRS* numerical rating scale
PACU indicates post-anesthetic care unit, values in median [Interquartile range]
Patient sample size at postoperative 6 months was 25 for both groups
* Significantly different at $P \leq 0.05$

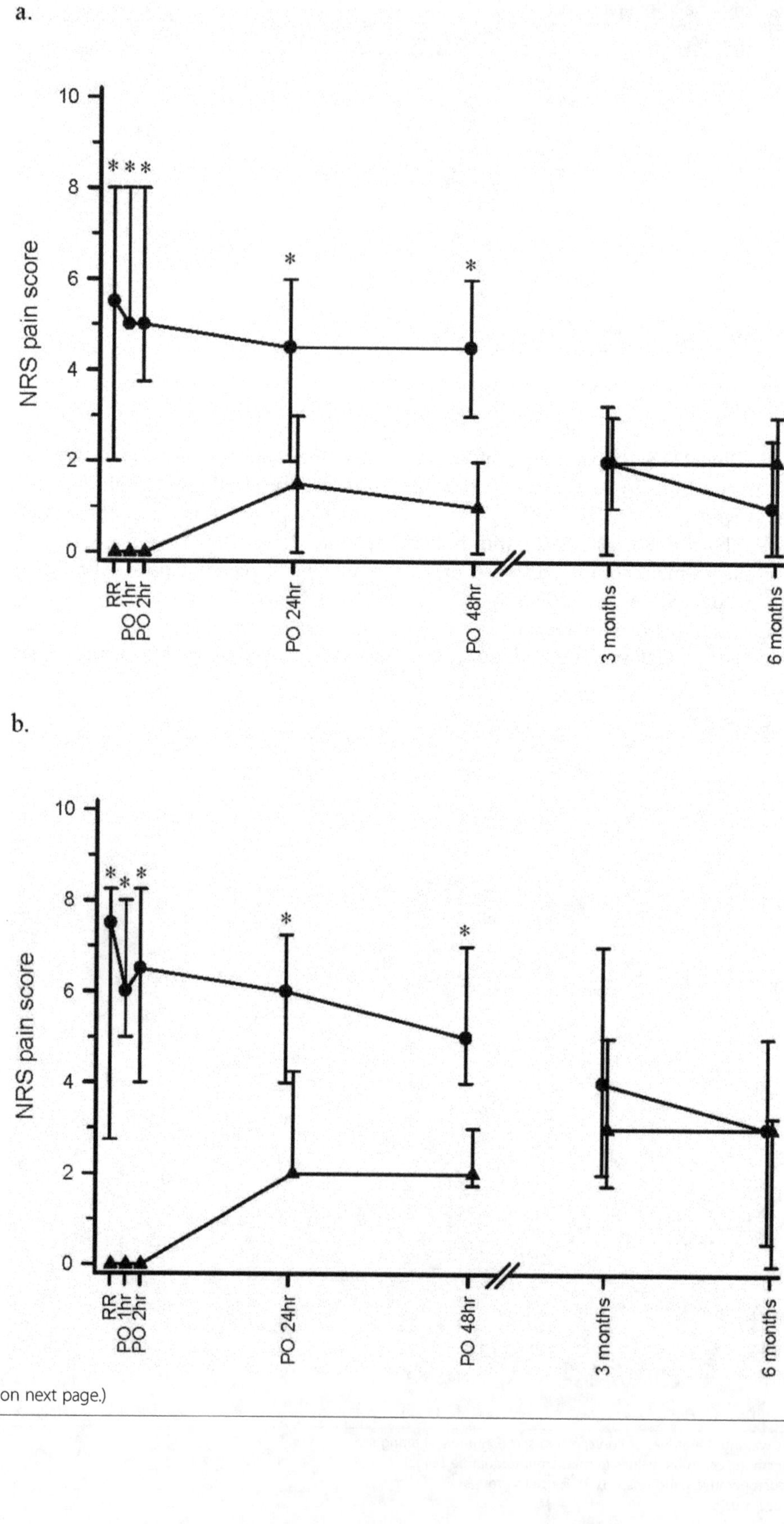

Fig. 2 (See legend on next page.)

(See figure on previous page.)
Fig. 2 Postoperative numerical rating scale (NRS) pain scores of patients given regional anesthesia with infraclavicular nerve block (RA) or general anesthesia (GA) at rest (**a**) and during movement of the operated upper limb (**b**) at each recording time point. RR indicates on arrival to the post-anesthetic care unit; PO1hr = 1 h after surgery, PO2hr = 2 h after surgery; PO24hr = 24 h after surgery; PO48hr = 48 h after surgery; 3 and 6 months = 3 and 6 months after surgery. Solid circle represents GA; solid triangle represents RA. Values expressed in median [Interquartile range] * Significantly different at $P \leq 0.05$. All differences in postoperative median NRS pain scores up to 48 h (at rest and with movement) remained statistically significant with adjusted $P \leq 0.05$ even after post hoc adjustment with Bonferroni multiple comparisons

types of upper limb surgery also did not demonstrate significant rebound pain [15, 17, 18]. All our patients were prescribed regular postoperative oral paracetamol which they took upon return to the ward before wearing off of the regional nerve block. Paracetamol taken regularly is recommended for postoperative pain control [19], and paracetamol is an effective analgesic medication [20, 21]. Since distal radial fracture surgery does not usually result in severe postoperative pain, regular oral paracetamol taken preventively was probably effective in controlling rebound pain. Unlike our study, standardized regular postoperative analgesic medication was not prescribed in the two clinical trials by Galos et al. and Rundgren et al. [7, 8]. In addition, our patients were also educated by ward staff about the possible experience of rebound pain and reinforced about the importance of taking regular analgesic medications, even in the absence of pain. Patient education was perhaps also useful in managing their expectations, which could affect their perception of pain. Our results suggest that regular preventive analgesic medications and patient education can attenuate rebound pain. This is in agreement with recommended strategies [11].

There are also other differences between our study and that of Galos et al. and Rundgren et al. that may have accounted for differences in our results. We examined both dynamic pain scores on movement of the upper limb and pain at rest, because we expected them to be distinctly different. In the clinical trials by Galos et al. and Rundgren et al., it is not clear whether pain scores assessed were at rest or with movement. The anesthetic technique was not standardized in the study

Table 3 Postoperative analgesic consumption and incidence of postoperative adverse effects

Postoperative analgesic consumption	GA ($n = 26$)	RA ($n = 26$)	P values
Morphine (mg)			
Morphine consumption in the PACU	2.3 (0–3)	0 (0–0)	< 0.001*
Oral Dihydrocodeine (mg) consumption			
Postoperative 2 h	0 (0–0)	0 (0–0)	1.000
Postoperative 24 h	0 (0–0)	0 (0–0)	0.149
Postoperative 48 h	0 (0–0)	0 (0–0)	0.719
Postoperative adverse effects			
Emergence agitation (Aono's four-point scale) in the PACU	1 (1–1)	1 (1–1)	0.057
Nausea	30.7% (13,49)	0.0% (NA)	0.004*
Vomiting	19.2% (4,34)	0.0% (NA)	0.050*
Dizziness	30.7% (13,49)	7.6% (−2,18)	0.075
Pruritus	0.0% (NA)	0.0% (NA)	1.000
Wound infection	0.0% (NA)	0.0% (NA)	1.000
Urinary retention	0.0% (NA)	3.8% (−4,12)	1.000
Others	11.5% (−1,25)	0.0% (NA)	0.235
Symptoms of the operated upper limb			
Paresthesia	23.1% (7,39)	11.5% (−1,25)	0.465
Tingling	23.1% (7,39)	7.7% (−2,18)	0.248
Abnormal sensation	19.2% (4,34)	3.8% (−4,12)	0.191
Weakness	30.8% (13,49)	7.7% (−2,18)	0.035*
Others	11.5% (−1,25)	0.0% (NA)	0.235

Values in median (IQR) or % (95% confidence interval)
PACU indicates post-anesthetic care unit; mg, milligram; *NA* not applicable
* Significantly different at $P \leq 0.05$

Table 4 Functional scores: Patient Rated Wrist Evaluation (PRWE) and Disabilities of the arm, shoulder and hand questionnaire (QuickDASH)

Patient Rated Wrist Evaluation (PRWE)	GA ($n = 26$)	RA ($n = 26$)	*P* values
Postoperative 3 months			
Pain [0–50]	14 (8.3–17.8)	15 (7–22)	0.986
Specific Activities [0–60]	11.5 (3.3–20.5)	23.5 (3.8–31.3)	0.312
Usual Activities [0–40]	8 (2–20.3)	12 (2.5–22)	0.525
Total score [0–100]	23 (11.9–40.6)	35 (11.4–46.6)	0.618
Postoperative 6 months	($n = 25$)	($n = 25$)	
Pain [0–50]	10 (4–6)	10.5 (3–19)	0.657
Specific Activities [0–60]	6 (1.5–21)	9 (3–18.8)	0.820
Usual Activities [0–40]	8 (0–13.5)	4 (0–10.8)	0.213
Total score [0–100]	12 (7–34.8)	18.8 (4.1–34.4)	0.959
Disabilities of the arm, shoulder and hand questionnaire (QuickDASH)	($n = 26$)	($n = 26$)	
Postoperative 3 months			
Disability/symptom score [0–100]	21.6 (11.4–47.7)	34.1 (10.8–50)	0.839
Postoperative 6 months			
Disability/symptom score [0–100]	22.5 (11.4–32.3)	13.6 (9.1–24.4)	0.276

Values in median (IQR)
PRWE Total score Pain score + (Specific activities score + Usual activities score)/2
* Significantly different at $P \leq 0.05$

by Galos et al. Differences in general anesthetic technique such as the choice of inhalational versus propofol total intravenous anesthesia can affect postoperative pain scores and opioid consumption [22–24]. Finally, 7 of the 44 patients had an inadequate block in the study by Rundgren et al., versus only 1 out of 26 patients in our study.

In this study, single shot infraclavicular nerve block was associated with improved postoperative analgesia for 48 h, which is beyond the pharmacological duration of the local anesthetic. This suggests that infraclavicular nerve block had preventive analgesic effects. Preventive analgesia is defined as a reduction in postoperative pain and/or analgesic consumption that persists longer than the clinical duration of the target drug (5.5 half-lives) [25]. We hypothesize that infraclavicular nerve block prevented central sensitization by inhibiting nociceptive input into the spinal cord, thereby producing preventive analgesia and prolonged analgesia [3, 26]. There have been some other clinical studies that also showed improved analgesia up to 48 h after surgery with single shot regional nerve blocks [27, 28].

We evaluated the opioid sparing effects of RA versus GA. Morphine consumption in the PACU was significantly lower in the RA group compared to the GA group, which is similar to other studies comparing RA versus GA for upper limb surgery [7, 15, 18]. However, no significant difference in oral dihydrocodeine consumption in the ward was observed. The absence of difference in rescue oral analgesic consumption may be because the pain scores after surgery were not very high. The median NRS pain scores at rest in the GA group were 4.5/10 at 24 and 48 h after surgery, which corresponds to pain of moderate intensity [29]. It was up to the patient whether or not to request oral dihydrocodeine. Although patients in the GA group experienced more pain, it may not have been severe enough to cause a significant difference in oral analgesic request. Patient satisfaction with anesthesia after surgery was significantly higher in the RA group on POD 1. This is probably due to better acute postoperative pain control and reduced nausea and vomiting in patients given RA. It has been shown that patient dissatisfaction is strongly associated with worse pain control as well as nausea and vomiting [30, 31]. Interestingly, patients in the RA group also had higher levels of satisfaction at 3 months after surgery, even though there was no difference in pain scores at that time point. Perhaps a trend towards better functional scores (PRWE and QuickDash) in the RA group contributed to higher levels of satisfaction. However, these differences were not statistically significant, and was probably not the only reason for this observation. In addition, although RA group patients had higher levels of satisfaction, the proportion of patients who would repeat the same anesthetic technique was similar between the two groups. Both GA and RA patients had good satisfaction scores (8.8 vs 7.3), and over 80% of both groups of patients would repeat the same anesthetic technique. The difference in patient satisfaction was probably not large enough to significantly affect this outcome. Another reason could be the concern of potential nerve block related complications.

We found no differences in longer-term outcomes between the 2 groups. This is in agreement with Galos et al. and Rundgren et al., which found no differences in pain, DASH, short musculoskeletal function assessment, PRWE, and EuroQol-5 Dimensions-3 Levels [7, 8]. On the other hand, an observational study involving 187 patients showed that RA was associated with reduced pain scores and higher upper limb functional scores (DASH) at 3 and 6 months after distal radial fracture fixation [32]. The relationship between RA and longer-term outcomes for distal radial fracture fixation remains unclear.

There were some limitations in this study. The patients were not blinded, and this can introduce bias. However, it was not possible to blind the patients in this study. The investigators performing patient assessment and data collection were blinded, and bias does not appear to be a significant issue when the observer is blinded [33]. Another limitation was that our study was not powered to look for differences in long-term pain score and functional outcomes at 3 and 6 months. The main focus of this study was to compare RA versus GA for acute postoperative pain control, but we recognize that long-term outcomes are also important. An additional limitation was that there may have been some variation in the amount of medication given to the two groups of patients intraoperatively, because the study protocol allowed the attending anesthetist to give medications within a given dose range. Airway management was also not standardized (laryngeal mask airway or endotracheal intubation was allowed). In addition, there was also some variation in the volume of local anesthetic used for the infraclavicular nerve block (between 15 and 20 ml), which could affect the quality of the block. However, the vast majority of the infraclavicular nerve blocks were sufficient for surgical anesthesia, indicating good block quality. There was 1 failed block in this study. This may have been reduced if a single anesthesiologist with special expertise in RA performed all the ultrasound guided infraclavicular nerve blocks. However, this was not done in order to make the results more generalizable to everyday clinical practice.

Conclusion

Our study suggests that RA improves acute postoperative pain control compared to GA for distal radial fracture fixation. RA was also associated with higher patient satisfaction, and less nausea and vomiting. Preventive regular analgesic medication in combination with RA is probably important to improve postoperative pain control and prevent rebound pain.

Abbreviations

AFPS: Aonos four point scale; ALT: Alanine aminotransferase; ASA: American Society of Anesthesiologist; AST: Aspartate aminotransferase; AUC: Area under curve; ECG: Electrocardiogram; GA: General anesthesia; HADS: Hospital Anxiety and Depression Scale; INR: International normalized ratio; MAC: Minimum alveolar concentration; NRS: Numerical rating scale; NSAIDs: Non-steroidal anti-inflammatory drugs; PACU: Post-anesthetic care unit; PO1hr: 1 hour after surgery; PO2hr: 2 hours after surgery ; PO24hr: 24 hours after surgery; PO48hr: 48 hours after surgery; POD: Postoperative day; PRWE: Patient Rated Wrist Evaluation; QuickDASH: Quick Disabilities of the Arm, Shoulder and Hand; RA: Regional anesthesia; RR: On arrival to the post-anesthetic care unit; SF12v2: Short Form 12 item (version 2) health survey

Acknowledgements

We would like to thank Dr. YF Chung for his assistance.

Authors' contributions

SSW conceived the study, helped design the study, conduct the study, analyze the data, draft the manuscript, and revise the manuscript. WSC helped analyze the data, draft the manuscript, and revise the manuscript. CF helped design the study, conduct the study, and revise the manuscript. CWC helped design the study and conduct the study. TWL helped conduct the study and revise the manuscript. FL helped conduct the study and revise the manuscript. CW Cheung helped design the study, analyze the data, and revise the manuscript. All authors had discussed the results and commented on the manuscript with final approval of the version to be published. SSW had full access to all of the data in the study and take responsibility for the integrity of the data and the accuracy of the data analysis.

Author details

[1]Laboratory and Clinical Research Institute for Pain, Department of Anaesthesiology, Li Ka Shing Faculty of Medicine, The University of Hong Kong, Queen Mary Hospital, Room 424, Block K, 102, Pokfulam Road, Hong Kong SAR, China. [2]Department of Orthopaedics and Traumatology, Li Ka Shing Faculty of Medicine, The University of Hong Kong, Hong Kong SAR, China. [3]Department of Anaesthesiology, Queen Mary Hospital, Hong Kong SAR, China. [4]Department of Orthopaedics and Traumatology, Queen Mary Hospital, Hong Kong SAR, China.

References

1. Rawal N. Current issues in postoperative pain management. Eur J Anaesthesiol. 2016;33(3):160–71.
2. Kehlet H. Postoperative pain, analgesia, and recovery-bedfellows that cannot be ignored. Pain. 2018;159(Suppl 1):S11–s16.
3. Barreveld A, Witte J, Chahal H, Durieux ME, Strichartz G. Preventive analgesia by local anesthetics: the reduction of postoperative pain by peripheral nerve blocks and intravenous drugs. Anesth Analg. 2013;116(5):1141–61.
4. Joshi G, Gandhi K, Shah N, Gadsden J, Corman SL. Peripheral nerve blocks in the management of postoperative pain: challenges and opportunities. J Clin Anesth. 2016;35:524–9.
5. Kessler J, Marhofer P, Hopkins PM, Hollmann MW. Peripheral regional anaesthesia and outcome: lessons learned from the last 10 years. Br J Anaesth. 2015;114(5):728–45.
6. Gabriel RA, Ilfeld BM. Peripheral nerve blocks for postoperative analgesia: from traditional unencapsulated local anesthetic to liposomes, cryoneurolysis and peripheral nerve stimulation. Best Pract Res Clin Anaesthesiol. 2019;33(3):293–302.
7. Galos DK, Taormina DP, Crespo A, Ding DY, Sapienza A, Jain S, Tejwani NC. Does brachial plexus blockade result in improved pain scores after distal radius fracture fixation? A randomized trial. Clin Orthop Relat Res. 2016; 474(5):1247–54.
8. Rundgren J, Mellstrand Navarro C, Ponzer S, Regberg A, Serenius S, Enocson A. Regional or general anesthesia in the surgical treatment of distal radial fractures: a randomized clinical trial. J Bone Joint Surg Am. 2019;101(13): 1168–76.
9. Chou R, Gordon DB, de Leon-Casasola OA, Rosenberg JM, Bickler S, Brennan T, Carter T, Cassidy CL, Chittenden EH, Degenhardt E, et al. Management of

Postoperative Pain: a clinical practice guideline from the American pain society, the American Society of Regional Anesthesia and Pain Medicine, and the American Society of Anesthesiologists' committee on regional anesthesia, executive committee, and administrative council. J Pain. 2016; 17(2):131–57.

10. Mariano ER, Schatman ME. A commonsense patient-centered approach to multimodal analgesia within surgical enhanced recovery protocols. J Pain Res. 2019;12:3461–6.
11. Lavand'homme P. Rebound pain after regional anesthesia in the ambulatory patient. Curr Opin Anaesthesiol. 2018;31(6):679–84.
12. Lam ET, Lam CL, Fong DY, Huang WW. Is the SF-12 version 2 health survey a valid and equivalent substitute for the SF-36 version 2 health survey for the Chinese? J Eval Clin Pract. 2013;19(1):200–8.
13. Lee EW, Chung MM, Li AP, Lo SK. Construct validity of the Chinese version of the disabilities of the arm, shoulder and hand questionnaire (DASH-HKPWH). J Hand Surg Br. 2005;30(1):29–34.
14. Wah JW, Wang MK, Ping CL. Construct validity of the Chinese version of the patient-rated wrist evaluation questionnaire (PRWE-Hong Kong version). J Hand Ther. 2006;19(1):18–26 quiz 27.
15. McCartney CJ, Brull R, Chan VW, Katz J, Abbas S, Graham B, Nova H, Rawson R, Anastakis DJ, von Schroeder H. Early but no long-term benefit of regional compared with general anesthesia for ambulatory hand surgery. Anesthesiology. 2004;101(2):461–7.
16. Cepeda MS, Africano JM, Polo R, Alcala R, Carr DB. What decline in pain intensity is meaningful to patients with acute pain? Pain. 2003;105(1–2):151–7.
17. Hadzic A, Arliss J, Kerimoglu B, Karaca PE, Yufa M, Claudio RE, Vloka JD, Rosenquist R, Santos AC, Thys DM. A comparison of infraclavicular nerve block versus general anesthesia for hand and wrist day-case surgeries. Anesthesiology. 2004;101(1):127–32.
18. O'Donnell BD, Ryan H, O'Sullivan O, Iohom G. Ultrasound-guided axillary brachial plexus block with 20 milliliters local anesthetic mixture versus general anesthesia for upper limb trauma surgery: an observer-blinded, prospective, randomized, controlled trial. Anesth Analg. 2009;109(1):279–83.
19. Wick EC, Grant MC, Wu CL. Postoperative multimodal analgesia pain management with nonopioid analgesics and techniques: a review. JAMA Surg. 2017;152(7):691–7.
20. Maund E, McDaid C, Rice S, Wright K, Jenkins B, Woolacott N. Paracetamol and selective and non-selective non-steroidal anti-inflammatory drugs for the reduction in morphine-related side-effects after major surgery: a systematic review. Br J Anaesth. 2011;106(3):292–7.
21. Ghaffarpasand F, Dadgostar E, Ilami G, Shoaee F, Niakan A, Aghabaklou S, Ghadimi M, Goudarzi S, Dehghankhalili M, Alavi MH. Intravenous acetaminophen (Paracetamol) for Postcraniotomy pain: systematic review and meta-analysis of randomized controlled trials. World Neurosurg. 2020; 134:569–76.
22. Wong SSC, Leung MYY, Cheung CW. The effect of total intravenous anaesthesia with propofol on postoperative pain after third molar surgery: A double-blind randomized controlled trial. Eur J Pain. 2019;23(5):884–93.
23. Wong SSC, Choi SW, Lee Y, Irwin MG, Cheung CW. The analgesic effects of intraoperative total intravenous anesthesia (TIVA) with propofol versus sevoflurane after colorectal surgery. Medicine. 2018;97(31):e11615.
24. Qiu Q, Choi SW, Wong SS, Irwin MG, Cheung CW. Effects of intra-operative maintenance of general anaesthesia with propofol on postoperative pain outcomes - a systematic review and meta-analysis. Anaesthesia. 2016;71(10): 1222–33.
25. Katz J, Clarke H, Seltzer Z. Review article: Preventive analgesia: quo vadimus? Anesth Analg. 2011;113(5):1242–53.
26. Strichartz GR. Novel ideas of local anaesthetic actions on various ion channels to ameliorate postoperative pain. Br J Anaesth. 2008;101(1):45–7.
27. Chan EY, Fransen M, Parker DA, Assam PN, Chua N. Femoral nerve blocks for acute postoperative pain after knee replacement surgery. Cochrane Database Syst Rev. 2014;(5):Cd009941. https://doi.org/10.1002/14651858.CD009941.pub2.
28. Buttner B, Mansur A, Hinz J, Erlenwein J, Bauer M, Bergmann I. Combination of general anesthesia and peripheral nerve block with low-dose ropivacaine reduces postoperative pain for several days after outpatient arthroscopy: a randomized controlled clinical trial. Medicine (Baltimore). 2017;96(6):e6046.
29. Breivik H, Borchgrevink PC, Allen SM, Rosseland LA, Romundstad L, Hals EK, Kvarstein G, Stubhaug A. Assessment of pain. Br J Anaesth. 2008;101(1):17–24.
30. Myles PS, Williams DL, Hendrata M, Anderson H, Weeks AM. Patient satisfaction after anaesthesia and surgery: results of a prospective survey of 10,811 patients. Br J Anaesth. 2000;84(1):6–10.
31. Benwu KM, Gebremedhin HG. A prospective study on elective surgical inpatient satisfaction with perioperative anaesthesia service at Ayder comprehensive specialized hospital, Mekelle, Ethiopia. BMC Anesthesiol. 2019;19(1):46.
32. Egol KA, Soojian MG, Walsh M, Katz J, Rosenberg AD, Paksima N. Regional anesthesia improves outcome after distal radius fracture fixation over general anesthesia. J Orthop Trauma. 2012;26(9):545–9.
33. Moustgaard H, Clayton GL, Jones HE, Boutron I, Jorgensen L, Laursen DRT, Olsen MF, Paludan-Muller A, Ravaud P, Savovic J, et al. Impact of blinding on estimated treatment effects in randomised clinical trials: meta-epidemiological study. BMJ. 2020;368:l6802.

17

Cerebrospinal fluid of chronic osteoarthritic patients induced interleukin-6 release in human glial cell-line T98G

Weiling Liu[1], Chunmei Li[2], Francis Chee Kuan Tan[1], Hong Jye Neo[1], Yiong Huak Chan[3], Chian-Ming Low[2,4] and Tat Leang Lee[1,2*]

Abstract

Background: Chronic osteoarthritic pain is not well understood in terms of its pathophysiological mechanism. Activated glial cells are thought to play a role in the maintenance of chronic pain. T98G glioblastoma cell line was previously observed to release higher amounts of interleukin-6 (IL-6) when treated with cerebrospinal fluid (CSF) from patients with another chronic pain condition, post-herpetic neuralgia. In this study, we investigated the ability of CSF from patients diagnosed with knee osteoarthritis suffering from chronic pain, to trigger the release of pro-inflammatory cytokines, IL-6, IL-1beta and tumour necrosis factor alpha (TNF-α) from T98G. Characterization of upstream signalling was also explored.

Methods: Fifteen osteoarthritis patients undergoing total knee replacement due to chronic knee pain and 15 patients without pain undergoing other surgeries with spinal anaesthesia were prospectively recruited. CSF was collected during anaesthesia. CSF were added to cultured T98G cells in the presence of lipopolysaccharide. IL-6, IL-1β and TNF-α release from T98G cells were measured using enzyme immunoassay. Antibody array and western blotting were performed using CSF-triggered T98G cell lysates to identify possible signalling targets. Age, gender and pain scores were recorded. Mann-Whitney U test was used to compare IL-6 release and protein expression between groups. Association between IL-6 and pain score was analysed using linear regression.

Results: Significant higher levels of IL-6 were released by T98G cells when induced by osteoarthritis patients' CSF in the presence of LPS. The IL-6 levels showed positive association with pain score (adjusted B estimate = 10.1 (95% Confidence Interval 4.3–15.9); $p = 0.001$). Antibody array conducted with 6 pooled T98G cell lysate induced with osteoarthritis pain patient CSF identified greater than 2-fold proteins including STE20-related kinase adaptor protein and spleen tyrosine kinase. Further validation done using western blotting of individual CSF-triggered T98G cell lysate showed non-significant increase.

(Continued on next page)

* Correspondence: analeetl@nus.edu.sg
[1]Department of Anaesthesia, National University Hospital, National University Health System, 5 Lower Kent Ridge Road, Singapore 119074, Singapore
[2]Department of Anaesthesia, Yong Loo Lin School of Medicine, National University of Singapore, 5 Lower Kent Ridge Road, Singapore 119074, Singapore

(Continued from previous page)
Conclusion: Higher IL-6 release from T98G when triggered by OA-CSF, in the presence of LPS, suggest the presence of "unknown molecule" in CSF that may be crucial in the maintenance phase of chronic pain in our osteoarthritis population. Further studies on the signalling pathways involved in pain and relevance of IL-6 release from T98G cells in other pain models are needed.

Keywords: Chronic pain, Osteoarthritis, Interleukin-6, Cytokine

Background

Osteoarthritis (OA) is a common joint degenerative disease affecting many patients worldwide. It is characterised by the progressive loss of articular cartilage, joint space narrowing, secondary bone hyperplasia and atrophy of joint muscles [1]. This disease affects weight-bearing joints and is more severe in the hips and knees. The hallmark symptom in OA frequently experienced by patients is localised chronic pain, which reduces their quality of life [2]. There is currently no cure for knee OA and the available treatments include use of medications, physical therapy or surgery that involves total joint replacement [3, 4]. Despite having medications to alleviate pain, chronic pain is still a major problem for OA patients.

There is a lack of understanding about the signalling pathways involved in pain. Mechanisms underlying chronic pain may involve activation of a series of signalling molecules leading to increased peripheral and/or central sensitisation. Some studies evaluated inflammatory cytokines such as tumour necrosis factor alpha (TNFα), interleukin-1 beta (IL-1β), IL-6 and IL-8 and IL-10 in patients with chronic pain-related diseases. For instance, IL-6 is elevated in cerebrospinal fluid (CSF) of patients with complex regional pain syndrome (CRPS) [5] and elevated IL-8 in patients with fibromyalgia [6].

Other studies showed chronic pain in OA being mediated by changes in neurotrophic factors, chemokines and interleukins as a response by chondrocytes or synovial cells at the joint in the synovial fluid [2]. Some showed glia activation related to pathogenesis of chronic pain [7]. Besides supporting neuronal cells, glial cells are found to have key roles in pain modulation. The exact role has not been elucidated [8].

Our group previously showed that CSF of post-herpetic neuralgia (PHN) chronic pain patients induced elevated IL-6 release from human glioblastoma T98G cells [9]. Therefore, we hypothesised that IL-6 is crucial in the maintenance phase of chronic pain signalling. In this study, we aimed to investigate whether CSF from a different chronic pain model (i.e. knee OA) could also induce the release of pro-inflammatory cytokines IL-6, IL-1β and TNFα from T98G cells. In addition, we also investigate possible signalling pathways involved in chronic OA pain.

Methods

Study design and patient population

The procedure for CSF collection was approved by our Institutional Ethics Board and written informed consent was obtained from each patient (DSRB Ref No. 2011/01710). Patients (both the pain group and the group without pain) were prospectively recruited by the attending anaesthesiologists prior to surgery. All patients recruited in the pain group satisfied the following inclusion criteria: (a) Confirmed OA of knees from history and x-ray of the knees by orthopaedic surgeons, (b) Numeric pain rating scale of more than 3 (0 being no pain; 10 being worst possible imaginable pain), (c) Knee pain of more than 6 months duration, (d) Scheduled for total knee replacement surgery under spinal anaesthesia, (e) Age of 21 years and above, (f) No other concurrent chronic pain conditions. Patients without pain (NP) and undergoing surgery with spinal anaesthesia served as the control group. The inclusion criteria for no pain (NP) group include: (a) Patients who do not have knee osteoarthritis, (b) No history of any type of chronic pain conditions over the past 1 year; (c) Patient consented for surgery below the umbilicus under a spinal anaesthesia, (d) Age of 21 years and above. Pregnant patients or patients with severe end-organ function impairment (e.g. heart, lungs, liver and kidneys) were excluded.

CSF was obtained during the conduct of spinal anaesthesia, where two-ml of CSF was withdrawn after the dura was punctured, before injecting local anaesthetic into the subarachnoid space to effect the spinal anaesthesia. A total of 15 chronic knee OA patients and 15 NP patients were recruited. CSF samples were then stored at − 80 °C. Patients' demographics such as gender and age were also recorded.

Measurement of pro-inflammatory cytokine release in cell culture

Human glioblastoma cell line T98G (ATCC-CRL1690, American Type Culture Collection, Manassas, VA) was cultured as previously described [9]. In brief, Eagle's Minimum Essential Medium (Gibco, Grand Island, New York) (EMEM) containing 10% fetal bovine serum (FBS) (HyClone, Utah, USA) and 1X antibiotic-anti-mycotic cocktail (HyClone, Utah, USA) was used.

T98G cells were grown to approximately 90% confluency in 12-well plates. CSF from patients were filtered using a 0.22 μm filter to remove any existing cells in the CSF prior to all subsequent experiments. Filtered CSF was added into cultured T98G cells. The culture medium was replaced with FBS-free EMEM medium before addition of 50 μl CSF along with 32 μg/ml lipopolysaccharide (LPS) from *Escherichia coli* 055:B5 (Sigma Aldrich, St Louis MO, USA) to the T98G cells. Cells were induced for 48 h at 37 °C and 5% CO_2 environment. LPS was used to enhance cytokine release from the cells [9, 10]. Each well with the trigger of 50 μl CSF was from individual patient. After 48 h, the medium containing "released cytokines" was collected and the amount of IL-6 in this supernatant was measured in duplicates using enzyme-linked immunosorbent assay (ELISA) according to manufacturer's instructions (DY206, R&D Systems, Minneapolis, USA). The detection range for the IL-6 standard used was between 9.38 pg/ml to 600 pg/ml.

Using supernatant from the above 48 h CSF-triggered T98G protocol, TNFα and IL-1β levels were also determined with ELISA assays- Human TNFα Duoset ELISA (DY210) and Human IL-1β/IL-1F2 Duoset (DY201) respectively (R&D Systems, Minneapolis, USA). Detection range of standards for TNFα was 15.6 pg/ml to 1000 pg/ml; and IL-1β was 3.91 pg/ml to 250 pg/ml.

Antibody array

Nuclear factor kappa light chain enhancer of activated B cells (NF-κB) phospho antibody array (PNK215, Fullmoon Biosystems, CA, USA) was used to screen for changes in protein expression and phosphorylation profile in our samples. This array applied an ELISA-based technique where samples were biotinylated before adding to the array slide containing the affixed antibodies. Biotin on samples upon interaction with dye-labelled streptavidin on array would generate the fluorescence signal. Patient CSF-triggered T98G cells, in the presence of LPS, were harvested and lysed with CelLytic MT Cell Lysis Reagent (C3228; Sigma Aldrich). Total protein from these T98G cell lysate were quantified using bicinchoninic acid (BCA) assay (Pierce BCA Protein Assay Kit, Thermo Scientific, USA). Due to limited amount of CSF drawn from each patient, and to obtain a minimum amount of protein for each antibody array, the triggered T98G cell lysates from OA pain samples ($n = 6$) were pooled in equal quantity and added to the antibody array slide. Similarly, the same amount of T98G cell lysates from NP samples (n = 6) were pooled and added to another antibody array slide. The assay was then performed according to manufacturer's instructions. Array image was captured using array scanner (GenePix 4000B; Molecular Probes, CA, USA). Analysis of array data was done using Genescan software. Comparison of signals between pooled OA pain sample and pooled NP sample was done after normalization with glyceraldehyde-3-phosphate dehydrogenase (GAPDH).

Western blot analysis

To validate the fold increase protein expression and phosphorylation changes as observed in the antibody array for OA triggered T98G cells, all individual OA and NP-CSF triggered T98G cell lysates ($n = 15$ each) were checked for protein expression level of targets with western blotting. Ten micrograms of each CSF-triggered T98G cell lysates were loaded per lane of 10% Tris-glycine gels and run using Sodium dodecyl sulphate polyacrylamide gel electrophoresis (SDS-PAGE). Proteins on gel were transferred onto Polyvinylidene difluoride (PVDF) membrane. 0.1% Tween-20 added into Tris-buffered saline (TBS-T) was used to wash membranes and prepare antibodies. Non-specific binding sites on the membranes were blocked in 5% w/v Bovine serum albumin (BSA)-TBS-T or milk-TBS-T. BSA was used when checking for spleen tyrosine kinase (Syk); while milk was used for STE20-related kinase adaptor protein (STRAD) and GAPDH. Primary antibodies used in this study are: STRAD (G-8) (Santa Cruz Biotechnology, CA, USA); Syk (D3Z1E) (Cell Signaling Technology Inc., MA, USA); and GAPDH (MAB374) (EMD Millipore, Darmstadt, Germany). GAPDH, with a molecular weight of 37 kDa, was used as the loading control for normalization. Membranes were imaged with ChemiDoc XRS+ system. Densitometry quantification was done with ImageLab software.

Statistical analysis

All data were analysed using GraphPad Prism v5.0 (GraphPad, La Jolla, CA, USA) and SPSS v24.0 (IBM SPSS, Armonk NY, USA). Cytokine levels was checked for normality and deemed not normally distributed, thus non-parametric Mann Whitney-U test was used. Mann-Whitney U test was also used to analyse STRAD and Syk protein levels from western blotting between groups. Simple and multivariate linear regression model analyses were used to study the relationship of pain score and cytokine level. A p-value of less than 0.05 was considered statistically significant.

Results

Patient demographics

The average age of patients in our cohort is 61 ± 13 years. Demographics of OA pain and NP patients are described in Table 1. The control group are patients without pain. The types of surgical procedures for the NP

Table 1 Patient demographics of study groups

Group	OA pain ($n = 15$)	No pain ($n = 15$)	p-value
Age (years)	60 ± 13	63 ± 14	0.618
Gender	7 male, 8 female	14 male, 1 female	0.014
Pain Score	7 ± 2	0	< 0.001
History of diabetes mellitus, yes	3 (20%)	5 (33.3%)	0.682
History of hypertension, yes	8 (53.3%)	8 (53.3%)	1
History of peripheral vascular disease, yes	0	0	–
History of hyperlipidaemia, yes	6 (40%)	8 (53.3%)	0.715

Data are presented as Mean ± standard deviation (SD) or number (percentage). p-value of 0.05 is considered statistically significant

group included transurethral resection of the prostate ($n = 7$), hernia repair ($n = 2$) and ligation of piles ($n = 6$).

IL-6 release from T98G cells

The IL-6 levels in the CSF samples from OA and NP patients were below the lowest detection limit of the ELISA kit (9.38 pg/ml) used. In order to detect IL-6 levels using the ELISA method, the additional induction methodology used in [9] were used to amplify the IL-6 changes. Briefly, CSF was used to induce T98G cells in the presence of LPS in order for the T98G cells to release IL-6 at levels measurable using the ELISA method.

In the absence of CSF, addition of LPS to T98G cells did not trigger detectable levels of IL-6 release [9]. When both patients' CSF and LPS were added to T98G cells, IL-6 release was detected in the cell culture media. 67.0 ± 17.7 pg/ml of IL-6 was detected when induced with OA-CSF ($n = 15$) whereas 23.7 ± 3.4 pg/ml of IL-6 was detected for NP-CSF group (n = 15). There was a statistically significant higher amount of IL-6 released from T98G cells triggered with OA-CSF as compared to NP-CSF (Fig. 1; Mann Whitney-U test, $p = 0.002$).

TNFα and IL-1β release from T98G cells

TNFα and IL-1β (lowest detection range of 15.6 pg/ml and 3.91 pg/ml respectively), were evaluated and found to be undetectable in T98G cell culture media when induced with CSF (OA/NP) and LPS, with their respective ELISA kits.

Relationship between IL-6 release and pain score

There was a significant positive relationship between pain score and IL-6 cytokine levels (unadjusted B estimate = 7.1 (95% Confidence Interval (C.I.) = 2.1–12.1); $p = 0.007$). After adjusting for age and gender in the multivariate model, the significant association persists (adjusted B estimate = 10.1 (95% CI = 4.3–15.9); $p = 0.001$).

Possible targets found in antibody array

The antibody array used consisted of 6 replicates of 215 antibodies for targets related to the NF-κB pathway. Forty microgram of T98G cell lysates, harvested from each of the 6 individual CSF samples trigger, in the presence of LPS, were pooled together to give a total 240 μg protein for the array testing. The 240 μg pooled OA-CSF triggered T98G cell lysate was added to one array slide; while pooled NP-CSF triggered T98G cell lysate was added to another slide. The fluorescence signal of all 6 antibody replicates within each array were recorded and the average was calculated. GAPDH was used to normalise the signal for both OA and NP samples. Those with a greater than 2-fold increase in OA-CSF triggered T98G cell lysate as compared to that of NP-CSF were noted. The more notable ones having greater than 3-fold increase were STRAD (4.25 fold), Syk (3.40 fold), lymphocyte-specific protein tyrosine kinase (3.30 fold) and IkappaB-alpha (3.07 fold) (Fig. 2). STRAD and Syk were chosen for further validation using western blotting.

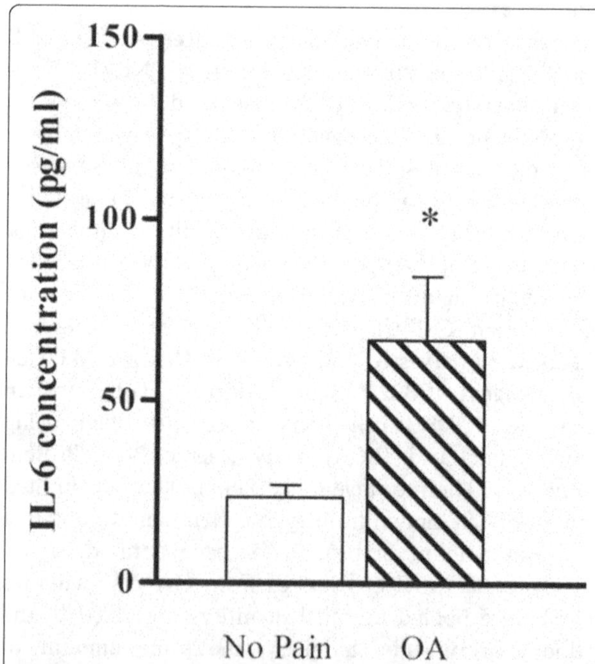

Fig. 1 Higher IL-6 release from OA pain CSF stimulated T98G cells, in the presence of LPS. Concentration of IL-6 release from T98G cells when triggered with 50 μl CSF of either OA-CSF or NP-CSF, in the presence of LPS. Bars are plotted as mean ± standard error of mean (15 patients per group), *$p < 0.05$ when using Mann Whitney-U test

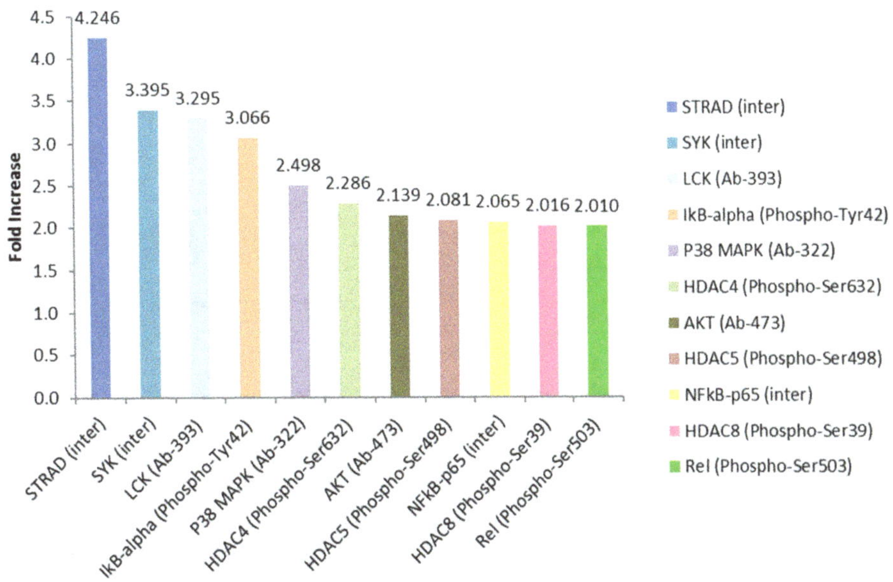

Fig. 2 Protein expression and phosphorylation changes in NF-κB related signalling pathways assayed using an antibody array. Pooled protein lysates from OA-CSF triggered T98G cell ($n = 6$) with the highest pain score and NP-CSF triggered T98G cell ($n = 6$) were assayed using the array. Proteins with expression or phosphorylation increase for more than 2-fold in OA-CSF triggered T98G lysate were plotted on the graph

Protein expression of STRAD and Syk

The molecular weight of STRAD is 48 kDa. For STRAD protein, there is a higher protein expression level in OA patients (1.26 ± 0.54; $n = 15$) as compared to NP patients (1.05 ± 0.42; n = 15). However, the difference was not statistically significant ($p = 0.298$) (Fig. 3).

Syk has a molecular weight of 72 kDa. Similarly, higher protein expression level was observed in OA patients (2.98 ± 2.9; n = 15) as compared to NP patients (1.96 ± 1.4; n = 15) for Syk protein. This higher protein expression in OA patients was not statistically significant ($p = 0.183$) (Fig. 4).

Discussion

IL-6 is a multi-functional protein cytokine known to play a role in the modulation of signalling in the central nervous system (CNS) such as those influencing immune responses, inflammation and wounds [11]. IL-6 has been implicated in various diseases related to pathological pain. It is generally believed that IL-6 release by the activated glial cells particularly the microglia and the astrocytes following painful stimuli [12]. Here, we showed that CSF obtained from a cohort of patients with chronic knee pain secondary to knee osteoarthritis when added together with LPS, was able to stimulate T98G cells to release IL-6. Whilst under similar condition, CSF obtained from a cohort of NP patients provoke significantly lesser IL-6 release. LPS alone did not stimulate T98G cells to release IL-6, and IL-6 was not detected in any CSF sample prior to the cell culture experiments. This is also supported by the positive correlation between

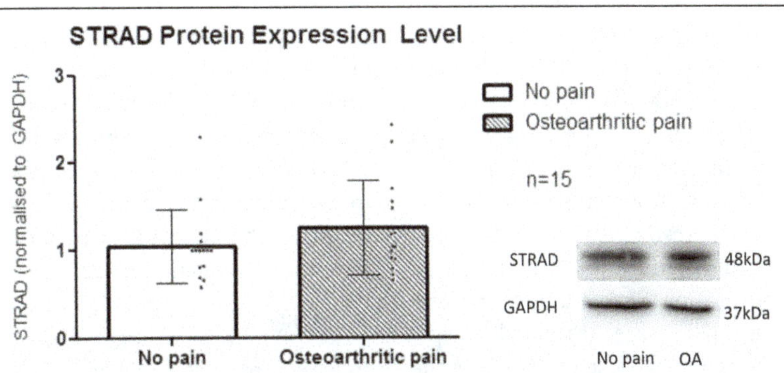

Fig. 3 Normalized STRAD protein expression level between the study groups. Western blotting was run and each dot represents STRAD protein expression of each sample of individual patient's CSF induction in T98G cells. Bars are plotted as mean ± SD (15 patients per group), *$p < 0.05$ when using Mann Whitney-U test

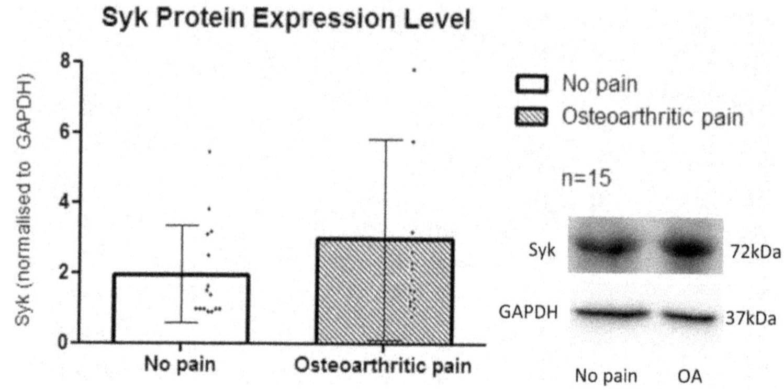

Fig. 4 Normalized Syk protein expression level between the study groups. Western blotting was run and each dot represents Syk protein expression of each sample of individual patient's CSF induction in T98G cells. Bars are plotted as mean ± SD (15 patients per group), $*p < 0.05$ when using Mann Whitney-U test

patient's numeric pain scores and the amount of IL-6 released. Taken together, our results suggest that CSF obtained from patients suffering from chronic OA knee pain, contain an as-yet-unknown molecule(s) which can trigger IL-6 release from cultured T98G cells. This result is also consistent with our previous published work using CSF obtained from another cohort of chronic pain patients (post-herpetic neuralgia).

We explored the signalling pathway upstream of IL-6 in our T98G model. Specifically, NF-κB explorer array was chosen as it is one of the common upstream molecular players of IL-6. Several protein targets were found to be elevated with greater than two-fold in OA-CSF triggered T98G cells as compared to NP-CSF triggered ones (Fig. 2), these targets could be important in delineating the chronic pain signalling mechanism.

Two protein targets which showed an increase of 4.2 and 3.4 fold in OA-CSF in the array were STRAD and Syk respectively. STRAD, predominantly found in CNS, is known to complex with serine/threonine kinase LKB1 and scaffold protein MO25α to activate AMP-activated protein kinase (AMPK) signalling pathway which includes release of pro-inflammatory cytokines [13]. Syk plays a role in signal transduction influencing cells of the immune system- both B and T cells [14]. NF-κB and IL-6 are downstream of AMPK [15]. Although both STRAD and Syk showed the highest expression among other potential target proteins in the pooled T98G cell lysate following exposure to CSF from 6 OA patients with the highest pain score, when all samples were further validated individually in western blotting, their differences were not statistically significant when compared with samples from the NP group (Figs. 3 and 4). Several possibilities to explain our result are: (a) small sample size, (b) wider range of patients' visual analog scale (VAS) pain scores in the 15 OA samples when tested in western blotting versus the pooled 6 OA samples with the highest VAS pain scores used on the array analysis.

The strength of our study is the use of human CSF to provide an objective evaluation of chronic pain. CSF, as compared to peripheral blood, has a more direct contact with the CNS environment. It bathes the CNS and therefore the contents in CSF may be crucial in understanding changes of the underlying disease associated with chronic knee pain [16]. Our findings may lead to better understanding of the pathogenesis of OA knee pain and future therapeutic approaches if the identity of the pain signalling molecule and the upstream signalling pathway(s) can be elucidated.

Although we found that a 48-h treatment time point for measuring IL-6 release provides sufficient signal strength in the ELISA, it may not be the peak protein expression or phosphorylation changes for STRAD and Syk, thus leading to overall lack of significance in western blotting results. Another limitation was that only a limited number of antibodies were tested.

Conclusion

In summary, CSF from chronic knee pain patients suffering from OA knees was able to induce higher levels of IL-6 release from T98G cells than NP-CSF in the presence of LPS. This finding suggests the presence of an as-yet-unknown molecule(s) in the CSF of patients with chronic pain which could potentially serve as clinically informative biomarker(s). Further studies are needed to investigate the relevance of IL-6 release by T98G glial cells in other chronic pain models and to evaluate any potential upstream players.

Abbreviations

AMPK: AMP-activated protein kinase; ATCC: American Type Culture Collection; BCA: Bicinchoninic acid; BSA: Bovine serum albumin; CI: Confidence Interval; CNS: Central Nervous System; CRPS: Complex Regional Pain Syndrome; CSF: Cerebrospinal fluid; ELISA: Enzyme-linked immunosorbent assay; EMEM: Eagle's minimum essential medium; F: Female; FBS: Fetal Bovine Serum; GAPDH: Glyceraldehyde-3-phosphate dehydrogenase; IL: Interleukin; LPS: Lipopolysaccharide; M: Male; NF-κB: Nuclear factor kappa light chain enhancer of activated B cells; NP: No pain; OA: Osteoarthritis; PHN: Post-herpetic Neuralgia; SD: Standard deviation; SDS-PAGE: Sodium dodecyl sulphate polyacrylamide gel electrophoresis; STRAD: STE20-related kinase adaptor protein; Syk: Spleen tyrosine kinase; TNFα: Tumour Necrosis Factor-alpha; VAS: Visual Analog Scale

Acknowledgements
Not applicable.

Authors' contributions
WL helped with conducting of study, data analysis and writing of manuscript. CL helped with conducting of study and preparation of manuscript. FCKT helped with data analysis and preparation of manuscript. HJN helped with collecting CSF samples and preparation of manuscript. YHC helped with data interpretation and preparation of manuscript. CML helped with study design and implementation, data interpretation and preparation of manuscript. TLL helped with study design and implementation, collecting CSF samples, data interpretation and preparation of manuscript. All authors approved the final manuscript.

Author details
[1]Department of Anaesthesia, National University Hospital, National University Health System, 5 Lower Kent Ridge Road, Singapore 119074, Singapore. [2]Department of Anaesthesia, Yong Loo Lin School of Medicine, National University of Singapore, 5 Lower Kent Ridge Road, Singapore 119074, Singapore. [3]Biostatistics Unit, Yong Loo Lin School of Medicine, National University of Singapore, Singapore, Singapore. [4]Department of Pharmacology, Yong Loo Lin School of Medicine, National University of Singapore, 16 Medical Drive, Singapore 117600, Singapore.

References
1. Dray A, Read SJ. Arthritis and pain. Future targets to control osteoarthritis pain. Arthritis Res Ther. 2007;9(3):212.
2. Miller RE, Miller RJ, Malfait A-M. Osteoarthritis joint pain: the cytokine connection. Cytokine. 2014;70(2):185–93.
3. Singapore Burden of Disease Study 2010. Ministry of Health Singapore. https://www.moh.gov.sg/docs/librariesprovider5/resources-statistics/reports/singapore-burden-of-disease-study-2010-report_v3.pdf. Accessed 22 April 2019.
4. Mushtaq S, Choudhary R, Scanzello CR. Non-surgical treatment of osteoarthritis-related pain in the elderly. Curr Rev Musculoskelet Med. 2011; 4(3):113–22.
5. Alexander GM, Rijn MAV, Hilten JJV, Perreault MJ, Schwartzman RJ. Changes in cerebrospinal fluid levels of pro-inflammatory cytokines in CRPS. Pain. 2005;116(3):213–9.
6. Bjurstrom MF, Giron SE, Griffis CA. Cerebrospinal fluid cytokines and Neurotrophic factors in human chronic pain populations: A comprehensive review. Pain Practice. 2014;16(2):183–203.
7. Loggia ML, Chonde DB, Akeju O, et al. Evidence for brain glial activation in chronic pain patients. Brain. 2015;138(3):604–15.
8. Sheridan C. Glial cells on the radar. Nat Biotechnol. 2009;27(2):114–6.
9. Tay AS, Liu EH, Lee TL, et al. Cerebrospinal fluid of postherpetic neuralgia patients induced interleukin-6 release in human glial cell-line T98G. Neurochem Int. 2013;63(5):517–21.
10. Grimaldi M, Navarra P, Pozzoli G, Preziosi P, Schettini G. Bacterial lipopolysaccharide increases Interleukin-6 and prostaglandin release in rat cortical type I astrocytes by different mechanisms: role of anti-inflammatory agents. Biochem Biophys Res Commun. 1998;250(3):798–804.
11. Choy E., Rose-John S. Interleukin-6 as a multifunctional regulator: inflammation, immune response, and fibrosis. J Scleroderma Relat Disord. 2017;2(no 2_suppl):S1–5.
12. Watkins LR, Milligan ED, Maier SF. Glial activation: a driving force for pathological pain. Trends Neurosci. 2001;24(8):450–5.
13. Hawley SA, Boudeau J, Reid JL, et al. Complexes between the LKB1 tumor suppressor, STRADα/β and MO25α/β are upstream kinases in the AMP-activated protein kinase cascade. J Biol. 2003;2(4):28.
14. Kyttaris VC. The role of Syk in osteoarthritis. Clin Immunol. 2012;144(3):283.
15. Salminen A, Hyttinen JM, Kaarniranta K. AMP-activated protein kinase inhibits NF-κB signaling and inflammation: impact on healthspan and lifespan. J Mol Med. 2011;89(7):667–76.
16. Sethuraman R, Lee TL, Tachibana S. Simple quantitative HPLC method for measuring physiologic amino acids in cerebrospinal fluid without pretreatment. Clin Chem. 2004;50(3):665–9.

18

Gradual withdrawal of remifentanil delays initial post-operative analgesic demand after thyroid surgery

Sarah Saxena[1,2*], Kimberly Gonsette[1], Willy Terram[1], Isabelle Huybrechts[1], Daniel A. Nahrwold[2,3], Matteo Cappello[4], Luc Barvais[1] and Edgard Engelman[1]

Abstract

Background: Mismanagement of remifentanil leads to severe side effects such as opioid-induced tolerance and hyperalgesia. Recently studies revealed an alternative withdrawal method to limit these side effects. A gradual withdrawal of remifentanil seems to be associated with less pain. The hypothesis of this double-blinded, randomized controlled trial was that a gradual withdrawal of remifentanil would be associated with less immediate post-operative pain compared to after an abrupt discontinuation of remifentanil in patients who underwent thyroid surgery.

Methods: This double-blinded, randomized controlled trial was conducted in a tertiary level hospital in Brussels (Belgium) from April until August 2017. 34 patients undergoing thyroid surgery were randomized and 29 patients completed the study. After randomization, patients undergoing thyroid surgery were allocated to two groups: one with an abrupt discontinuation of remifentanil after surgery and one with a gradual withdrawal of remifentanil after surgery. The primary outcome was the initial post-operative demand of analgesic medication.

Results: Gradual withdrawal of remifentanil was associated with a delayed initial post-operative demand of analgesic medication ($P = 0.006$). The first morphine bolus was given after 76.3 +/− 89.0 min in the group with a gradual withdrawal of remifentanil versus after 9.0 +/− 13.5 min in the group with an abrupt discontinuation of remifentanil.
However, overall morphine consumption, numeric rating scale scores, Ramsay Sedation Scale scores, and quality of recovery scores (QoR-40) were similar in both groups ($P > 0.05$).

Conclusion: Though overall morphine consumption, numeric rating scale scores, Ramsay Sedation Scale scores, and quality of recovery scores (QoR-40) are not altered, a gradual withdrawal of remifentanil after thyroid surgery is safe and associated with a delayed initial post-operative demand of analgesic drugs. The withdrawal process does, however, require vigilance and training.

* Correspondence: sarah.saxena@ulb.ac.be
[1]Department of Anesthesia and Perioperative Care, CUB Erasme University Hospital, Université Libre de Bruxelles, 808, Route de Lennik, 1070 Brussels, Belgium
[2]Department of Anesthesia and Perioperative Care, Zuckerberg San Francisco General Hospital & Trauma Center, University of California, San Francisco, USA

Background

Over the last decade, remifentanil has been subjected to bad press [1, 2]. Initially, this drug was hailed for its benefits which included being an ultra short-acting phenylpiperidine opioid analgesic with high lipid solubility, having a rapid onset of action, and being rapidly metabolized by non-specific blood and tissue esterases. For these reasons, many anesthesiologists became accustomed to using remifentanil. It can be given in high doses, is easily titratable, and leads to predictable, rapid recoveries.

However, the mismanagement of remifentanil can lead to a wide range of side effects including opioid-induced tolerance and hyperalgesia. Additionally, due to its rapid elimination, a bridge to post-operative analgesia is a necessity when administering this drug.

Opioid tolerance is defined as an increase in the dose required to maintain analgesia in patients receiving opioids for pain relief in the clinical setting. Opioid-induced hyperalgesia is a state of nociceptive sensitization and is defined as increased pain from a stimulus that normally provokes pain [3]. While clear definitions are accepted, the underlying mechanisms behind these concepts are still widely misunderstood and remain under investigation.

Recently, studies have been published about an alternative withdrawal method of remifentanil. Albrecht et al. demonstrated that immediate discontinuation of remifentanil after digestive surgery is associated with increased postoperative pain levels [4].

A gradual withdrawal of remifentanil may be associated with less pain in a rodent population [5]. Several research groups have evaluated this hypothesis in healthy human volunteers and have seemingly confirmed the theory that a gradual withdrawal of remifentanil is associated with less pain [6, 7].

Our group wanted to put this theory into practice within the perioperative period. The hypothesis of this double-blinded, randomized controlled trial was that a gradual withdrawal of remifentanil would be associated with less immediate post-operative pain compared to after an abrupt discontinuation of remifentanil in patients undergoing thyroid surgery.

Methods

Ethics

This study was designed adhering to the Declaration of Helsinki and the CONSORT checklist, and was approved by the internal review board (03/30/2017; P2017/074; Comité Ethique, Erasme hospital, Brussels; Chairman: Jean-Marie Boeymans). The trial was registered on clinicaltrials.gov (NCT03110653; PI: Luc Barvais; date of registration: 03/31/2017). Written informed consent was obtained from each patient participating in the study.

Inclusion criteria were the following: male or female patients aged 18–65 undergoing thyroid surgery at the Erasme hospital, Brussels, ASA physical status of I-III, and a knowledge of French, English, or Dutch.

Exclusion criteria were the following: pregnancy, hypo or hyperthyroidism, gastro-duodenal ulcer, allergy or contraindications to one of the study drugs, renal insufficiency, liver insufficiency, neuropsychiatric disturbance, BMI > 30, history of drug and alcohol abuse, and pre-operative analgesic drug use.

The main objective of this study was to evaluate immediate post-operative pain levels in patients who underwent two types of remifentanil withdrawal methods. The timing of the first demand of post-operative analgesic was compared in both groups. In parallel, post-operative morphine consumption was also compared between both groups, as well as numeric rating scale (NRS) values at rest and after a small head flexion. In this way, pain was evaluated after 0, 15, 30, 45, 60, 75, 90, 105, 120 min, and 4 h after admission to the post-anesthesia care unit (PACU), as well as 24 h post-operatively. A quality of recovery (QoR-40) questionnaire was given to each patient pre- and post-operatively to evaluate patient satisfaction [8]. In the PACU, sedation was assessed in both groups via the Ramsay Sedation Scale [9].

Patients were randomized to one or the other group using a computer-generated randomization list (QuickCalcs program-GraphPad Software Inc., La Jolla, USA). For premedication, all patients received alprazolam (0.5 mg P.O.) one hour pre-operatively. Multi-parameter monitoring was used according to our institution's protocol (ECG, pulse oximetry, non-invasive blood pressure every three minutes, Bispectral Index (BIS), and neuromuscular blockade monitoring utilizing the train-of-four ratio). In the case of blood pressure dropping 20% or more from initial baseline measurement, a bolus of intravenous ephedrine was administered.

Anesthesia was induced intravenously in both groups with remifentanil TCI (Minto model; 5 ng ml^{-1}; approximately 0.15 mcg kg^{-1} min^{-1}) and propofol TCI (Schnider model; starting at 3 mcg ml^{-1}; adjusted to BIS levels between 45 and 55). Rocuronium (0.6 mg kg^{-1}) was then administered to facilitate tracheal intubation. After tracheal intubation, but pre-incision, remifentanil levels were lowered to 2 ng ml^{-1} (approximately 0.065 mcg kg^{-1} min^{-1}). Just before incision, remifentanil levels were increased to 5 ng ml^{-1}, and acetaminophen (1000 mg), diclofenac (1 mg kg^{-1}) and morphine (0.15 mg kg^{-1}) were administered as co-analgesics. Dexamethasone (10 mg) was administered to both groups. By the end of the surgery, ondansetron (4 mg) was given to all patients. Upon skin closure, remifentanil levels were progressively lowered to 3.5 ng ml^{-1} (approximately 0.13 mcg kg^{-1} min^{-1}). By the end of the surgery, propofol TCI was discontinued and remifentanil was kept at 2 ng ml^{-1}. Tracheal extubation was accomplished after adequate spontaneous ventilation was ensured, as well as the patient's responsiveness to verbal commands.

The patients were then transferred to the PACU with the remifentanil TCI infusion pump running at 2 ng ml^{-1}. Back check valves and continuous saline infusion were used in the IV line in order to avoid backflow, dead space syndrome, or unintentional bolus.

According to pre-operative randomization, the remifentanil infusion syringe was then switched in the PACU to a new syringe, which was prepared by a colleague (WT) who was independent of the study. This post-operative syringe was either remifentanil diluted to 20 mcg/ml or NaCl 0.9%. PACU nurses and the primary anesthesiologist did not know whether their patients had received a newly prepared remifentanil or NaCl 0.9% syringe.

A gradual decrease of this infusion was then started in the PACU according to the following protocol: a reduction in infusion rate of 30% every 15 min (2 - > 1.4 - > 1 - > 0.7- > 0.5 - > 0.35 - > 0.25 - > 0 ng ml^{-1}). This gradual decrease was achieved in two hours.

While in the PACU, intravenous morphine (2 mg every five minutes) was administered if a patient's pain was more than 3/10 on the NRS. All patients were monitored and under immediate medical surveillance, and therefore no limit was imposed on total morphine consumption. Additionally, acetaminophen (1000 mg every 6 h) and diclofenac (1 mg kg^{-1} every 12 h) were administered to all patients. Patients stayed a minimum of four hours in the PACU and were discharged from the PACU once they were comfortable (e.g. NRS < 3/10, no post-operative nausea and vomiting, Ramsay scores of 2–3, no hematoma at the surgical site).

The total quantities of each drug used, as well as the different timings (induction, incision, end of surgery, and extubation times), were recorded. The primary anesthesiologist collected data pre-operatively and post-operatively (the first 24 h post-operation).

Statistical analysis

As the primary outcome of the study was to compare the first post-operative demand of analgesic drugs, we considered a difference of 35 min or more to be of clinical relevance. With a two-sided alpha level of 0.05 and power of 90% (standard deviation (SD) of 27 min), the study needed to be conducted on 26 patients with each group consisting of 13 patients.

Statistix 9.0 (Analytical Software, Tallahassee, USA) was used for statistical analyses. The results were presented as mean ± standard deviation. P values < 0.05 were considered to be statistically significant. The Mann-Whitney U test was used for the analysis of the first demand of analgesic drug data, morphine consumption data, QoR-40 data, and NRS score data at 24 h. NRS values and Ramsay scale scores in the PACU were analyzed using a two-way ANOVA for repeated measures.

Results

Thirty-four patients were randomized from April to August 2017 (Fig. 1). Three patients were excluded from analysis due to missing data. Additionally, the protocol was not adhered to in two patients. Therefore, 29 patients were analyzed with 15 in the remifentanil group and 14 in the control group.

Patient characteristics are described in Table 1. Age, weight, BMI, gender, and ASA scores were collected for both groups pre-operatively. Our primary outcome measure was the timing of the initial demand of post-operative analgesic drug, and our data analysis revealed a statistically significant difference between the two groups ($P = 0.006$). The first morphine bolus was given 76.3 ± 89.0 min post-operatively in the remifentanil group and 9.0 ± 13.5 min in the control group (Table 2).

A statistically significant difference in morphine consumption was not observed while patients were in the PACU ($P = 0.251$). In addition, there was no difference in overall (intra- and post-operative) morphine consumption ($P = 0.325$; Table 2). Examination of NRS values in the PACU showed no statistically significant between-group differences both at rest ($P = 0.358$) and during head flexion ($P = 0.418$; Table 3; Fig. 2). Review of these same NRS values 24 h post-operatively on the ward did not demonstrate any statistically significant between-group differences ($p = 0.113$; Table 2). Furthermore, analysis of the QoR-40 scores exhibited no differences between the groups ($P = 0.513$; Table 2). Ramsay scores, indicating the patient's sedation level, were not different between the groups ($P = 0.337$; Table 4).

Discussion

This double-blinded, randomized controlled trial showed that a gradual decrease of remifentanil levels is associated with a delayed initial demand of post-operative analgesic drug. This corresponds with what others have already described in healthy volunteers [6, 7].

Remifentanil-induced hyperalgesia remains a misunderstood concept, with multiple theories attempting to find its cause. One interesting cellular model for pain amplification and hyperalgesia after opioid withdrawal is referred to as the long-term potentiation (LTP) of synaptic strength in nociceptive pathways. Opioid withdrawal LTP has been described as the following: "A brief application of remifentanil *in vivo* leads to acute depression of synaptic strength in C-fibers. Upon withdrawal, synaptic strength not only quickly returns to normal, but becomes potentiated for prolonged periods of time" [10]. A study on spinal dorsal horns from rats showed that

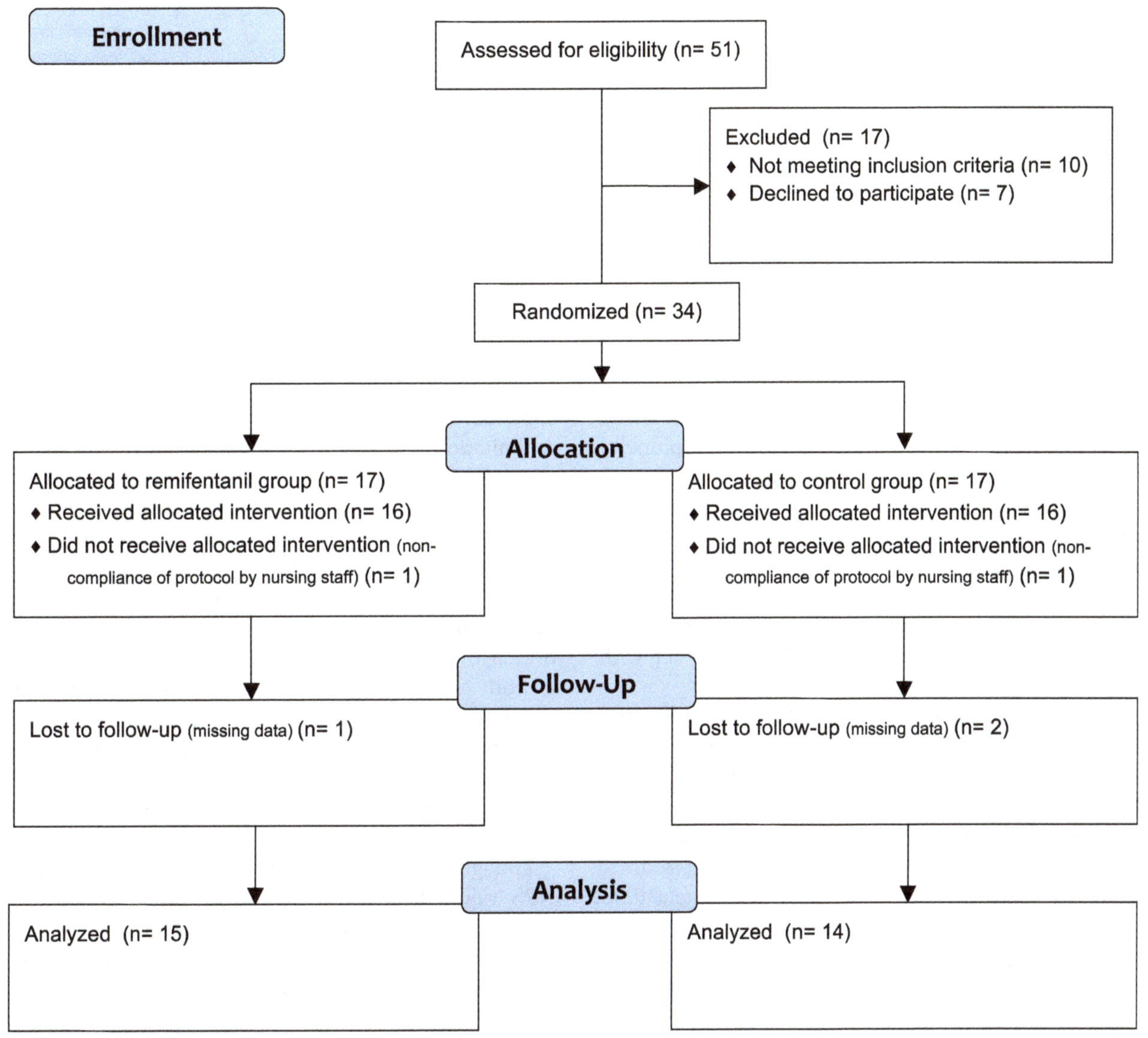

Fig. 1 Flow diagram

withdrawal LTP may be prevented by tapering of the remifentanil infusion instead of abrupt withdrawal [5]. This LTP could indeed explain why a gradual withdrawal of remifentanil was associated with a delayed initial post-operative analgesic demand.

Table 1 Demographic data

	Remifentanil group	Control group	*P* value
Age (years)	42.0 ± 10.3	44.6 ± 12.2	0.50
Weight (kg)	72.5 ± 13.3	78.1 ± 20.5	0.56
BMI (kg/m^2)	26.5 ± 4.7	27.2 ± 5.8	0.91
Gender (F/M)	14 / 1	12 / 2	0.60
ASA score (1/2)	2 / 13	0 / 14	0.48

Data as Mean ± SD or number of patients – Analysis by Mann-Whitney U test or Fisher exact test

Another theory explaining remifentanil-induced hyperalgesia is the activation of the N-methyl-D-aspartate (NMDA) receptor, which counteracts its analgesic effects. Indeed, blocking NMDA receptors can prevent this development by decreasing the activation of pronociceptive systems that are triggered by opioids [11].

In our study, remifentanil was administered in conjunction with propofol. Propofol, by inhibiting the NMDA subtype of the glutamate receptor, may have a preventative effect on remifentanil-induced hyperalgesia [1, 12].

The administration mode of remifentanil was based on the Minto model, which is relatively standard for most European countries. A TCI mode of remifentanil seems to be associated with less hyperalgesia [13].

The analgesia protocol of this trial was designed to prevent post-operative pain as much as possible [3]. A

Table 2 Initial demand of post-operative analgesic, morphine consumption, QoR-40 scores, NRS values (24 h)

	Remifentanil group	Control group	*P* value for difference between groups
Time to administration of the first iv morphine bolus (min)	76.3 ± 89.0 (45.0)	9.0 ± 13.5 (3.5)	0.006
Supplementary postoperative morphine during the first 4 post-operative hours (mg)	6.4 ± 5.1 (6.0)	8.3 ± 3.9 (8.0)	0.251
Supplementary morphine, including the administration at the beginning of surgery, during the first 4 post-operative hours (mg)	16.6 ± 4.9 (17.0)	18.0 ± 4.2 (18.5)	0.325
Numeric rating scale score for pain at rest 24 h after surgery	1.85 ± 1.46 (2.5)	0.91 ± 1.37 (0.0)	0.113
QoR-40 score	173.4 ± 16.3 (176.0)	179.0 ± 10.8 (178.5)	0.513

Data as Mean ± SD (median) - Analysis by Mann-Whitney U test

multimodal analgesia regimen (consisting of NSAIDS, acetaminophen, and timely administered morphine) is standard practice in our institution and was therefore applied to this study. This allowed us to keep remifentanil levels relatively low (at maximum 5 ng ml^{-1} or approximately 0.15 mcg kg^{-1} ml^{-1}).

In this study, remifentanil was gradually withdrawn in the PACU over the course of two hours, though at present, no consensus exists regarding the exact withdrawal method of remifentanil.

As mentioned, mismanagement of remifentanil administration leads to severe side effects. This study was conducted with extreme caution and required training of the nursing and anesthesia staff in order to avoid accidental boluses, especially during transport from the operating room to the PACU. In this way, episodes of respiratory depression and apnea were nonexistent (SP02 remained > 95% at all times). Sedation levels were the same in both groups, and all patients underwent anesthesia and the subsequent 24 h post-operative period uneventfully.

Limitations

A limitation of our study was that hyperalgesia was not properly assessed through pain threshold tests at the surgical site. Pain was evaluated through the NRS, total morphine consumption, and initial post-operative demand of an analgesic.

Even though this initial demand of an analgesic was delayed through a gradual withdrawal of remifentanil, overall morphine consumption was quite low and equal in both groups (16.6 ± 4.9 mg in the remifentanil group versus 18.0 ± 4.2 mg in the control group). This could be explained by the fact that a well-timed multimodal analgesia plan was applied to both groups. Additionally, our study may not have been powered to show a difference in morphine consumption.

Though the difference in immediate post-operative NRS values between both groups was not statistically significant, some interesting observations can be made. While both groups benefitted from the same perioperative multimodal analgesia strategy, raw NRS values

Table 3 Numeric Rating Scale (NRS) Values for Pain

	PACU arrival	PACU + 15 min	PACU + 30 min	PACU + 45 min	PACU + 60 min	PACU + 75 min	PACU + 90 min	PACU + 105 min	PACU + 120 min	PACU + 240 min
NRS value for pain at rest										
Remifentanil group	2.53 ± 2.32	2.60 ± 2.19	3.06 ± 2.57	2.86 ± 1.99	3.26 ± 1.94	2.73 ± 1.71	2.93 ± 1.58	2.66 ± 1.54	2.06 ± 1.33	1.86 ± 1.72
Control group	4.53 ± 2.93	5.23 ± 2.86	5.15 ± 2.44	4.46 ± 2.22	3.46 ± 2.25	2.46 ± 1.94	2.07 ± 1.70	1.84 ± 1.34	1.61 ± 1.04	1.30 ± 1.25
	P value for difference between groups: 0.358 *P* value for difference between times: < 0.001 P value for interaction: < 0.001									
NRS value for pain during head flexion										
Remifentanil group	2.80 ± 2.33	2.93 ± 2.21	3.40 ± 2.66	3.33 ± 2.02	3.80 ± 1.93	3.26 ± 1.79	3.46 ± 1.50	3.13 ± 1.59	2.66 ± 1.75	2.60 ± 2.06
Control group	5.00 ± 3.13	5.69 ± 2.84	5.30 ± 2.84	4.61 ± 2.72	4.00 ± 2.76	3.15 ± 2.51	2.76 ± 2.42	2.61 ± 2.39	2.38 ± 2.32	1.84 ± 1.62
	P value for difference between groups: 0.418 *P* value for difference between times: < 0.001 *P* value for interaction: < 0.001									

Data as Mean ± SD - Analysis by 2-way ANOVA for repeated measures

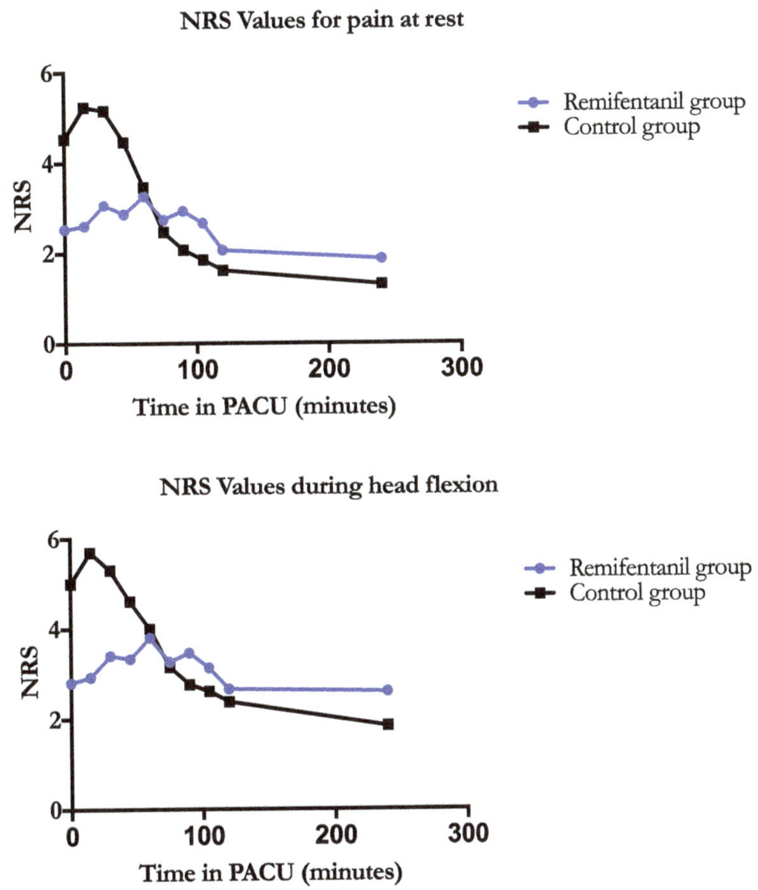

Fig. 2 **a** Illustrates the Numeric Rating Scale (NRS) values in both groups during their stay in the PACU while at rest. Pain evaluation was done upon arrival to the PACU and every 15 min during the first 2 h post-operatively, as well as after 4 h. Patients evaluating their pain as > 3/10 on the NRS received a morphine bolus (2 mg every 5 min as needed). Values are Means ± SD. 2 way-ANOVA for repeated measures. *P* value for difference between both groups: 0.358; *P* value for difference between times: < 0.001; *P* value for interaction: < 0.001. **b** Illustrates the Numeric Rating Scale (NRS) values in both groups during their stay in the PACU during a light head flexion. Upon arrival and every 15 min during the first 2 h post-operatively, as well as after 4 h, patients were asked to do a light head flexion. During this moment, NRS values were recorded. Values are Means ± SD. 2 way-ANOVA for repeated measures. *P* value for difference between both groups: 0.418; *P* value for difference between times: < 0.001; *P* value for interaction: < 0.001

showed a remarkably different trajectory (Fig. 2). The control group ($n = 14$) had declining NRS values starting relatively high, whereas the remifentanil group ($n = 15$) had zigzag values centered around 3/10. A likely explanation for this is that the remifentanil group still received an opioid, remifentanil, in addition to morphine, and was therefore less prone to experiencing pain. However, the remifentanil concentrations were quite low, especially in the second hour of the withdrawal phase, and consequently may not completely explain the observed differences in NRS values. Again, it could also be that our study was not powered adequately to fully examine NRS values.

Though the study demonstrated a delayed initial post-operative analgesic demand after a gradual withdrawal of

Table 4 Ramsay Sedation Scale score

	PACU arrival	PACU + 15 min	PACU + 30 min	PACU + 45 min	PACU + 60 min	PACU + 75 min	PACU + 90 min	PACU + 105 min	PACU + 120 min	PACU + 240 min
Remifentanil group	2.46 ± 0.91	2.46 ± 0.64	2.53 ± 0.64	2.53 ± 0.64	2.40 ± 0.63	2.33 ± 0.61	2.33 ± 0.61	2.47 ± 0.74	2.47 ± 0.74	2.06 ± 0.25
Control group	2.21 ± 0.57	2.07 ± 0.47	2.07 ± 0.47	2.14 ± 0.36	2.14 ± 0.36	2.37 ± 0.63	2.28 ± 0.46	2.42 ± 0.75	2.35 ± 0.74	2.21 ± 0.57
	P value for difference between groups: 0.337 *P* value for difference between times: 0.224 *P* value for interaction: 0.047									

Data as Mean ± SD - Analysis by 2-way ANOVA for repeated measures remifentanil, another limitation was that it was conducted on patients who underwent relatively minor thyroid surgeries. Larger studies must be done in major surgeries in order to see whether the results from this study can be reproduced in patients who experience greater noxious stimuli and further our understanding of some of the NRS interactions revealed in our study.

Conclusion

Though overall morphine consumption, numeric rating scale scores, Ramsay Sedation Scale scores, and quality of recovery scores (QoR-40) are not altered, a gradual withdrawal of remifentanil after thyroid surgery is safe and associated with a delayed initial post-operative demand of analgesic drugs. The withdrawal process does, however, require vigilance and training.

Abbrevations

LTP: Long term potentiation; NMDA: N-methyl-D-aspartate; NRS: Numeric Rating Scale; PACU: Post-anesthesia care unit; QoR: quality of recovery; TCI: Target controlled infusion

Acknowledgements

The authors thank the nursing staff of the Erasme hospital, Brussels. Data from this study were presented at the IARS annual conference (Chicago 2018).

Authors' contributions

All authors have read and approved the manuscript. SS: patient recruitment, data collection, writing up draft of the paper. KG: patient recruitment, data collection. WT: study material preparation, study design. IH: patient recruitment, data collection. DN: revision of draft of the paper. MC: patient recruitment, data collection. LB: study design, supervision. EE: data analysis and interpretation, supervision.

Author details

[1]Department of Anesthesia and Perioperative Care, CUB Erasme University Hospital, Université Libre de Bruxelles, 808, Route de Lennik, 1070 Brussels, Belgium. [2]Department of Anesthesia and Perioperative Care, Zuckerberg San Francisco General Hospital & Trauma Center, University of California, San Francisco, USA. [3]Department of Anesthesiology, H. Lee Moffitt Cancer Center & Research Institute, University of South Florida, Tampa, USA. [4]Department of Cardiothoracic Surgery, CUB Erasme University Hospital, Université Libre de Bruxelles, Brussels, Belgium.

References

1. Fletcher D, Martinez V. Opioid induced hyperalgesia in patients after surgery: a systematic review and a meta-analysis. Br J Anaesth. 2014;112: 991–1004.
2. Guignard B, Bossard AE, Coste C, et al. Acute opioid tolerance: intraoperative remifentanil increases postoperative pain and morphine requirement. Anesthesiology. 2000;93:409–17.
3. Yu EHY, Tran HD, Lam SW, Irwin MG. Remifentanil tolerance and hyperalgesia: short-term gain, long term pain? Anaesthesia. 2016;71:1347–62.
4. Albrecht S, Fechner J, Geisslinger G, et al. Postoperative pain control following remifentanil-based anaesthesia for major abdominal surgery. Anaesthesia. 2000;55:315–22.
5. Didla R, Gassner M, Gingl E, Sandkuhler J. Induction of synaptic long-term potentiation after opioid withdrawal. Science. 2009;325:207–10.
6. Comelon M, Raeder J, Stubhaug A, Nielsen CS, Draegni T, Lenz H. Gradual withdrawal of remifentanil infusion may prevent opioid induced hyperalgesia. Br J Anaesth. 2016;116:524–30.
7. Sprenger C, Eichler IC, Eichler L, Zollner C, Buchel C. Altered signaling in the descending pain modulatory system after short-term infusion of the mu-opioid agonist remifentanil. J Neurosci. 2018;38:2454–70.
8. Myles PS, Weitkamp B, Jones K, Melick J, Hensen S. Validity and reliability of a postoperative quality of recovery score: the QoR-40. Br J Anaesth. 2000;84:11–5.
9. Ramsay MA, Savege TM, Simpson BR, Goodwin R. Controlled sedation with alphaxolone-alphadalone. BMJ. 1974;2:656–9.
10. Sandkühler J, Gruber-Schoffnegger D. Hyperalgesia by synaptic long-term potentiation (LTP): an update. Curr Opin Pharmacol. 2012;12:18–27.
11. Richebé P, Cahana A, Rivat C. Tolerance and opioid-induced hyperalgesia. Is a divorce imminent. Pain. 2012;153:1547–8.
12. Lee M, Silverman SM, Hansen H, Patel VB, Manchikanti L. A comprehensive review of opioid-induced hyperalgesia. Pain Physician. 2011;14:145–61.
13. Richebé P, Pouquet O, Jelacic S, et al. Target-controlled dosing of remifentanil during cardiac surgery reduces postoperative hyperalgesia. J Cardiothorac Vasc Anesth. 2011;25:917–25.

19

Efficacy and safety of pulsed radiofrequency as a method of dorsal root ganglia stimulation for treatment of non-neuropathic pain

Ivana Vuka[1], Svjetlana Došenović[2], Tihana Marciuš[1], Lejla Ferhatović Hamzić[3], Katarina Vučić[4], Damir Sapunar[1,5†] and Livia Puljak[5*†]

Abstract

Background: We systematically reviewed the evidence on the efficacy and safety of dorsal root ganglion (DRG) targeted pulsed radiofrequency (PRF) versus any comparator for treatment of non-neuropathic pain.

Methods: We searched MEDLINE, CINAHL, Embase, PsycINFO, clinicaltrials.gov and WHO clinical trial register until January 8, 2019. All study designs were eligible. Two authors independently conducted literature screening. Primary outcomes were pain intensity and serious adverse events (SAEs). Secondary outcomes were any other pain-related outcome and any other safety outcome that was reported. We assessed the risk of bias using the Cochrane tool and Risk of Bias In Non-randomized Studies of Interventions (ROBINS-I). We conducted narrative evidence synthesis and assessed the conclusiveness of included studies regarding efficacy and safety.

Results: We included 17 studies with 599 participants, which analyzed various pain syndromes. Two studies were randomized controlled trials; both included participants with low back pain (LBP). Non-randomized studies included patients with the following indications: LBP, postsurgical pain, pain associated with herpes zoster, cervicogenic headache, complex regional pain syndrome type 1, intractable vertebral metastatic pain, chronic scrotal and inguinal pain, occipital radiating pain in rheumatoid arthritis and chronic migraine. In these studies, the PRF was usually initiated after other treatments have failed. Eleven studies had positive conclusive statements (11/17) about efficacy; the remaining had positive inconclusive statements. Only three studies provided conclusiveness of evidence statements regarding safety – two indicated that the evidence was positive conclusive, and one positive inconclusive. The risk of bias was predominantly unclear in randomized and serious in non-randomized studies.

(Continued on next page)

* Correspondence: livia.puljak@gmail.com; livia.puljak@unicath.hr
†Damir Sapunar and Livia Puljak contributed equally to this work.
[5]Center for Evidence-Based Medicine and Health Care, Catholic University of Croatia, Ilica 242, 10000 Zagreb, Croatia

(Continued from previous page)
Conclusion: Poor quality and few participants characterize evidence about benefits and harms of DRG PRF in patients with non-neuropathic pain. Results from available studies should only be considered preliminary. Not all studies have reported data regarding the safety of the intervention, but those that did, indicate that the intervention is relatively safe. As the procedure is non-destructive and early results are promising, further comparative studies about PRF in non-neuropathic pain syndromes would be welcomed.

Keywords: Chronic pain, Non-neuropathic pain, Pulsed radiofrequency, Dorsal root ganglion

Background

Chronic pain is one of the major public health issues worldwide and is one of the leading causes of years lived with disability [1]. Estimates on the prevalence of chronic pain in the general population vary, ranging from 11% [2] up to 64% [3]. These different estimates are mostly due to differences in the definition of chronic pain regarding the duration of symptoms (3 vs. 6 months) and the wording of questions used for assessing chronic pain [4]. Besides its major clinical impact and costs for the healthcare system, chronic pain impairs patients' quality of life, as well as their ability to work and function, causing massive indirect socioeconomic costs worldwide [5]. Chronic pain asserts this major impact on individuals, health systems and society because of inadequate treatment modalities.

Pulsed radiofrequency (PRF) emerged as a therapeutic treatment for various painful conditions, including both neuropathic and non-neuropathic pain [6–8]. PRF has been described as "a non-neurodestructive therapy in pain management "[9]. PRF is a minimally invasive intervention, which involves the application of pulses of electric current, created at the tip of an electrode, without a harmful increase in the temperature [9].

It has been suggested that a dorsal root ganglion (DRG) is a desirable target for the treatment of pain [10]. PRF application close to dorsal root could alleviate neuropathic pain [11]. However, we have observed an increasing number of studies on chronic pain, reporting use of DRG targeted PRF treatment of non-neuropathic pain in humans. Therefore, we aimed to conduct a systematic review about the evidence on the efficacy and safety of DRG targeted PRF treatment of non-neuropathic pain.

Methods

Study design

We published a systematic review protocol a priori in the PROSPERO database (registration number: CRD42017076502). Since the original protocol covered extremely wide scope and heterogeneous interventions, subsequently we divided the original protocol into a separate assessment of DRG targeted electrical field stimulation (EFS) [12] and PRF. The systematic review was performed following the PRISMA statement and Center for Reviews and Dissemination (CRD) manuals.

Eligibility criteria

Participants, intervention and study designs

We included primary studies with participants suffering from various painful conditions which are not currently classified as purely of neuropathic origin (i.e. non-neuropathic pain). In case that condition was defined of both origins, neuropathic and non-neuropathic, such as post-surgical pain or low back pain we included such condition. We excluded studies where PRF treatment was used for neuropathic pain as it is defined in the guidelines of the International Association for the Study of Pain (IASP). We used the IASP classification of chronic pain for ICD-11. We chose to include both randomized controlled trials (RCTs) as well as non-randomized study designs (NRSDs) because we expected a few RCTs in this research area, and we wanted to provide a comprehensive picture of evidence in this field of research. We used Cochrane Handbook for Reviews of Interventions to define the design of included studies. Manuscripts that included more than 10 participants were classified as case series, while those that included less than 10 participants were defined as case reports [13]. We only included studies where PRF treatment was directed to the DRG, including a combination of PRF with other therapies. If the study only reported results about efficacy, and safety was not reported, we still included such a study to get comprehensive evidence synthesis regarding efficacy.

Outcome measures

Primary outcomes were: pain intensity and serious adverse events (SAEs). For primary outcome, we reported any outcome measures, as reported in included manuscripts. Secondary outcomes for efficacy were any other pain-related outcomes, and for safety any other safety data, including non-serious adverse events and other complications regarding tested intervention.

Search strategy and information source

We searched four databases: MEDLINE via Ovid, Embase via Ovid, CINAHL and PsycINFO via

EBSCOhost (Supplementary Table 1). Databases were searched from the date of inception until January 8, 2019 with no restriction regarding the language. Records were then exported to the EndNote X5 citation software (Clarivate Analytics, Boston, MA, USA) and duplicates removed. Furthermore, reference lists of all included studies and their citations were downloaded from Web of Science and screened to find additional eligible studies. ClinicalTrials.gov and World Health Organization's International Clinical Trial Registry Platform (WHO ICTRP) were searched to identify ongoing studies.

Study selection

Reviewers independently screened each title/abstract of retrieved records as well as full-texts of retrieved studies for possible inclusion (authors LFH, IV, TM and SD participated in screening). Discrepancies were resolved by another author (DS).

Data extraction

Independent data extraction was performed by two authors for each data point (authors: IV, and TM or KV). We extracted the following data: the surname of the first author, year of publication, study design, details about intervention (treatment protocol and device used), comparator, inclusion and exclusion criteria, number of participants, baseline characteristics of participants, follow-up period, DRG level treated and outcomes about efficacy and safety.

Risk of bias assessment

We used the Cochrane Risk of Bias (RoB) tool (version from 2011) to assess RoB in RCTs and the Risk of Bias In Non-randomized Studies of Interventions (ROBINS-I) tool for cohort type studies. RoB was analyzed independently by two authors (IV, and SD or KV). Discrepancies were resolved by another author (LP).

Synthesis of results

Due to the heterogeneity of included studies, it was not possible to conduct a meta-analysis, even though we have planned to do it in our study protocol. For this reason, we conducted a narrative and tabular synthesis of results. We also conducted an analysis of conclusiveness about efficacy and safety of the treatment in the abstracts of included studies. We divided conclusiveness statements into five categories: positive conclusive (favorable conclusion in favor of PRF), positive inconclusive (favorable conclusion, but with a note about insufficient or low quality evidence), negative conclusive (PRF not beneficial), negative inconclusive (PRF not beneficial, but with a note about insufficient or low quality evidence) and not reported.

Results

The flow chart in Fig. 1 shows the number of records analyzed in each screening phase. We screened 63 manuscripts in full text, and we finally included 17 manuscripts in this systematic review. Excluded studies, and reasons for their exclusion, are listed in Supplementary Table 2. The characteristics of the included studies are detailed in Table 1.

Among 17 included studies there were two randomized controlled trials [14, 15] and 15 non-randomized studies (Table 1). The total number of participants in these studies was 599; the median number of participants was 28 (range: 1 to 127) (Table 1). Both RCTs included participants with low back pain (LBP) [14, 15]. Non-randomized studies included patients with the following indications: LBP [16–18], postsurgical pain [19–21], pain associated with herpes zoster [6], cervicogenic headache [22, 23], complex regional pain syndrome type 1 [24, 25], intractable vertebral metastatic pain [26], chronic scrotal and inguinal pain [27], occipital radiating pain in rheumatoid arthritis [28] and chronic migraine [29] (Table 1). These studies had highly heterogeneous parameters of stimulation (Table 2). Detailed information about inclusion and exclusion criteria, as well as baseline characteristics of included participants, are listed in Table 3.

Low back pain

In this group, there were 5 studies with a total of 328 participants, including two RCTs with 28 participants in one [14] and 60 participants in another one [15], one retrospective cohort study including 29 participants [16], and two before and after comparisons with 84 participants in one [17] and 127 participants in another [18].

Trial by Holanda et al. [14] included 28 participants which were randomized in three groups: PRF treatment group with the probe directed through the needle in the second lumbar intervertebral foramen ($N = 11$), lidocaine injection group ($N = 7$) and laser irradiation treatment group ($N = 10$). All participants from the lidocaine injection group and laser irradiation group reported a 100% reduction in visual analogue scale (VAS) scores immediately after the treatment, while participants from the PRF group reported a 62.5% reduction in pain. At 1-month follow-up laser irradiation group had a 55.5% reduction in pain; lidocaine injection group 62.5% reduction and PRF group only 20% [14].

An RCT by Lee et al. [15] analyzed predictive value and cost-effectiveness of the use of diagnostic blocks before PRF treatment. They included 60 participants suffering from LBP with or without lower-limb pain, randomized into two groups. In one group ($N = 30$) participants received DRG blocks with 1 ml of 2% bupivacaine and 1 ml of 2% triamcinolone, and those who had at least 50% improvement were scheduled for PRF

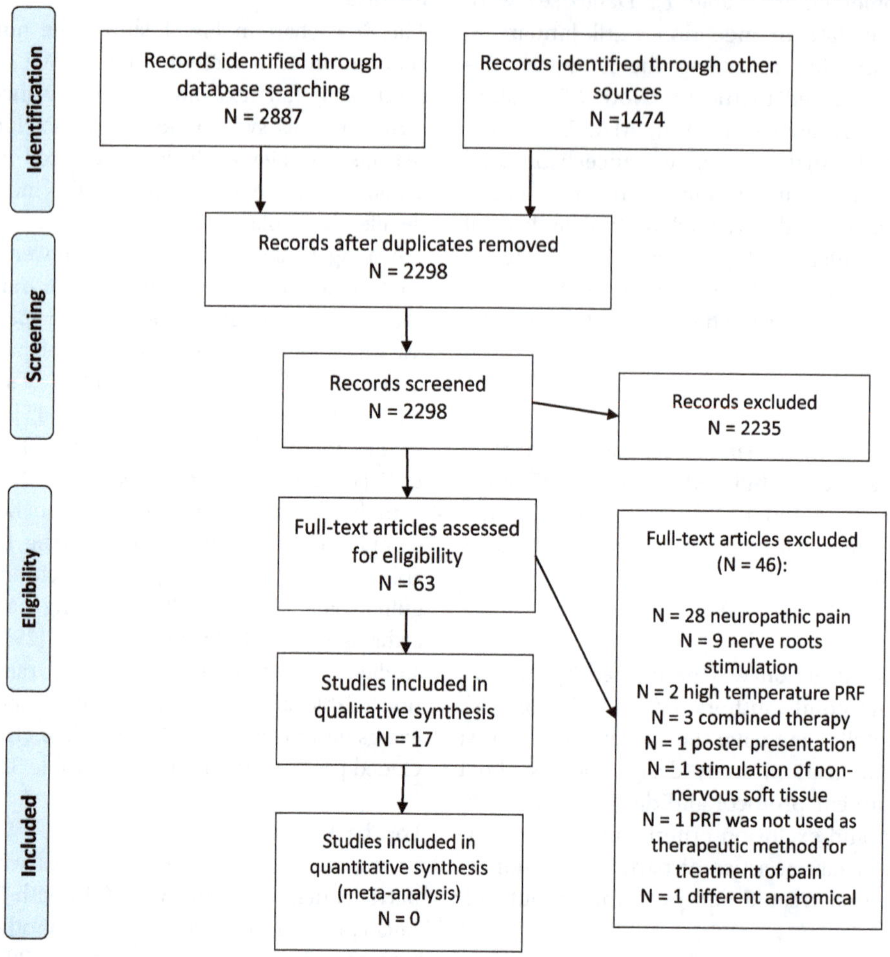

Fig. 1 Flow chart of study inclusion

treatment. The other group ($N = 30$) received only PRF treatment without DRG blocks. Limited low back pain was treated with DRG block or PRF applied to the L2 DRG; lower -limb pain was treated with PRF applied to the L3–S1 DRG. The authors concluded that DRG blocks had no statistically significant impact on the results of PRF treatment, while their application resulted in overall higher medical costs [15].

Yang et al. [16] reported results of a retrospective cohort study that aimed to develop a patient-mounted navigated intervention (PaMNI) system for spinal diseases to evaluate the success of the PRF treatment. The study also included a pilot clinical trial were the new PaMNI system ($N = 16$) was compared to conventional fluoroscopy ($N = 13$). In all patients, PRF treatment was delivered on the L4 DRG. Both groups showed a reduction in VAS scores 1 month after the treatment with no statistically significant difference between groups ($P = 0.238$). However, the study showed the feasibility and efficacy of the PaMNI system [16].

Before and after comparison by Hsu et al. [17] followed 84 participants up to 3 years to investigate the correlation between different types of lumbar lordosis with the outcomes of PRF treatment applied to L2 DRG in chronic low back pain. The analysis showed that after 3-year follow-up participants had a statistically significant reduction in low back pain, regardless of the type of lumbar lordosis [17]. The study by Tsou et al. [18], also followed participants for up to 3 years. They included participants who had low back pain with lower -limb pain ($N = 78$) or without it ($N = 49$). LBP was treated with PRF applied to the L2 DRG and lower-limb pain was treated with PRF applied to the L3–S1 DRG. Percentage of participants achieving at least 50% improvement in VAS scores was similar in both groups at 1-year follow-up, with 20 out of 45 participants (44.44%) in the group without lower -limb pain and 34 out of 74 participants (45.95%) in the group with lower -limb pain [18].

None of the studies reported serious adverse events. Two studies reported minor complications: mild discomfort

Table 1 Characteristics about efficacy and safety of included studies

Author and year/Study design (Cochrane handbook and study authors)	Interventions prior to PRF treatment	Number of participants (for each pain condition treated)	Follow-up	Outcome measures	Results: efficacy for pain intensity	Conclusion statement about efficacy	Results: serious adverse events	Results: any other safety data	Conclusion statement about safety
Low back pain (LBP)									
Holanda 2016 [14] RCT / pilot study	No other intervention	PRF treatment group $n = 11$; lidocaine injection group $n = 7$; laser irradiation treatment group $n = 10$	5 min and 1 month	1. Lumbar pain intensity by VAS presented as percentage of relative difference 2. Chronic LBP relief by PRS	**PRF group:** VAS relative difference at 5 min: 62.5% VAS relative difference at 1 month: 20% **Lidocaine injection group:** VAS relative difference at 5 min: 100% VAS relative difference at 1 month: 62.5% **Laser treatment group:** VAS relative difference at 5 min: 100% VAS relative difference at 1 month: 55%	Positive conclusive	No SAEs occurred	Some patients experienced only mild discomfort during procedure	Not reported
Lee 2018 [15] RCT / randomized, prospective, and comparative study	Diagnostic block + PRF group received diagnostic block with 1 ml of 2% bupivacaine and 1 ml of 2% triamcinolone.	Diagnostic block + PRF group ($n = 30$); PRF group ($n = 30$)	2 weeks, 1, 3 and 6 months	1. Pain intensity by NRS 2. Functional disabilities by ODI	**Diagnostic block + PRF group:** Baseline NRS: 8 (range 5–9); NRS at 2 weeks: 2 (range 1–7); NRS at 1 month: 2 (range 1–8); NRS at 3 months: 3 (range 1–8); NRS at 6 months: 4 (range 1–8). **PRF alone group:** Baseline NRS: 7.5 range (3–10); NRS at 2 weeks: 2 (range 1–9); NRS at 1 month: 2 (range 1–9); NRS at 3 months: 3 (range 1–9); NRS at 6 months: 4 (range 1–9). *P* values comparison between groups: NRS at 2 weeks: $P = 0.302$ NRS at 1 month: $P = 0.690$ NRS at 3 moths: $P = 0.957$	Positive inconclusive	Not reported	Not reported	Not reported

Table 1 Characteristics about efficacy and safety of included studies *(Continued)*

Author and year/Study design (Cochrane handbook and study authors)	Interventions prior to PRF treatment	Number of participants (for each pain condition treated)	Follow-up	Outcome measures	Results: efficacy for pain intensity	Conclusion statement about efficacy	Results: serious adverse events	Results: any other safety data	Conclusion statement about safety
					NRS at 6 months: $P = 0.673$				
Yang 2010 [16] RCS / in vivo clinical trial	No other intervention	PaMNI system $n = 16$; conventional fluoroscopy $n = 13$	1 month	1. Pain intensity by VAS	**PaMNI group:** Baseline VAS: 5.8 (±2.3); VAS at 1 month: 4.1 (± 2.1). $P = 0.005$. **Fluoroscopy group:** Baseline VAS: 6.5 (±2.2); VAS at 1 month: 5.3 (± 2.8). $P = 0.067$. No statistical difference between groups at 1 month ($P = 0.238$).	Positive conclusive	Not reported	Not reported	Not reported
Hsu 2017 [17] BA / retrospective study	No other intervention	84	1 week after the treatment and at 3, 6, 9, 12 months and yearly postoperatively (for 3 years in total)	1. Pain intensity by VAS 2. Functional disabilities by ODI	Analysis of VAS scores for pain indicated significant reductions of low back pain during the 3-year follow-up for patients with all 4 types of lumbar lordosis.	Positive conclusive	No SAEs occurred	Cerebral spinal fluid leaking from the cannulas of two patients while the needle was being directed toward the DRG. This leakage ceased immediately after adjusting the location of the needle tip.	Specific adverse events mention, no overall conclusion about safety
Tsou 2010 [18] BA / not stated	No other intervention	Group A (CLBP without lower-limb pain) $n = 49$; Group B (CLBP with lower-limb pain) $n = 78$	From 1 week up to 3 years post-operatively	1. Pain intensity by VAS 2. Adverse events	**Group A, L2 treatment:** ≥50% VAS improvement: at 1 week: 25/49 (51.02%); at 3 months: 27/49 (55.1%); at 1 year 20/45 (44.44%). **Group B, L2 treatment:** ≥50% VAS improvement: at 1 week: 34/78 (43.59%); at 3 months: 37/78 (47.44%); at 1 year: 34/74 (45.95%).	Positive conclusive	No SAEs occurred	No obvious complications were observed	Positive conclusive
Postsurgical pain									
Albayrak 2017 [19]	In the PRF	PRF group (TENS +	15 days and 1-	1. Pain intensity by	**PRF group activity:**	Positive	No SAEs	No	Not reported

Table 1 Characteristics about efficacy and safety of included studies *(Continued)*

Author and year/Study design (Cochrane handbook and study authors)	Interventions prior to PRF treatment	Number of participants (for each pain condition treated)	Follow-up	Outcome measures	Results: efficacy for pain intensity	Conclusion statement about efficacy	Results: serious adverse events	Results: any other safety data	Conclusion statement about safety
PCS / retrospective study of prospectively collected data	group participants received prognostic diagnostic block prior to involvement.	exercise + PRF) $n = 22$; TENS group (TENS + exercise) $n = 17$	month post treatment and following last control examination. The mean follow-up time was 253.8 ± 109 days; for TENS group: 217 ± 114 days and for PRF group: 282.2 ± 97 days	VAS 2. Degree of neuropathic pain reduction by DN4 3. Change in knee flexion by ROM 4. Functional status by WOMAC 5. Patient satisfaction Success was defined as at least 50% reduction to the VAS (activity, rest, night)	baseline VAS: 6.6 (±1.5); VAS at 15 days: 3 (±1.4); VAS at 1 month: 3.9 (±2); VAS at last control: 3.5 (±2.4). **PRF group rest:** baseline VAS: 4.3 (±1.7); VAS at 15 days: 1.8 (± 0.9); VAS at 1 month: 2.6 (± 1.5); VAS at last control: 2 (± 1.6). **PRF group night:** baseline VAS: 3.8 (±2.2); VAS at 15 days: 1.5 (± 1.1); VAS at 1 month: 2.1 (± 1.4); VAS at last control: 1.7 (±1.4). **TENS group activity:** baseline VAS: 5.9 (±1.9); VAS at 15 days: 3.8 (± 2.2); VAS at 1 month: 4.3 (± 2.2); VAS at last control: 4.4 (±2.1). **TENS group rest:** baseline VAS: 5 (±2.4); VAS at 15 days: 2.6 (± 2.4); VAS at 1 month: 3.4 (± 2.5); VAS at last control: 2.8 (±2.1). **TENS group night:** baseline VAS: 4.3 (±2.6); VAS at 15 days: 2.1 (± 2.7); VAS at 1 month: 2.7 (± 2.6); VAS at last control: 2.6 (±1). Significant difference achieved in an improvement of at least 50% on the VAS scores at activity following the	conclusive	occurred	complications were observed	

Table 1 Characteristics about efficacy and safety of included studies *(Continued)*

Author and year/Study design (Cochrane handbook and study authors)	Interventions prior to PRF treatment	Number of participants (for each pain condition treated)	Follow-up	Outcome measures	Results: efficacy for pain intensity	Conclusion statement about efficacy	Results: serious adverse events	Results: any other safety data	Conclusion statement about safety
					last control examination between the two groups ($P = 0.006$), but not on the VAS scores at rest and night ($P > 0.05$).				
Cohen 2006 [20] RCS / retrospective data analysis	No other intervention	PRF DRG group $n = 13$; PRF ICN group $n = 15$; MM group $n = 21$	6 weeks, 3 months	1. Pain intensity by VAS 2. Answers to 2 questions evaluating patient satisfaction and functional improvement Successful was defined as ≥50% pain reduction on VAS and affirmative answer to 2 questions	No separate VAS scores shown in manuscript, success was achieved as follows: **PRF DRG group:** 6 weeks: 61.5% 3 months: 53.8% **PRF ICN group:** 6 weeks: 21.4% 3 months: 6.7% **MM group:** 6 weeks: 27.3% 3 months: 19.9% Effect did not reach statistical significance at 6 weeks ($P = 0.12$). At 3 months, success rate for PRF DRG group was significantly greater than for those patients treated with PRF ICN ($P = 0.01$), and approached significance when compared with MM ($P = 0.06$).	Positive conclusive	Small incidental pneumothorax was found during a routine scan of the lung fields after PRF DRG. This patient was not symptomatic and was treated conservatively with observation.	No other complications occurred	Not reported
Fam 2018 [21] BA / single arm intervention study	Steroid injections with 1 ml of bupivacaine 0.25% and 1 ml of dexamethasone 4 mg in a total volume of 2 ml immediately after PRF procedure.	$n = 100$	1 week, 1, 3 and 6 months	1. Pain intensity by VAS 2. Quality of life by QOLS 3. Change in use of pain medication 4. Adverse effects 5. Patient satisfaction	Baseline VAS: 7.48 ± 1.46 (median: 8); VAS at 1 week: 5.01 ± 2.61 (median: 5) ($P = 0.032344$); VAS at 1 month: 3.26 ± 2.37 (median: 3) ($P < 0.0001$); VAS at 3 months: 4.44 ± 2.8 (median: 4) ($P = 0.00139$); VAS at 6 months: 4.7 ± 2.88 (median: 4) ($P = 0.0057$).	Positive inconclusive	No SAEs occurred	Pain at the needling site, fever of unknown etiology at the night of intervention, mild to moderate elevation of glucose level in portion of diabetic participants	Positive inconclusive
Pain associated with herpes zoster									
Kim 2017 [6] RCS / retrospective	No other intervention	PRF group $n = 20$; continuous	1, 3 and 6 months	1. Pain intensity by NRS	**PRF group:** baseline NRS: 6.30 ± 0.98	Positive conclusive	No SAEs occurred	1 patient complained of	Not reported

Table 1 Characteristics about efficacy and safety of included studies *(Continued)*

Author and year/Study design (Cochrane handbook and study authors)	Interventions prior to PRF treatment	Number of participants (for each pain condition treated)	Follow-up	Outcome measures	Results: efficacy for pain intensity	Conclusion statement about efficacy	Results: serious adverse events	Results: any other safety data	Conclusion statement about safety
cohort study		epidural group (ropivacaine) $n = 22$		2. Dose of anticonvulsants and analgesics	**Continuous epidural group:** baseline NRS: 6.73 ± 0.88 NRS values were significantly lower in PRF group from 1 to 3 months and 6 months after the procedure ($P = 0.029$) than those in continuous epidural group.			pain at the procedure site, and it improved within few days	
Cervicogenic headache									
van Zundert 2003 [22] BA / clinical audit	Diagnostic block prior to involvement. Participants with > 50% pain relief received PRF.	$n = 14$	2 months and 6 months after the last patient were included. Mean follow-up was 19.4 months (±8.9 months), maximum 2.5 years.	1.Satisfactory pain relief (GPE: defined as a score of 6 or 7 points on the Likert scale; at least 50% pain relief 2. Duration of the effect 3. Other treatments 4. Change in use of pain medication	Data about pain relief (GPE): 9/14 patients (64%) reported successful pain reduction (6 or 7 points on the GPE Likert scale).	Positive conclusive	No SAEs occurred	No other complications observed	Positive conclusive
Zhang 2011 [23] CR/CR	Diagnostic blocks with 1.5% lidocaine. Positive response was considered as 90% pain relief lasting for 30 min.	$n = 2$	6 months	1. Pain intensity by NRS	**Patient 1:** Baseline NRS: 5; NRS at 6 months: 0. **Patient 2:** Baseline NRS: 4; NRS at 6 months: 0.	Positive inconclusive	No significant complications occurred	No significant complications occurred	Not reported
Complex regional pain syndrome									
Albayrak 2016 [24] CR / CS	No other intervention	$n = 2$	1 and 3 days after PRF, 2 and 5 or 10 months (different last follow-up time point for 2 patients)	1. Pain intensity by VAS 2. ROM degree	**Patient 1:** Baseline VAS during movement: 80; VAS at 3 days: 30; VAS at 2 and 10 months: 20. **Patient 2:** Baseline VAS during movement: 100; VAS at 3 days: 30; VAS at 2 months: 20; VAS at 5 months: 10.	Positive inconclusive	No SAEs occurred	No complications were observed	Not reported
Apiliogullari 2015 [25] CR / CR	No other intervention	$n = 1$	1 day after treatment (2	1. Pain intensity by VAS	Baseline VAS: 100; VAS at 1 day (PRF on	Positive inconclusive	No SAEs occurred	No significant complications	Not reported

Table 1 Characteristics about efficacy and safety of included studies *(Continued)*

Author and year/Study design (Cochrane handbook and study authors)	Interventions prior to PRF treatment	Number of participants (for each pain condition treated)	Follow-up	Outcome measures	Results: efficacy for pain intensity	Conclusion statement about efficacy	Results: serious adverse events	Results: any other safety data	Conclusion statement about safety
			weeks after first PRF the treatment was repeated), 6 months		L5): 50; VAS at 2 weeks (after repeated PRF on L4): 10. The patient had symptoms relief for over 6 months.			occurred	
Intractable vertebral metastatic pain									
Arai 2015 [26] CS / CR	No other intervention	n = 15	0, 1, 7, 21, 28, 35 and 42 days	1. Pain intensity by NRS at rest and while moving	**NRS at rest:** baseline NRS: from 1 to 4 (median 3); NRS at day 1: median 2; NRS at day 7: median 1; NRS at day 21: median 1. Significant decrease in 3 weeks ($P < 0.0001$). **NRS while moving:** baseline NRS from 5 to 10 (median 8); NRS at day 1: median 4; NRS at day 7: median 4; NRS at day 21: median 3. Significant decrease in 3 weeks ($P < 0.0001$).	Positive conclusive	No SAEs occurred	No other complications occurred	Not reported
Chronic scrotal and inguinal pain									
Hofmeester 2013 [27] CR / CR	Diagnostic block with 1 ml of levobupivacaine 0.25%	n = 1	12 months	1. Pain intensity by VAS	Baseline VAS scores: 7–8; VAS initially after intervention: 4; VAS at 12 months: 0–1.	Positive conclusive	Not reported	Not reported	Not reported
Occipital radiating pain in rheumatoid arthritis									
Lee 2015 [28] CR / CR	Diagnostic block with 0.3 ml of 0.75% levobupivacaine and 1 mg triamcinolone	n = 1	6 months	1. Pain intensity by VAS	Baseline VAS: 10; VAS at 6 months: 0.	Positive conclusive	Not reported	Not reported	Not reported
Chronic migraine									
Li 2018 [29] CR / CR	Diagnostic block with 1 ml of 2% lidocaine	n = 1	1 year	1. Pain intensity by VAS	Baseline VAS: 8; VAS at 1 year: complete pain relief.	Positive inconclusive	Not reported	Not reported	Not reported

Abbreviations: BA before and after, *CR* case report, *CS* case series, *CLBP* chronic low back pain, *DRG* dorsal root ganglion, *GPE* global perceived effect, *ICN* intercostal nerves, *MM* medical management, *NRS* numerical rating scale, *ODI* Oswestry disability index, *PaMNI system* patient-mount navigated intervention, *PRF* pulsed radiofrequency, *PRS* pain relief scale *QOLS* quality of life scale, *RCS* retrospective cohort study, *ROM* range of motion, *TENS* transcutaneous electrical nerve stimulation, *SAEs* serious adverse events, *VAS* visual analogue scale, *WOMAC* functional status by Western Ontario and McMaster universities osteoarthritis index

Table 2 Parameters of pulsed radiofrequency treatment of dorsal root ganglion

Author and year	Comparator	Protocol used for treatment	Device used	Position of the electrode
Low back pain				
Holanda 2016 [14]	PRF treatment and lidocaine injection vs. laser irradiation	Pulse width: 20 ms with wash-out period of 480 ms; Frequency: 50 Hz; Amplitude: 45 V; Duration: 5 min (with wash out periods of 300 ms); Temperature: 42 °C	150 mm RF probe with 5 mm active tip (company is not specified); COSMAN G4 pulse generator (Cosman Medical, Burlington, MA, USA).	L2
Lee 2018 [15]	Diagnostic block + PRF	Amplitude: 100 V; Duration: 240 s; Temperature: 40–42 °C	20-gauge cannula and Cosman Four-Electrode Radiofrequency Generator (G4) (Cosman Medical, Burlington, MA, USA).	L2 - L5 and S1
Yang 2010 [16]	2 implantation techniques	No stimulation parameters given	22-gauge, SMK-C10 (Radionics Inc., Burlington, MA, USA). RF generator not specified.	L4
Hsu 2017 [17]	No comparator	Frequency: 2 Hz; Amplitude: 45 V; Duration: 120 s; Temperature: 42 °C	10-cm 22-gauge sliced-tip cannula with 1 cm active tip (company is not specified); RF generator (Baylis Medical Company, Montreal, Canada).	L2
Tsou 2010 [18]	No comparator	Frequency: 2 Hz; Amplitude: 45 V; Duration: 120 s; Temperature: 42 °C	10-cm, 22-gauge, curved-tip cannula with a 1 cm active tip electrode (company not specified); RF generator (Baylis Medical Co., Montreal, Canada).	L2-L5 and S1
Postsurgical pain				
Albayrak 2017 [19]	TENS + exercise vs. TENS + exercise + PRF	Pulse width: 20 ms active and 480 ms silent periods; Frequency: 2 Hz; Amplitude: 45 V; Duration: 120 s; Temperature: 42 °C	22-gauge cannula (OWL RF cannula 100 mm) with 5 mm active tip electrode (Diros Technology Inc., Canada); NeuroTherm 1100 RF generator (NeuroTherm, Wilmington, MA, USA).	L4
Cohen 2006 [20]	Intercostal nerve stimulation and medical management	Pulse width: 20 ms in 1 s cycle; Frequency: 2 Hz; Amplitude: 45 V; Duration: 120 s; Temperature: 42 °C. The procedure was repeated 4 times, for a total duration of 8 min.	10 cm electrode with a 5 mm active tip (PMC22–100-5, Baylis Medical, Montreal, Quebec, Canada); PMG-115-TD, V2.0A RF generator (Baylis Medical Company, Montreal, Canada).	Exact DRGs are not specified
Fam 2018 [21]	No comparator	Duration: 120 s; Temperature: 42 °C 2 cycles performed	22-gauge, 10 cm, curved cannula with 10 mm active tip (Baylis Medical Company, Montreal, Canada). RF generator used not reported.	T2 and T3
Pain associated with herpes zoster				
Kim 2017 [6]	Continuous epidural block (ropivacaine)	Pulse width: 20 ms; Frequency: 2 Hz; Amplitude: 45 V; Duration: 360 s; Temperature: 42 °C	22-gauge 10 cm electrode with 10 mm active tip (Radionics Inc., Burlington, MA, USA); RF generator not specified.	Cervical, thoracic, lumbosacral (exact DRGs not specified)
Cervicogenic headache				

Table 2 Parameters of pulsed radiofrequency treatment of dorsal root ganglion *(Continued)*

Author and year	Comparator	Protocol used for treatment	Device used	Position of the electrode
van Zundert 2003 [22]	No comparator	Pulse width: 20 ms; Amplitude: 45 V; Duration: 120 s (20 ms current and 480 ms without current); Temperature: 42 °C	54 mm, 22-gauge SMK Pole needle with 4 mm active tip (Cotop International BV, Amsterdam, Netherlands); RFG 3C Plus RF generator (Radionics Inc. Burlington, MA, USA).	Cervical DRG
Zhang 2011 [23]	No comparator	Duration: 360 s; Temperature: 42 °C	Information not given.	C2
Complex regional pain syndrome				
Albayrak 2016 [24]	No comparator	Pulse width: 20 ms active and 480 ms silent periods; Frequency: 2 Hz; Amplitude: 40 V; Duration: 120 s; Temperature: 42 °C	22-gauge cannula (OWL RF cannula 54 mm) with 4 mm active tip electrode (Diros Technology Inc., Canada); NeuroTherm 1100 RF generator (NeuroTherm, Wilmington, MA, USA).	C5 and C6
Apiliogullari 2015 [25]	No comparator	Pulse width: 20 ms active and 480 ms silent periods; Frequency: 2 Hz; Amplitude: 45 V; Duration: 120 s; Temperature: 42 °C	22-gauge cannula (OWL RF cannula 54 mm) with 4 mm active tip electrode (Diros Technology Inc., Canada); NeuroTherm 1100 RF generator (NeuroTherm, Wilmington, MA, USA).	L4 and L5
Intractable vertebral metastatic pain				
Arai 2015 [26]	No comparator	Pulse width: 20 ms active and 480 ms silent periods; Frequency: 2 Hz; Amplitude: 40 V; Duration: 120 s; Temperature: 42 °C	5 mm active tip KT, guiding needle (Hakko Co. Ltd., Tokyo, Japan); RF generator JK-3 NeuroTherm (Morgan Automation Ltd., Liss, UK).	On each metastatic vertebral body, L1–5 and Th 7, 9–12
Scrotal and inguinal pain				
Hofmeester 2013 [27]	No comparator	Pulse width: 8 ms; Frequency: 2 Hz; Amplitude: 45 V; Duration: 480 s; Temperature: 42 °C	Information not given.	T12, L1 and L2
Occipital radiating pain in rheumatoid arthritis				
Lee 2015 [28]	No comparator	Duration: 120 s, three cycles performed; Temperature: 42 °C	21-gauge 10 cm insulated needle (company is not specified); RF generator not specified.	C2
Chronic migraine				
Li 2018 [29]	No comparator	Pulse width: 20 ms; Frequency: 2 Hz; Amplitude: 45 V; Duration: 900 s; Temperature: 42 °C	22-gauge needle, RF generator G4 (Cosman Medical, Burlington, MA, USA).	C2

Abbreviations: DRG dorsal root ganglion; *PRF* pulsed radiofrequency; *RF* radiofrequency

Table 3 Inclusion and exclusion criteria and baseline characteristics of participants

ID	Inclusion criteria / Previous treatment	Exclusion criteria	Baseline characteristics
Low back pain			
Holanda 2016 [14]	- low back pain for > 3 months	- cancer in lumbar region - coagulation disturbance - infection - neurologic deficits	**PRF treatment group:** - 2 males, 9 females - age range: 42–86 years - pain duration range: 3–144 months **Lidocaine injection group:** - 3 males, 4 females - age range: 33–82 years - pain duration range: 3–48 months **Laser treatment group:** - 3 males, 7 females - age range: 35–84 years - pain duration range: 14–120 months
Lee 2018 [15]	- age 20 years or older - predominantly axial low back pain for > 3 months - medication therapy for > 3 months without benefit - physical rehabilitation for > 3 months without benefit	- an identified etiology of low back pain (i.e., grade II or III spondylolisthesis) - positive response to previous spine interventions such as epidural steroids or sacroiliac joint blocks - previous facet interventions, lumbar spine fusion - untreated coagulopathy - concomitant medical (e.g., unstable angina or degenerative osteoarthritis of knee), or psychiatric conditions - concurrent lumbar pain generator (i.e., muscular/fascial pain, or organs within the abdominal cavity) that could confound the diagnosis of low back pain	**TFESI DRG block + PRF treatment group:** - median age: 74 years, range 53–90 years - median duration of symptoms: 26 months, range: 3–58 months **PRF treatment alone group:** - median age: 75 years, range 33–93 years - median duration of symptoms: 25 months, range: 3–125 months
Yang 2010 [16]	- chronic LBP with focal neurologic symptoms for > 3 months	- spinal disorders - coagulopathy - concomitant medical or psychiatric illness	**PaMNI group:** - 5 males, 11 females - mean age: 55.5 ± 13.9 years **Fluoroscopy group:** - 2 males, 11 females - mean age: 57.2 ± 14.7 years
Hsu 2017 [17]	- age 20 years or older - LBP for > 6 months that worsened upon prolonged sitting or standing - failed to improve after at least 3 months of conservative treatment	- sagittal imbalance - spinal listhesis - infection - tumor - stenosis - disc herniation causing nerve root compression	- 29 males, 55 females - mean age: 56.03 ± 9.04 years
Tsou 2010 [18]	- chronic LBP with or without lower-limb pain for > 6 months - conservative treatment for > 3 months without benefit - participants with symptoms of nerve root compromise due to mild or moderate bulging disc also included	Not given	**LBP without lower limb pain group:** - 26 males, 23 females - men age: 62.94 ± 12.39 years - level treated: L2: 49 **LBP with lower limb pain group:** - 33 males, 45 females - men age: 63.88 ± 14.00 years - levels treated: L2: 78, L3: 14, L4: 33, L5: 72, S1: 21

Table 3 Inclusion and exclusion criteria and baseline characteristics of participants *(Continued)*

ID	Inclusion criteria / Previous treatment	Exclusion criteria	Baseline characteristics
Postsurgical pain			
Albayrak 2017 [19]	- VAS score of ≥3 during activity - pain lasting for ≥2 months - no improvement with physical medicine and rehabilitation - refractory to pharmacological therapies including paracetamol 2 g/day and the maximum tolerable dose of nonsteroidal anti-inflammatory drugs for 1 week and pregabalin 300 mg/day for 2 weeks	- any pathological features, such as acute strain or sprain - stroke/central nervous system disease - serious psychiatric disorders - sciatic pain - fibromyalgia - mental impairment affecting ability to understand tests/measures	**PRF + TENS + exercise group:** - 2 (9.1%) males, 20 (90.9%) females - mean age: 62.1 ± 4.9 years **TENS + exercise group:** - 2 males (11.8%), 15 (88.2%) females - mean age: 65.8 ± 6.5 years
Cohen 2006 [20]	- age 18 years or older - duration of pain ≥3 months - VAS score ≥ 5 - pain deemed to be of neuropathic origin based on history and physical examination	- presence of pathology that could account for a majority of persistent symptoms (e.g. recurrent cancer) - untreated coagulopathy - unstable medical or psychiatric condition	**PRF treatment group:** - 6 males, 7 females - mean age: 45.8 ± 4.7 years **Intercostal nerve stimulation:** - 7 males, 8 females - mean age: 50.8 ± 4.0 years **Medical management group:** - 9 males, 12 females - mean age: 48.6 ± 2.4 years
Fam 2018 [21]	- between 18 and 65 years - refractory to morphine sulfate (MST) and pregabalin	- bleeding tendency - local infection at the site of the intervention - psychological disorders - disturbed anatomy (congenital, traumatic, and postsurgical) - allergy to used medication (local anesthetics and contrast) - inability to lie comfortably during the intervention as the cardiopulmonary distress	Not given
Pain associated with herpes zoster			
Kim 2017 [6]	- participants who underwent the procedure between 30 and 180 days after zoster onset	- trigeminal-nerve-involved zoster - follow-up loss within 6 months after the procedure - participants who did not receive appropriate antiviral treatment during the acute phase of herpes zoster - cases where both procedures were performed between 30 and 180 days of zoster onset	**PRF treatment group:** - 11 males, 9 females - mean age: 68.10 ± 7.99 years - days from zoster onset: 68.20 ± 40.53 **Continuous epidural block group:** - 6 males, 16 females - mean age: 70.41 ± 10.25 years - days from zoster onset: 74.09 ± 44.50
Cervicogenic headache			
van Zundert 2003 [22]	- 18 years or older - chronic pain in the cervical region for > 6 months - pharmacotherapy, physical or manual therapy, TENS, and/or rehabilitation program without benefit - temporary pain relief of at least 50% on 7-point Likert scale after a diagnostic segmental nerve block - ability to understand the information provided - informed consent	- systemic disease - tumor - clinically demonstrable neurologic deficit - signs of radicular compression	- 5 males, 13 females - age range: 27–77 years - duration of pain prior to treatment: < 1–40 years - DRG level treated: C2: 4, C3: 2, C4: 2, C5: 4, C6: 3, C7: 3

Table 3 Inclusion and exclusion criteria and baseline characteristics of participants *(Continued)*

ID	Inclusion criteria / Previous treatment	Exclusion criteria	Baseline characteristics
Zhang 2011 [23]	- initial diagnostic selective the greater occipital nerve blocks with 1.5% lidocaine - pain relief of 90% or more lasting for at least 30 min.	NA	**Patient 1:** - 40-years-old woman - pain lasting for 5 years **Patient 2:** - 66-years-old women - pain lasting for 1 year
Complex regional pain syndrome			
Albayrak 2016 [24]	- no improvement with the combined use of medical therapy, physical therapy, and the rehabilitation program	NA	**Patient 1**: - 69-years-old women - 9 months of previous pain **Patient 2:** - 48-years-old women
Apiliogullari 2015 [25]	NA	NA	16-years-old girl
Intractable vertebral metastatic pain			
Arai 2015 [26]	- confirmed to have vertebral metastases by bone scintigraphy, computed tomography, and magnetic resonance imaging - systemic analgesics did not provide a sound pain relief	- neurological deficit - coagulopathy - significant cardiovascular disease	- 9 males, 6 females - age range: 34–82 years
Scrotal and inguinal pain			
Hofmeester 2013 [27]	- an orchidopexy performed - test block of the relevant DRG with 1 ml of levobupivacaine 0.25%	NA	- 13-years-old boy
Occipital radiating pain in rheumatoid arthritis			
Lee 2015 [28]	- right 3rd occipital and right 4th, - 5th, and 6th cervical medial branch blocks with levobupivacaine (0.3 mL; 0.75%) and triamcinolone (1 mg) were injected at each level	NA	- 74-years-old female - pain lasting for 2–3 years
Chronic migraine			
Li 2018 [29]	- failure of pharmacological therapy and stellate ganglion block - diagnostic C2 block with 1 mL of 2% lidocaine with 75–100% pain relief for only 4 days	NA	- 34-years-old female - 10 years of chronic migraine

Abbreviations: ***DRG*** **dorsal root ganglion,** ***LBP*** **low back pain,** ***NA*** **not applicable,** ***PaMNI system*** **patient-mount navigated intervention,** ***PRF*** **pulsed radiofrequency,** ***RF*** **radiofrequency,** ***TENS*** **transcutaneous electrical nerve stimulation,** ***TFESI*** **transforaminal epidural steroid injection,** ***VAS*** **visual analogue scale**

during the procedure [14] and leakage of the cerebrospinal fluid [17]. One study reported that there were no complications [18]. Two studies from this group did not report any outcomes regarding safety [15, 16], but one of them provided a general warning about the radiation dose exposure [16].

In this group all studies reported positive statements regarding the efficacy of the treatment, four studies had positive conclusive statements [14, 16–18] while one study had positive inconclusive statement [15]. Only one study reported a positive conclusive statement about safety [18], one reported only specific adverse events that occurred [17], while others did not report any conclusion statements (Table 1 and Supplementary Table 3).

Post-surgical pain

Three studies explored PRF in postsurgical pain, with a total of 188 participants. In a cohort study of Albayrak et al. [19] there were 39 participants with postsurgical pain after total knee arthroplasty. In another cohort study, Cohen et al. [20] included 49 participants suffering from thoracic postsurgical pain. Fam et al. [21] included 100 women suffering from intercostobrachial neuralgia (ICBN) postmastectomy in a study designed as before and after comparison. Despite different etiology of postsurgical pain the majority of participants experienced a reduction in pain after the treatment (details are given in Table 1).

One participant from the study of Cohen et al. [20] had a serious adverse event that could not be related to procedure or treatment. Small pneumothorax was found during a routine scan after the PRF procedure. This participant was treated conventionally and monitored [20]. Pain at the site of the procedure was reported as a mild complication [21]. The third study reported that complications were not observed [19].

Two studies from this group reported positive conclusive statement for efficacy, while the conclusion for safety was not reported [19, 20]. The study by Fam et al. [21] reported positive inconclusive statements for both efficacy and safety [21] (Table 1 and Supplementary Table 3).

Pain associated with herpes zoster

A retrospective cohort study by Kim et al. [6] with 42 participants addressed PRF of DRG for pain associated with herpes zoster but before post-herpetic neuralgia (PHN) was established. The study analyzed two groups of participants; one received continuous epidural block ($N = 22$), and the other received PRF treatment ($N = 20$) after the acute phase of herpes zoster, but before it was well established, meaning between 30 and 180 days of the herpes zoster diagnosis. Participants from the continuous epidural block group received 0.187% ropivacaine at the rate of 1 ml per hour, while concentration and rate of administration depended on pain relief and adverse effects (mean concentration of ropivacaine and infusion rates used were $0.22 \pm 0.07\%$ and 1.82 ± 0.65 ml/hr). When satisfactory pain relief was achieved catheter was removed. Reduction in pain was significantly higher in the PRF group compared to a continuous epidural block group ($P = 0.029$) up to 6 months after the treatment [6]. From the safety aspect, only procedural pain was reported [6]. The study abstract had a positive conclusive statement about efficacy, while safety conclusion was not reported [6] (Table 1 and Supplementary Table 3).

Cervicogenic headache

The before and after comparison by van Zundert et al. [22] included 18 participants, of which 14 had pain related to non-neuropathic origin (their characteristics were reported separately in Table 1). Participants were followed for a mean time of 19.4 months (maximum follow-up time 2.5 years) [22]. Before study inclusion, participants received diagnostic nerve blocks with 0.5 mL of 2% lidocaine. Treatment outcomes were scored using a 7-point Likert scale.

Participants who had at least 50% pain relief were included in the study and received PRF treatment. Successful PRF treatment was defined as 6 (≥ 50% improvement) or 7 (≥ 75% improvement) points on 7-point Likert scale (Global Perceived Effect good or very good). Participants from the group of non-neuropathic pain origin had successful treatment in 9 cases while treatment was not successful in 5 cases. The case report by Zhang et al. [23] described 2 participants who reported 100% pain relief lasting for 6 months after the treatment. Both studies reported that no complications occurred (Table 1).

The study by van Zundert et al. [22] reported positive conclusive statements about both, safety and efficacy, while Zhang et al. [23] reported positive inconclusive statement about efficacy, while safety was not reported (Table 1 and Supplementary Table 3).

Complex regional pain syndrome

This group included only two case reports [24, 25] with three participants included. Albayrak et al. [24] reported cases of two women with post-stroke complex regional pain syndrome (CRPS). Both patients used multiple treatment modalities before the PRF treatment, including medical therapy, physical therapy, rehabilitation program and transcutaneous electrical nerve stimulation (TENS). After PRF treatment, both participants had an immediate resolution of their symptoms that lasted up to 5 and 10 months which were final follow-up time points [24].

Apiliogullari et al. [25] reported a case of a 16-year-old girl suffering from CRPS due to sequelae of poliomyelitis, who did not respond to non-steroidal anti-inflammatory drugs. However, after two PRF treatments (first applied at L5 and repeated after 2 weeks at L4 DRG) she reported immediate pain relief, with VAS scores going from 100 points down to 10, this effect remained for over 6 months of follow-up [25]. Both studies reported that no complications occurred (Table 1).

Both studies from this group reported positive inconclusive statements about efficacy, while the conclusion about safety was not reported [24, 25] (Table 1 and Supplementary Table 3).

Intractable vertebral metastatic pain

The case series of Arai et al. [26] included 15 cases with vertebral metastatic pain, which demonstrated pain relief, defined as a 50% pain reduction from baseline values. Values on the numerical rating scale (NRS), measured during rest and upon movement, were significantly lower 3 weeks after the PRF treatment ($P <$ 0.0001) [26]. From the safety aspect, there were no SAEs or other complications (Table 1). The study reported positive conclusive statements about efficacy, while conclusion about safety was not reported [26] (Table 1 and Supplementary Table 3).

Chronic scrotal and inguinal pain

Hofmeester et al. [27] reported the first case of using PRF to treat scrotal and inguinal pain after orchidopexy in a 13-year boy. PRF was performed at three levels (T12 -L2) after other treatment modalities have failed. The PRF of DRG led to an immediate and lasting pain alleviation of more than 70% as reported by the patient [27]. Information about safety was not reported. The study reported positive conclusive statements about efficacy, while the conclusion about safety was not reported [27] (Table 1 and Supplementary Table 3).

Occipital radiating pain in rheumatoid arthritis

Lee et al. [28] reported PRF of the C2 DRG to treat occipital radiating headache in a 74-year old woman with rheumatoid arthritis. The patient has not complained of any occipital radiculopathy for 6 months, and the posterior neck pain has since been reduced to a visual analogue scale (VAS) score of three, from initial 6/10. Information about safety were not reported [28]. This study also reported positive conclusive statements about efficacy, while the conclusion about safety was not reported [28] (Table 1 and Supplementary Table 3).

Chronic migraine

Li et al. [29] reported a case of a 34-year old woman who suffered from chronic migraine with occipital pain. She underwent PRF treatment after the failure of other treatment modalities. The patient had complete pain relief with no symptoms 1 year after the treatment [29]. Details are given in Table 1. The study did not report conclusion about safety, while the conclusion about efficacy was positive inconclusive [29] (Table 1 and Supplementary Table 3).

Parameters of PRF treatment

Low back pain was a painful condition which had the most different treatment parameters among included studies, with a range of different values for amplitude (45 and 100 V), frequency (2 and 50 Hz) and duration of treatment (120, 240 and 300 s). Pulse width was only reported in one study [14] (Table 2). In other studies parameters were similar, the majority had a pulse width of 20 ms, the amplitude of 45 V, frequency of 2 Hz and duration of 120 s (Table 2). The temperature at the electrode tip was constant parameter, same in all studies, and set to 42 °C in order to avoid tissue damage.

Participants' inclusion criteria

More than a half of included studies were before and after comparisons, case series or case reports where participants were included and scheduled for PRF treatment after failure of other treatment modalities and as a last treatment option (Table 3). On the other side, higher-quality studies, such as RCTs and cohort type studies had clearly defined inclusion and exclusion criteria as well as described participants' baseline characteristics (Table 3).

Summary on the conclusiveness of the evidence

Among 17 included studies, 11 studies had positive conclusive statements about efficacy; the remaining had positive inconclusive statements. The majority of the studies did not provide conclusive statements regarding safety in the manuscript abstracts. Only three studies provided safety conclusiveness statements – two indicated that the evidence was positive conclusive, and one positive inconclusive (Table 1 and Supplementary Table 3).

Risk of bias

Analysis of two included RCTs, with Cochrane Rob tool, indicated that the majority of the domains were judged with unclear RoB due to insufficient information about the used methodology (Supplementary Table 4, Fig. 2). Four non-randomized studies were eligible for assessment with ROBINS-I. The most common judgment for analyzed domains (12 domains out of 28 domains judged

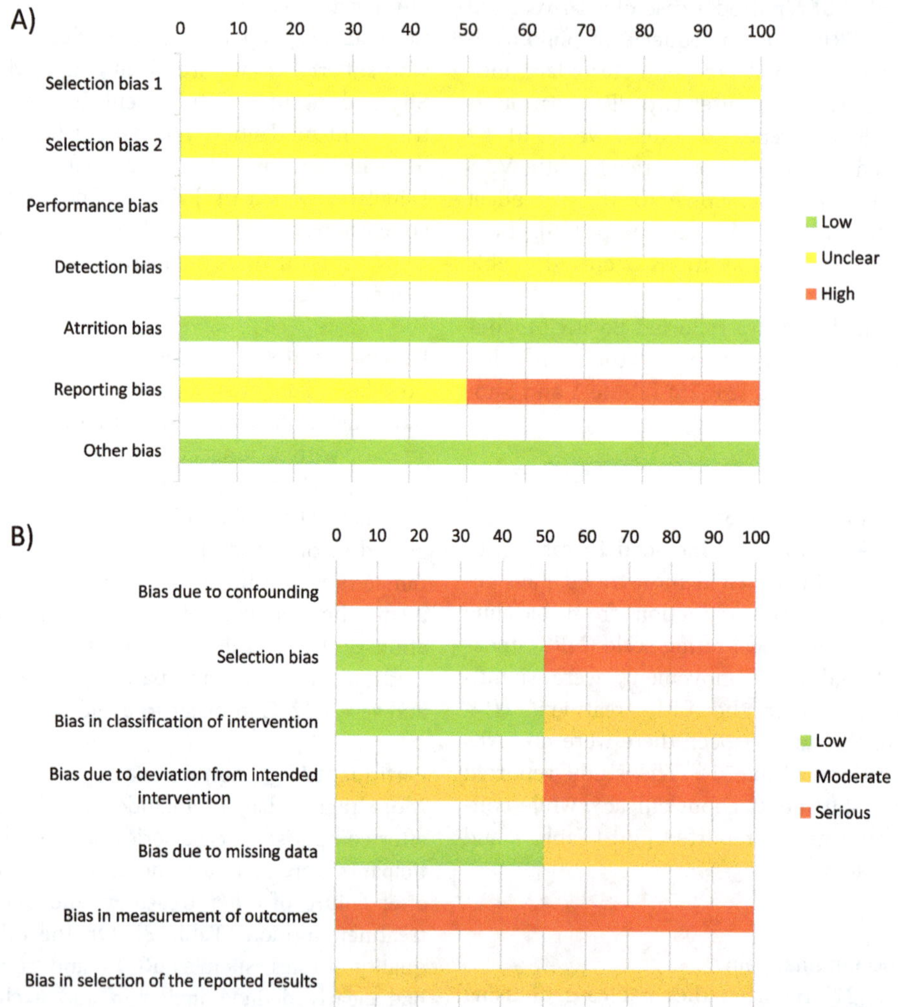

Fig. 2 Risk of bias assessment for randomized controlled studies and cohort type studies

for these four studies) was serious RoB. Ten domains were judged with moderate RoB, and only 6 domains with low RoB (Supplementary Table 5, Fig. 2).

Studies awaiting classification

One RCT, which aims to study DRG thermal RF versus PRF for metastatic pain in the thoracic vertebral body on 69 participants, is classified as completed on July 30, 2018. Results were reported to Clinical Trials.gov but were returned to the authors after the quality control review so results are still not publicly available (NCT03204942). A trial that aimed to study superior hypogastric plexus block versus PRF for chronic pelvic cancer pain on 40 participants is classified as 'Not yet recruiting' since June 26, 2018 (NCT03228316). Studies awaiting classification are described in Supplementary Table 6.

Discussion

In this systematic review, we included 17 studies about the treatment of several non-neuropathic chronic pain conditions with PRF directed to DRG. All studies presented positive conclusions (both conclusive and inconclusive) about the efficacy of the treatment. However, the studies were mostly non-randomized, with small sample sizes, and issues related to the risk of bias. Therefore, their results should only be considered as preliminary.

PRF was developed as a less destructive pain relief modality alternative to conventional radiofrequency (CRF) which can selectively block delta and C fibers [30]. The first report about the clinical effects of PRF on DRG was published relatively recently, in 1998. Due to its theoretical benefits, it was postulated that PRF could be particularly helpful in neuropathic pain [31]. However, we have observed in the literature that clinicians and researchers apply PRF to non-neuropathic chronic pain as well.

Despite the number of studies found in the literature about the treatment of non-neuropathic chronic pain in humans with PRF, their findings cannot be generalized. In the studies that we have found, the PRF was usually initiated after other treatments have failed. We reported a similar issue in our recent systematic review in which we studied the efficacy and safety of EFS of DRG [12]. In that systematic review, we found only one RCT among 29 included studies; most of the studies were low-level of evidence – non-randomized study designs, including case series and case reports. The review about EFS of DRG also included few participants, with a median of 6 participants per study [12]. In this systematic review there were 17 included studies, with a median of 28 participants.

The paucity of large and high-quality studies in the field of DRG neuromodulation is likely due to the relative novelty of this approach for the treatment of pain. In this systematic review, about PRF of DRG in non-neuropathic pain, only two of 17 included studies were RCTs, and RoB judgment for the majority of their methodological aspects was unclear. Likewise, the most common assessment in non-randomized studies assessed with the ROBINS-I tool was that there was a serious risk of bias. Besides their suboptimal methodological reporting, the analyzed studies were relatively small. Even the two included randomized controlled trials were small; one included a total of 28 patients in 3 groups, and the other one included 60 patients in two groups.

The highest number of studies was found for the low back pain indication. However, we were not able to perform a meta-analysis due to clinical heterogeneity of the studies, as can be seen from characteristics of included studies, different comparators used in included trials, and different stimulation parameters. Differences in treatment approaches can result in different clinical outcomes.

Despite the low level of evidence, all of the analyzed studies sent positive conclusions to the research community in their abstracts. The majority of these conclusions were conclusive, i.e. they did not mention the need to conduct further studies on this subject. Despite the authors' positive conclusions regarding the tested interventions, caution is needed when advising DRG targeted PRF to chronic pain patients, because of the paucity of high-quality and high-level evidence. This intervention should be tested in large-scale, high-quality RCTs to truly test whether the intervention has expected benefits and harms. Until then, these studies should be treated as preliminary evidence only.

A broad focus of this systematic review could be considered as a limitation of this review, as we included any pain condition that fits the IASP criteria of non-neuropathic pain. Furthermore, we acknowledge that the examined studies included patients with various clinical conditions, and thus there is a possibility that the effectiveness of the treatment depends on underlying pathogenic mechanisms. However, as can be observed from our results, there were very few studies in each group of indications; the highest number of studies (five) was found for low back pain. Therefore, focusing on every single one of these indications in a separate systematic review would result in a high number of systematic reviews, with minimal results included. Furthermore, with this approach, we are giving readers a very wide and informative picture of all the non-neuropathic pain conditions that were reported in the literature as treated with DRG targeted PRF.

We have used IASP classification for definitions of non-neuropathic pain; these classifications are evolving and changing, so the included conditions may be categorized differently, depending on the time of categorization and reference classification used. Previous versions of chronic pain classification were to some extent insufficient for chronic neuropathic pain conditions since some conditions were not defined properly or were missing so we decided to use the updated version of classification since it is crucial to get the comprehensive evidence synthesis. According to the newest IASP classification that we used (ICD-11) when deciding about study inclusion we might have included some studies that in previous versions of classification were classified either as neuropathic pain or as the pain of mixed origin. We have included CRPS 1 [25], which is not considered neuropathic pain. In the study of Kim et al. [6] the authors studied the effects of DRG PRF beyond the acute phase of zoster, bur before PHN was well established (from 30 days to 180 days after zoster onset). The study of van Zundert [22] has excluded "signs of radicular compression".

It has been questioned before what is the value of systematic review including poor evidence and small studies [32]. However, such systematic reviews are valuable because they are highlighting the paucity of evidence and the low quality of available information [33]. Our systematic review is such a case. We even included two case reports with only one participant which may be considered anecdotal rather than firm evidence. It could be argued that such studies should not even be included in systematic reviews; however, we did not set any restrictions regarding number of participants in our study eligibility criteria. By showing that many clinicians and researchers have published small studies, with low-level evidence, about potential benefits of PRF in chronic non-neuropathic pain, we hope that trialists will be inspired to explore this intervention in studies that are considered high-level evidence.

Conclusion

Even though PRF of DRG was primarily studied for neuropathic pain, we have found as many as 17 published studies that have reported the use of DRG targeted PRF in non-neuropathic pain conditions. Although all of these studies reported positive information regarding the analyzed interventions, considerable caution is needed when interpreting these results as anything more than preliminary. The quality of evidence is low, as there were only two randomized controlled trials among included studies, and the risk of bias was predominantly unclear in RCTs and severe among non-randomized studies. The majority of studies included patients that have failed other therapies so these results cannot be generalized. PRF treatment needs to be tested in new, high-quality and large-scale trials, to confirm the efficacy of this intervention.

Supplementary information

Additional file 1: Supplementary Table 1. Search strategies for four bibliographic databases searched.

Additional file 2: Supplementary Table 2. Characteristics of excluded studies.

Additional file 3: Supplementary Table 3. Conclusion statements presented in the abstracts of included studies.

Additional file 4: Supplementary Table 4. Individual Cochrane risk of bias judgments for randomized controlled trials.

Additional file 5: Supplementary Table 5. Individual ROBINS judgments for non-randomized studies.

Additional file 6: Supplementary Table 6. Details about studies awaiting classification.

Abbreviations

AEs: adverse events; BA: before and after comparison; CLBP: chronic low back pain; CR: case report; CRPS: complex regional pain syndrome; CRD: center for reviews and dissemination; CS: case series; DRG: dorsal root ganglion; EFS: electrical field stimulation; GPE: global perceived effect IASP – International Association for the Study of Pain; ICN: intercostal nerves; LBP: low back pain; MM: medical management; NA: not applicable; NRS: numeric rating scale; NRSD: non-randomized study designs; ODI: Oswestry disability index; PaMNI: patient-mounted navigated intervention; PHN: post-herpetic neuralgia; PRF: pulsed radiofrequency; QOLS: quality of life scale; RCS: retrospective cohort study; RCT: randomized controlled trial; RoB: risk of bias; ROBINS-I: Risk of Bias In Non-randomized Studies of Interventions; ROM: range of motion; SAEs: serious adverse events; TENS: transcutaneous electrical nerve stimulation; TFESI: transforaminal epidural steroid injection; VAS: visual analogue scale; WHO ICTRP: World Health Organization's International Clinical Trial Registry Platform; WOMAC: functional status by Western Ontario and McMaster universities osteoarthritis index

Acknowledgements

We are very grateful to Ms. Ana Utrobicic, expert librarian, for reviewing our search strategies and providing valuable advice.

Authors' contributions

IV, SD, DS, LP: study design. IV, TM, SD, LFH, KV: data collection and analysis. IV, TM, SD, LFH, KV, DS, LP: manuscript writing, approval of final version of the manuscript

Author details

[1]Laboratory for Pain Research, University of Split School of Medicine, Šoltanska 2, 21000 Split, Croatia. [2]Department of Anesthesiology, Reanimatology and Intensive Care, University Hospital Split, Spinčićeva 1, 21000 Split, Croatia. [3]Center for Translational and Clinical Research, Department of Proteomics, University of Zagreb School of Medicine, Šalata 3, 10000 Zagreb, Croatia. [4]Department for Safety and Efficacy Assessment of Medicinal Products, Agency for Medicinal Products and Medical Devices, Ksaverska cesta 4, 10000 Zagreb, Croatia. [5]Center for Evidence-Based Medicine and Health Care, Catholic University of Croatia, Ilica 242, 10000 Zagreb, Croatia.

References

1. Vos T, Flaxman AD, Naghavi M, et al. Years lived with disability (YLDs) for 1160 sequelae of 289 diseases and injuries 1990-2010: a systematic analysis for the global burden of disease study 2010. Lancet. 2012;380(9859):2163–96.
2. Goldberg DS, Mcgee SJ. Pain as a global public health priority. BMC Public Health. 2011;11:770.
3. Harstall C, Ospina M. How prevalent is chronic pain? Pain Clinical Updates. 2003;11:1–4.
4. Landmark T, Romundstad P, Dale O, Borchgrevink PC, Kaasa S. Estimating the prevalence of chronic pain: validation of recall against longitudinal reporting (the HUNT pain study). Pain. 2012;153(7):1368–73.
5. Breivik H, Eisenberg E, O'brien T. The individual and societal burden of chronic pain in Europe: the case for strategic prioritisation and action to improve knowledge and availability of appropriate care. BMC Public Health. 2013;13:1229.
6. Kim ED, Lee YI, Park HJ. Comparison of efficacy of continuous epidural block and pulsed radiofrequency to the dorsal root ganglion for management of pain persisting beyond the acute phase of herpes zoster. PLoS ONE. 2017; 12(8):e0183559. https://doi.org/10.1371/journal.pone.0183559.
7. Chang MC, Cho YW, Ahn SH. Comparison between bipolar pulsed radiofrequency and monopolar pulsed radiofrequency in chronic lumbosacral radicular pain: a randomized controlled trial. Medicine. 2017; 96(9):e6236.
8. Lin WL, Lin BF, Cherng CH, et al. Pulsed radiofrequency therapy for relieving neuropathic bone pain in cancer patients. J Med Sci (Taiwan). 2014;34(2): 84–7.
9. Snidvongs S, Mehta V. Pulsed radio frequency: a non-neurodestructive therapy in pain management. Current Opinion Supportive Palliative Care. 2010;4(2):107–10.
10. Sapunar D, Kostic S, Banozic A, Puljak L. Dorsal root ganglion - a potential new therapeutic target for neuropathic pain. J Pain Res. 2012;5:31–8.
11. Vuka I, Marcius T, Dosenovic S, Ferhatovic Hamzic L, Vucic K, Sapunar D, Puljak L. Efficacy and safety of pulsed radiofrequency of the dorsal root ganglia in patients with neuropathic pain: a systematic review. Pain Med. https://doi.org/10.1093/pm/pnaa141.
12. Vuka I, Marcius T, Dosenovic S, et al. Neuromodulation with electrical field stimulation of dorsal root ganglion in various pain syndromes: a systematic review with focus on participant selection. J Pain Res. 2019;12:803–30.
13. Higgins JPT, Green S (editors). Cochrane Handbook for Systematic Reviews of Interventions Version 5.1.0 [updated March 2011]. London: The Cochrane Collaboration; 2011. Available from https://training.cochrane.org/handbook/archive/v5.1/.
14. Holanda VM, Chavantes MC, Silva DF, et al. Photobiomodulation of the dorsal root ganglion for the treatment of low back pain: a pilot study. Lasers Surg Med. 2016;48(7):653–9.
15. Lee CC, Chen CJ, Chou CC, et al. Lumbar dorsal root ganglion block as a prognostic tool before pulsed radiofrequency: a randomized, prospective, and comparative study on cost-effectiveness. World Neurosurgery. 2018;112: e157–64.
16. Yang CL, Yang BD, Lin ML, Wang YH, Wang JL. A patient-mount navigated intervention system for spinal diseases and its clinical trial on percutaneous pulsed radiofrequency stimulation of dorsal root ganglion. Spine. 2010; 35(21):E1126–32.
17. Hsu HT, Chang SJ, Huang KF, Tai PA, Li TC, Huang CJ. Correlation between lumbar lordosis and the treatment of chronic low back pain with pulsed radiofrequency applied to the L2 dorsal root ganglion. Formosan J Surg. 2017;50(4):125–30.
18. Tsou H-K, Chao S-C, Wang C-J, et al. Percutaneous pulsed radiofrequency

applied to the L-2 dorsal root ganglion for treatment of chronic low-back pain: 3-year experience clinical article. J Neurosurg-Spine. 2010;12(2):190–6.
19. Albayrak I, Apiliogullari S, Dal CN, Levendoglu F, Ozerbil OM. Efficacy of pulsed radiofrequency therapy to dorsal root ganglion adding to TENS and exercise for persistent pain after Total knee Arthroplasty. J Knee Surg. 2017; 30(2):134–42.
20. Cohen SP, Sireci A, Wu CL, Larkin TM, Williams KA, Hurley RW. Pulsed radiofrequency of the dorsal root ganglia is superior to pharmacotherapy or pulsed radiofrequency of the intercostal nerves in the treatment of chronic postsurgical thoracic pain. Pain Physician. 2006;9(3):227–35.
21. Fam BN, El-Sayed GGE, Reyad RM, Mansour I. Efficacy and safety of pulsed radiofrequency and steroid injection for intercostobrachial neuralgia in postmastectomy pain syndrome - a clinical trial. Saudi J Anaesth. 2018;12(2): 227–34.
22. Van Zundert J, Lame IE, De Louw A, et al. Percutaneous pulsed radiofrequency treatment of the cervical dorsal root ganglion in the treatment of chronic cervical pain syndromes: a clinical audit. Neuromodulation. 2003;6(1):6–14.
23. Zhang J, Shi D-S, Wang R. Pulsed radiofrequency of the second cervical ganglion (C2) for the treatment of cervicogenic headache. J Headache Pain. 2011;12(5):569–71.
24. Albayrak I, Apiliogullari S, Onal O, Gungor C, Saltali A, Levendoglu F. Pulsed radiofrequency applied to the dorsal root ganglia for treatment of post-stroke complex regional pain syndrome: a case series. J Clin Anesth. 2016; 33:192–7.
25. Apiliogullari S, Aydin BK, Onal O, Kirac Y, Celik JB. Pulsed radiofrequency of dorsal root ganglia for the treatment of complex regional pain syndrome in an adolescent with poliomyelitis sequel: a case report. Pain Med. 2015;16(7): 1369–72.
26. Arai Y-CP, Nishihara M, Yamamoto Y, et al. Dorsal root ganglion pulsed radiofrequency for the management of intractable vertebral metastatic pain: a case series. Pain Med. 2015;16(5):1007–12.
27. Hofmeester I, Steffens MG, Brinkert W. Chronic scrotal and inguinal pain after orchidopexy in a 13-year-old boy, treated by pulsed radiofrequency of the dorsal ganglia. J Pediatric Urol. 2013;9(6 Pt B):e155–6.
28. Lee SY, Jang DI, Noh C, Ko YK. Successful treatment of occipital radiating headache using pulsed radiofrequency therapy. J Korean Neurosurgical Society. 2015;58(1):89–92.
29. Li J, Yin Y, Ye L, Zuo Y. Pulsed radiofrequency of C2 dorsal root ganglion under ultrasound guidance for chronic migraine: a case report. J Pain Res. 2018;11:1915–9.
30. Letcher FS, Goldring S. The effect of radiofrequency current and heat on peripheral nerve action potential in the cat. J Neurosurg. 1968;29(1):42–7.
31. Byrd D, Mackey S. Pulsed radiofrequency for chronic pain. Curr Pain Headache Rep. 2008;12(1):37–41.
32. Roberts I, Ker K. How systematic reviews cause research waste. Lancet. 2015; 386(10003):1536.
33. Handoll HH, Langhorne P. In defence of reviews of small trials: underpinning the generation of evidence to inform practice. Cochrane Database Systematic Reviews doi:https://doi.org/10.1002/14651858. ED000106(11), ED000106 (2015).

Doxapram alleviates low SpO_2 induced by the combination of propofol and fentanyl during painless gastrointestinal endoscopy

Zhengfeng Gu, Lian Xin*, Haoxing Wang, Chunxiao Hu, Zhiping Wang, Shunmei Lu, Jingjing Xu, Yiling Qian and Jun Wang

Abstract

Background: Painless gastrointestinal endoscopy under intravenous propofol anesthesia is widely applied in the clinical scenario. Despite the good sedation and elimination of anxiety that propofol provides, low SpO_2 may also result. Doxapram is a respiratory stimulant with a short half-life. The primary aim of this study was to investigate the effects of doxapram on alleviating low SpO_2 induced by the combination of propofol and fentanyl during painless gastrointestinal endoscopy.

Methods: In this prospective study, patients scheduled for painless gastrointestinal endoscopy were randomly assigned to group D or S with 55 patients per group. Initially, both groups received a combination of propofol and fentanyl. Patients in group D received 50 mg doxapram after propofol injection, while patients in group S received an equal volume of saline. Vital signs of the patients, propofol dose, examination duration, and incidences of low SpO_2 were recorded.

Results: There were no statistical differences in propofol consumption and examination duration between the two groups. Twenty-six patients in group S experienced low SpO_2 versus 10 in group D ($P = 0.001$). Nineteen patients in group S underwent oxygenation with a face mask in contrast to 8 in group D ($P = 0.015$). Eighteen patients in group S were treated with jaw lifting compared to 5 in group D ($P = 0.002$). Four patients in group S underwent assisted respiration compared to 2 in group D (without statistical difference). The average oxygen saturation in group S was significantly lower than that in group D at 1, 2 and 3 min after propofol injection ($P < 0.001$, $P = 0.001$ and $P = 0.020$, respectively). There were no statistical differences in oxygen saturation at other time points. There were no statistical differences in MAP and HR (except for the time point of 1 min after the induction) between the two groups.

Conclusions: Low dose of doxapram can effectively alleviate low SpO_2 in painless gastrointestinal endoscopy with intravenous propofol, without affecting propofol consumption, examination duration, MAP, or HR.

Keywords: Propofol, Doxapram, Respiratory depression, Painless gastrointestinal endoscopy, MAP, HR, SpO_2

* Correspondence: tomytomytomy123@sohu.com
Department of Anesthesiology, Wuxi People's Hospital Affiliated to Nanjing Medical University, 299 Qingyang Road, Wuxi 214023, Jiangsu, China

Background

Painless gastrointestinal endoscopy is increasingly applied in Class-A Tertiary Hospitals in China. Many patients prefer painless gastrointestinal endoscopy under sedation with analgesia for the pain resulting from mesenteric traction maneuvers, colonic distension by gas insufflations, and winding of the device within the intestinal tract. Accordingly, propofol, combined with analgesics, is commonly used for these procedures [1–3]. This method reduces anxiety and discomfort, improves tolerability and patient satisfaction, and provides better effects for the procedure.

The advantages of propofol include earlier onset, shorter examination duration and quicker emergence. However, in the case of intravenous administration, low SpO_2 and circulatory inhibition may occur. Low SpO_2 resulting from propofol, especially in combination with an analgesic, such as fentanyl, can potentially render risk to patients undergoing painless gastrointestinal endoscopy, in which case anesthesia with intravenous administration of propofol requires rigorous supervision by an experienced anesthesiologist. Doxapram is a respiratory stimulant with a short duration and fast onset [4]. Low-dose doxapram may excite the respiratory center by stimulating the chemoreceptor of the carotid sinus, whereas large dose of doxapram can directly excite medullar respiratory center, spinal cord and brainstem, which could lead to increased tidal volume [5]. As per the pharmacological mechanism, we postulated that doxapram should well alleviate low SpO_2 induced by propofol during painless gastrointestinal endoscopy, without affecting the quality of anesthesia. The primary aim of this study was to investigate the effects of doxapram on alleviating low SpO_2 induced by the combination of propofol and fentanyl during painless gastrointestinal endoscopy. Our prospective study specifically compared the administration of propofol and fentanyl with or without doxapram for painless gastrointestinal endoscopy performed by anesthesiologists.

Methods

Patients scheduled for painless gastrointestinal endoscopy were recruited for this prospective, randomized, double-blind study. The trial was conducted at the Department of Gastroenterology, Wuxi People's Hospital from August 2018 through January 2019. It was approved by the institutional Ethics Committee of Clinical and New Technology of Wuxi People's Hospital (KYLLH2018029) and registered in the Chinese Clinical Trial Register (ChiCTR) (ChiCTR1800017832). The trial mainly aimed to evaluate the effects of doxapram on propofol-induced low SpO_2 when combined with fentanyl analgesia. Secondly, we evaluated the total consumption of propofol, examination duration, mean arterial pressure (MAP), and heart rate (HR). The study adheres to consolidated standards of reporting trials.

All patients over 18 years of age scheduled for a diagnostic gastrointestinal endoscopy were included in this study, after submission of written informed consent. The exclusion criteria included medical history such as medication of diazepam, neuroleptics, and anticonvulsants that interfere with heart rate; anaphylaxis to drugs used in the study; cardiovascular diseases such as hypertension, arrhythmia, abnormal electrocardiogram (ECG); abnormal liver and/or kidney functions; lung disease, such as chronic obstructive pulmonary disease (COPD); abdominal laparotomy; body mass index above 30 $kg \cdot m^{-2}$; age over 75 years or below 18 years; clinical suspicion of intestinal subocclusion or stenosis; colorectal tumors; psychiatric patients; and requirement for complex therapeutic procedures during diagnostic colonoscopy.

Sample size calculation was performed with a probability of type I error (α) at 0.05, a power (1-β) of 0.90, a low SpO_2 of 80 and 50% in the control and intervention groups, respectively. Thus, 52 patients were required in each group. Considering an approximately 5% loss to follow-up, we included 55 patients in each group.

An anesthetist nurse prepared the same volume of doxapram or saline as per the randomization by the computer in the envelope. Both the patients and the anesthesiologists in charge of anesthesia were blinded to the allocation. All patients were monitored with pulse oximetry, continuous ECG, and noninvasive blood pressure assessed every 1 min in the first 5 min and then at a 5-min interval after doxapram or saline administration. The outcome was assessed and recorded by another anesthetist nurse who was blinded to study group assignment. Each patient in Group D received intravenous infusion (IV) of fentanyl 0.05 mg and propofol 1–2 $mg \cdot kg^{-1}$ sequentially, followed by IV doxapram 50 mg, and patients in Group S individually received sequential IV fentanyl 0.05 mg and propofol 1–2 $mg \cdot kg^{-1}$, followed by IV saline (same volume as doxapram in group D). In both groups, anesthesia was induced with propofol 1–2 min after IV fentanyl, and the total dose was slowly infused within 60 s, or limited to the drooping eyelid with loss of corneal-palpebral reflex (Ramsay Score 6). An additional dose of 0.5 $mg \cdot kg^{-1}$ was given in the event of signs of motor function. In both groups, oxygenation was applied with a nasal tube (3 L/min). Gastrointestinal endoscopy was performed by the same endoscopist using an Olympus OEV262H video system with gastroscopic tubes from the GIF-H290 series and colonoscopic tubes from the CF-H2901 series. The endoscopists performed gastroscopy and colonoscopy sequentially.

The primary aim of the study was to investigate the effects of doxapram on low SpO_2. Low SpO_2 was considered significant when SpO_2 was < 90% [6]. A face mask covering the patient's nose and mouth was applied when the $SpO_2 < 90\%$. The method of jaw lifting would be applicable when the SpO_2 was still less than 90% 10 s after face mask application. Assisted ventilation with a simple breathing balloon would be performed immediately in the case of the SpO_2 still below 90% 10 s after jaw lifting.

Patients were transferred to the post-anesthesia care unit (PACU) under the care of an experienced anesthetist nurse on completion of the endoscopy. After 30 min in the PACU, we evaluated the satisfaction scores of the endoscopists and patients using a visual analog scale (VAS, 0 = dissatisfaction, and 10 = full satisfaction). Patients were considered eligible for discharge with a score ≥ 9, according to the modified Aldrete–Kroulik index [7].

Statistical analyses were performed using Medcalc software (version 15, Medcalc Software bvba, Ostend, Belgium) [8]. Age, weight, and height of patients, total examination duration, total propofol consumption, BP, HR, and SpO_2 were recorded, together with profiles as low SpO_2, face mask use, jaw lifting, and assisted ventilation. Study outcomes included the development of low SpO_2 (< 90%) and the necessity of the following managements by minutes. The variations of MAP and HR were compared as well as the satisfaction of both endoscopists and patients. The gender proportions and cases of low SpO_2 were compared with a Pearson Chi-squared test. Levels of outcome parameters were compared with independent samples t-test after checking for normal distribution. Mann-Whitney test (independent samples) was employed if the parameters presented an abnormal distribution. $P < 0.05$ was considered statistically significant.

Results

A total of 110 patients rated as ASA I-II were enrolled in this study. All patients underwent a complete gastrointestinal endoscopy. Table 1 showed study data with no statistical differences, with respect to gender, age, weight, and height. The dosages of propofol consumption, examination duration, and satisfaction VAS of endoscopists and patients were also similar between the two groups.

As shown in Fig. 1, SpO_2 was significantly higher in group D than in group S at 1, 2, and 3 min after propofol injection ($P < 0.001$, $P = 0.007$, and $P = 0.020$, respectively). There were no statistical differences in SpO_2 at other time points (Fig. 1). MAP decreased after propofol administration in both groups. There were no statistical differences in MAP at any time point between the two groups. HR measurements, at 1 min after propofol infusion, were significantly lower in group S compared to group D (72.4 ± 14.8 vs. 82.5 ± 11.1, $P = 0.001$). No other side effects of doxapram were observed throughout the experiment.

Table 1 Demographics, propofol, examination duration, and satisfaction of VAS

Parameter	Group D ($n = 55$)	Group S ($n = 55$)	Statistics	P
Gender (f/m)	33/22	30/25	1.200	0.273
Age (yr)	46.2 ± 11.50	50.0 ± 10.10	1.839	0.069
Weight (kg)	60.8 ± 10.10	63.0 ± 10.10	1.107	0.271
Height (cm)	164.1 ± 7.40	165.5 ± 8.10	0.936	0.351
BMI ($kg{\cdot}m^{-2}$)	22.5 ± 2.80	22.9 ± 2.30	0.788	0.433
Propofol (mg)	262.3 ± 53.70	244.0 ± 60.60	−1.681	0.096
Duration (s)	810.1 ± 243.60	781.6 ± 284.60	−0.566	0.573
VAS (endoscopist)	9.7 ± 0.20	9.6 ± 0.20	−0.130	0.898
VAS (patient)	9.8 ± 0.20	9.8 ± 0.20	0.170	0.866

Note: data presented as mean ± standard deviation (SD)

Patients in group S had a higher incidence of low SpO_2 compared to those in group D ($P = 0.001$), as shown in Table 2. There were significantly lower incidences of face mask use and jaw lifting in group D compared to those in group S ($P = 0.015$ and $P = 0.002$, respectively). Four patients in group S and 2 in group D underwent assisted ventilation, with insignificant statistical difference.

Discussion

Gastrointestinal endoscopy is a common procedure for prevention, diagnosis, and treatment of a variety of symptoms and diseases of the stomach and lower digestive tract. Sedation or anesthesia is an important means to increase comfort and decrease anxiety, discomfort and pain during the endoscopic maneuver [9]. Propofol is a satisfactory intravenous anesthetic due to its short half-life, fast emergence from anesthesia, and low incidence of nausea and vomiting. It is widely used in outpatient gastrointestinal endoscopic procedures for sedation and/ or anesthesia without increasing cardiopulmonary adverse events compared to conventional agents [10]. It has a very narrow therapeutic window, which can easily progress from moderate to deep sedation or general anesthesia without a reversal agent [11]. Thus, anesthetists must be meticulous for the side effects of propofol, including injection pain, hypotension, bradycardia, and low SpO_2 [12]. In our study, the administration of intravenous propofol combined with fentanyl, as the anesthetic agent, resulted in a high incidence of low SpO_2 (34.5%). Despite the respiration-assisted techniques and airway management available to ensure patients' safety, decreasing the incidence of low SpO_2 without affecting the quality of anesthesia is of interest to clinicians [13]. Intravenous propofol is routinely combined with a small dose of fentanyl and/or midazolam to assist in sedation and analgesia during colonoscopies on the grounds of its short analgesic effects [14–16]. Fentanyl, a synthetic opioid analgesic, has good analgesic effects at small doses. It is fast-acting

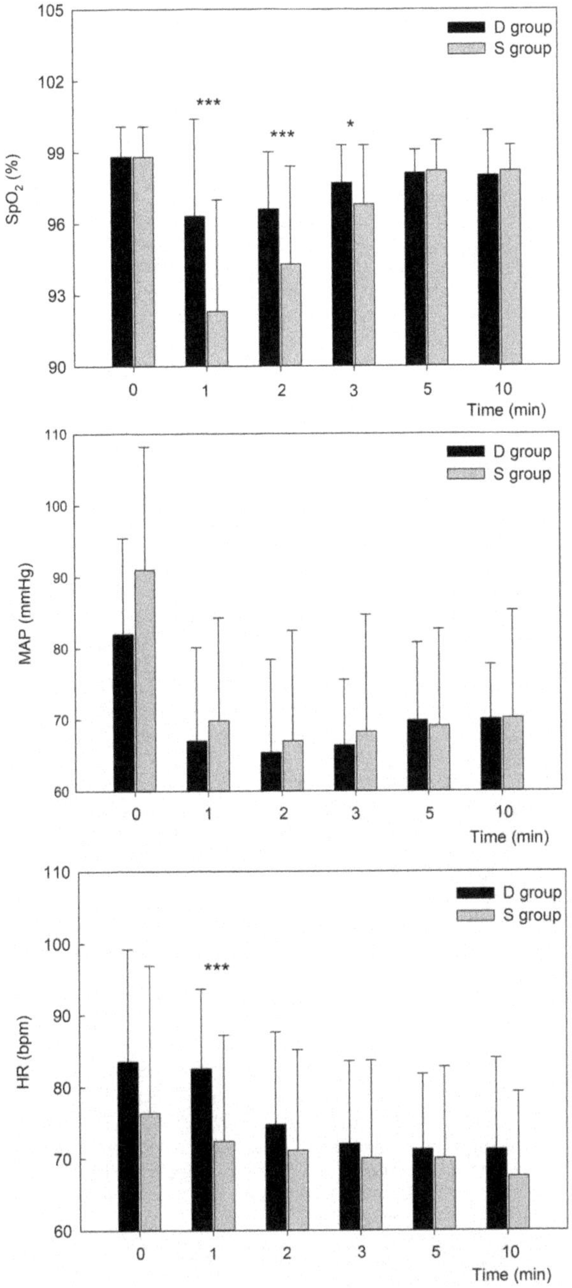

Fig. 1 Variation of SpO_2, MAP, and HR between group D and group S at different time points ($n = 55$ per group). Note: data are presented as mean ± standard deviation (SD). * represents significant differences at $P < 0.05$

Table 2 Cases of respiratory depression and therapy

	S ($n = 55$)	D ($n = 55$)	χ^2	P
Low SpO_2	26	10	10.5706	0.001*
Inhaling of oxygen with a face mask	19	8	5.9393	0.015*
Jaw lifting	18	5	9.2904	0.002*
Assisted ventilation	4	2	0.7051	0.401

* represents significant differences at $P < 0.05$

and results in fewer low SpO_2. Fentanyl is often administered in outpatient painless colonoscopy in combination with propofol to reduce propofol consumption, promote emergence and abridge theater stay. Unfortunately, both propofol and fentanyl may result in low SpO_2. Thus, the combined application may render patients at increased risk of low SpO_2. On the contrary, doxapram, a fast and short-acting respiratory stimulant, may reduce the incidence of low SpO_2 from propofol and fentanyl [17], and is frequently applicable to low SpO_2 due to anesthesia or central inhibition [18]. Moreover, doxapram can also serve as an analeptic after general anesthesia, such as sevoflurane inhalation [19].

Our results revealed that SpO_2 was significantly increased at 1, 2, and 3 min subsequent to propofol injection in the group treated with doxapram compared to the saline-treated group. We also observed a decreased incidence of low SpO_2, oxygen inhalation with a face mask and jaw lifting in the group treated with doxapram compared to the saline-treated group. These outcomes may be related to the effect of respiratory stimulation of doxapram and its action duration. Doxapram can reflexively stimulate the respiratory center via chemical receptors in the carotid body at low doses. At large doses, however, doxapram directly stimulates the respiratory center in the medulla oblongata [20]. S. Kruszynski et al. [21] attributed that part of the stimulatory effects of doxapram to the direct input on brainstem centers with differential effects on the rhythm generating kernel (Pre-Bötzinger Complex) and the downstream motor output. Propofol acts as an agonist of γ-aminobutyric acid (GABA) receptor. $GABA_B$ activates the channel of K^+ on postsynaptic membrane and leads to hyperpolarization of the latter. Doxapram blocks the K^+ channel on postsynaptic membrane via Ca^{2+}-dependent K^+ conductance [22]. We speculated that this action might be one of the mechanisms underlying doxapram antagonizing the side effect of propofol. Our study demonstrated that doxapram could effectively alleviate the occurrence of low SpO_2 during gastrointestinal endoscopy, thus providing improved safety of patients.

Despite the alleviation of low SpO_2 by doxapram, precautions should be taken against the side effects whereby. Doxapram may induce headache, dyspnea, arrhythmia, diarrhea, nausea, vomiting, chest pain, and hypertension, etc., among which arrhythmia, dyspnea and hypertension are the most relevant and severe side effects. Notwithstanding the absence of adverse effects as arrhythmia, dyspnea and hypertension in this study, our small sample size did not suffice to reach a compelling conclusion for a risk-benefit balance of doxapram. Consequently, larger trials are required in order to verify the definite role of doxapram during general anesthesia for gastrointestinal endoscopy.

The development of hypotension and bradycardia in anesthesia is probably attributable to the effects of vascular dilation and myocardial inhibition by propofol on the gamma-aminobutyric acid receptors and the atrial muscarinic cholinergic receptors [23]. Doxapram causes transient tachycardia (1 min after injection), which may be related to the stimulation of catecholamine release via β_1-receptor stimulation. In our study, even in the event of hypotension and bradycardia, doxapram may not have adequately exerted its reversive effects largely due to the relatively low dosage.

Doxapram is occasionally applied to promote emergence from volatile anesthesia, such as sevoflurane [19]. Our findings demonstrated that regardless of doxapram administration, all the 110 patients were discharged with a modified Aldrete–Kroulik index >9 within 30 min, which indicated that doxapram did not affect the time required for emergence from anesthesia. We speculated that the inefficacy on emergence timing was due to the doxapram administered at the commencement rather than the denouement of anesthesia, as in the study by HL Wang et al. using total intravenous anesthesia with dexmedetomidine, propofol and remifentanil [24].

There are some limitations in our study. First, our results would have been more accurate provided that propofol delivery had been guided by the monitoring of anesthetic depth, as with a bispectral index for instance. Despite the same dose of doxapram we adopted for each patient, questions still remained as to whether the dose should be administered as per body weight. Second, we did not monitor $ETCO_2$ as an element of respiratory depression and moreover we did not increase the flow rate of oxygen prior to application of face mask/jaw lifting or ventilation with constant flow rate for each patient, either. Furthermore, we did not employ SpO_2/FiO_2 ratio to evaluate respiratory depression, and we did not monitor for postoperative pulmonary complications for the patients in PACU. Nonetheless, with respect to the care of outpatients, early safe discharge from PACU is of importance for the improved medical efficiency and the medical care system at large, thus awaiting more profound investigations as to whether doxapram could decrease the emergence time in scenario of PACU.

Conclusion

With the addition of 50 mg of doxapram in intravenous anesthesia with propofol and fentanyl for gastrointestinal endoscopy, the incidence of hypoxemia and the necessity of respiratory assistance following anesthetic induction were significantly reduced for the initial 3 min. The medication of doxapram did not affect the satisfaction scores of the endoscopists and has little effect on MAP and HR at the 50 mg dose.

Abbreviations

HR: Heart rate; IV: Intravenous injection; MAP: Mean arterial pressure; PACU: Post anesthesia care unit; SpO2: Oxygen saturation; VAS: Visual analogue scale

Acknowledgments

The authors sincerely appreciate our team in the successful operation.

Authors' contributions

ZFG: conception of the trial design, acquisition of data, drafting of original manuscript; HXW: acquisition of data; CXH: interpretation of data; ZPW: interpretation of data; SML: data processing and software operation; JJX: formal analysis of data; YLQ: analysis of data; JW: acquisition of data; LX: drafting and revision of manuscript. All authors have read and approved the manuscript and ensure that this is the case.

References

1. Zhang L, Bao Y, Shi D. Comparing the pain of propofol via different combinations of fentanyl, sulfentanil or remifentanil in gastrointestinal endoscopy. Acta Cir Bras. 2014;29:675–80.
2. Zhao YJ, Liu S, Mao QX, Ge HJ, Wang Y, Huang BQ, Wang WC, Xie JR. Efficacy and safety of remifentanil and sulfentanil in painless gastroscopic examination: a prospective study. Surg Laparosc Endosc Percutan Tech. 2015;25:e57–60.
3. Rudner R, Jalowiecki P, Kawecki P, Gonciarz M, Mularczyk A, Petelenz M. Conscious analgesia/sedation with remifentanil and propofol versus total intravenous anesthesia with fentanyl, midazolam, and propofol for outpatient colonoscopy. Gastrointest Endosc. 2003;57:657–63.
4. Kruszynski S, Stannitis K, Brandes J, Poets CF, Koch H. Doxapram stimulates respiratory activity through distinct activation of neurons in the nuleus hypoglossus and the pre-Bötzinger complex. J Neurophysiol. 2019;121: 1102–10.
5. Yost CS. A new look at the respiratory stimulant doxapram. CNS Drug Rev. 2006;12:236–49.
6. Deng C, Wang X, Zhu Q, Kang Y, Yang J, Wang H. Comparison of nalbuphine and sufentanil for colonoscopy: a randomized controlled trial. PLoS One. 2017;12:e0188901.
7. Júnior OG, Serralheiro FC, Fonseca FL, Junior RO, Adami F, Christofolini DM, et al. Randomized double-blind clinical trial comparing two anesthetic techniques for ultrasound-guided transvaginal follicular puncture. Einstein. 2016;14:305–10.
8. Gu Z. J Yang LX, J Xu, Y Yang, Z Wang. Dose-dependent effects of dexmedetomidine during one-lung ventilation in patients undergoing lobectomy. Int J Clin Exp Med. 2017;10:5216–21.
9. Neves JFNPD, Araújo FDP, Ferreira CM, Duarte FBN, Pace FH, Ornellas LC, et al. Colonoscopy sedation: clinical trial comparing propofol and fentanyl with or without midazolam. Braz J Anesth. 2016;66:231–6.
10. Wadhwa V, Issa D, Garg S, Lopez R, Sanaka MR, Vargo JJ. Similar risk of cardiopulmonary adverse events between propofol and traditional anesthesia for gastrointestinal endoscopy: a systematic review and meta-analysis. Clin Gastro Hepat. 2016;15:194.
11. Goulson DT, Fragneto RY. Anesthesia for gastrointestinal endoscopic procedures. Periop Nurs Clin. 2009;4:421–35.
12. Agostoni M, Fanti L, Gemma M, Pasculli N, Beretta L, Testoni PA. Adverse events during monitored anesthesia care for GI endoscopy: an 8-year experience. Gastrointest Endosc. 2011;74:266–75.
13. Usha P, Kate L, Audrey SE, Paul M, Silbert BS. Early cognitive impairment after sedation for colonoscopy: the effect of adding midazolam and/or fentanyl to propofol. Anesth Analg. 2009;109:1448–55.
14. Lovett P, Gómez V, Hodge DO, Ladlie B. Propofol versus midazolam/fentanyl sedation for colonoscopy in the elderly patient population. J Perianesth Nurs. 2017;32:210.
15. Eberl S, Polderman JAW, Preckel B, Kalkman CJ, Fockens P, Hollmann MW. Is "really conscious" sedation with solely an opioid an alternative to every day used sedation regimes for colonoscopies in a teaching hospital? Midazolam/fentanyl, propofol/alfentanil, or alfentanil only for colonoscopy: a randomized trial. Tech Coloproctol. 2014;18:745–52.
16. Hsu CD, Huang JM, Chuang YP, Wei HY, Su YC, Wu JY, et al. Propofol target-controlled infusion for sedated gastrointestinal endoscopy: a comparison of propofol alone versus propofol fentanyl midazolam. Kaohsiung J Med Sci. 2015;31:580–4.

17. Owen-Falkenberg AP. Doxapram hydrochloride. Treatment of postoperative hypoventilation caused by fentanyl. Ugeskr Laeger. 1980;142:2488.
18. Dahan A, van der Schrier R, Smith T, Aarts L, van Velzen M, Niesters M. Averting opioid-induced respiratory depression without affecting Analgssia. Anesthesiology. 2018;128:1027–37.
19. Wu CC, Mok MS, Chen JY, Wu GJ, Wen YR, Lin CS. Doxapram shortens recovery following sevoflurane anesthesia. Can J Anaesth. 2006;53:456–60.
20. Li GC, Jiao YG, Wu ZH, Fang F. Effect of doxapram on the respiratory rhythmical discharge activity in the brainstem slice of neonatal rats. J Southern Med Univ. 2010;30:245–8.
21. Kruszynski S, Stanaitis K, Brandes J, Poets CF, Koch H. Doxapram stimulates respiratory activity through distinct activation of neurons in the nucleus Hypoglossus and the PreBötzinger complex. J Neurophysiol. 2019;121:1102–10.
22. Osaka Y, Onimaru H, Kotani S, Kashiwagi M, Morisaki H, Takeda J. The effects of doxapram on medullary respiratory neurones in brainstem-spinal cord preparations from newborn rats. Anaesthesia. 2014;69:468–75.
23. Aguero REP, Pascuzzo-Lima C, Granado AED, Cabarcas RAB. Propofol-induced myocardial depression: possible role of atrial muscarinic cholinergic receptors. Rev Esp Anestesiol Reanim. 2008;55:81–5.
24. Wang HL, Tang SH, Wang XQ, Gong WH, Liu XM, Lei WF. Doxapram hastens the recovery following total intravenous anesthesia with dexmedetomidine, propofol and remifentanil. Exp Ther Med. 2015;9:1518–22.

21

Intrathecal morphine is associated with reduction in postoperative opioid requirements and improvement in postoperative analgesia in patients undergoing open liver resection

Jefferson Tang[1], Leonid Churilov[2], Chong Oon Tan[1], Raymond Hu[1], Brett Pearce[1], Luka Cosic[1], Christopher Christophi[3] and Laurence Weinberg[1,3*]

Abstract

Background: Our study aimed to test the hypothesis that the addition of intrathecal morphine (ITM) results in reduced postoperative opioid use and enhanced postoperative analgesia in patients undergoing open liver resection using a standardized enhanced recovery after surgery (ERAS) protocol with multimodal analgesia.

Methods: A retrospective analysis of 216 adult patients undergoing open liver resection between June 2010 and July 2017 at a university teaching hospital was conducted. The primary outcome was the cumulative oral morphine equivalent daily dose (oMEDD) on postoperative day (POD) 1. Secondary outcomes included postoperative pain scores, opioid related complications, and length of hospital stay. We also performed a cost analysis evaluating the economic benefits of ITM.

Results: One hundred twenty-five patients received ITM (ITM group) and 91 patients received usual care (UC group). Patient characteristics were similar between the groups. The primary outcome - cumulative oMEDD on POD1 - was significantly reduced in the ITM group. Postoperative pain scores up to 24 h post-surgery were significantly reduced in the ITM group. There was no statistically significant difference in complications or hospital stay between the two study groups. Total hospital costs were significantly higher in the ITM group.

Conclusion: In patients undergoing open liver resection, ITM in addition to conventional multimodal analgesic strategies reduced postoperative opioid requirements and improved analgesia for 24 h after surgery, without any statistically significant differences in opioid-related complications, and length of hospital stay. Hospital costs were significantly higher in patients receiving ITM, reflective of a longer mandatory stay in intensive care.

Keywords: Analgesia, Liver resection, Hospital costs, Intrathecal morphine, Enhanced recovery after surgery

* Correspondence: laurence.weinberg@austin.org.au
[1]Department of Anaesthesia, Austin Health, Heidelberg, Victoria, Australia
[3]Department of Surgery, University of Melbourne, Austin Health, Heidelberg, Victoria, Australia

Background

Perioperative analgesia is critical for maximising patient satisfaction and recovery outcomes in surgery. The optimal postoperative analgesic technique for patients undergoing open liver resection is controversial. Continuous thoracic epidural analgesia has been considered the cornerstone analgesic modality, however limitations of its use in this setting include risk of epidural haematoma (in the context of coagulopathy associated with postoperative hepatic insufficiency), prolonged motor block limiting mobilisation, urinary retention, and hypotension [1–3]. Epidural analgesia is furthermore a labor intensive and more technically complicated intervention. Indeed, a large international and multicenter landmark randomized controlled trial (RCT) found that most adverse morbid outcomes in high-risk patients undergoing major abdominal surgery are not reduced by the use of epidural analgesia [4]. The Enhanced Recovery After Surgery (ERAS) Society guidelines now strongly advocate that routine thoracic epidural analgesia cannot be recommended in open liver surgery for ERAS patients and that intrathecal opiates can be good alternatives when combined with multimodal analgesia [5].

Single shot intrathecal morphine (ITM) has recently emerged as a promising alternative practice yielding better patient outcomes [6–8]. Intrathecal anaesthesia is a simpler and quicker alternative neuraxial technique with a lower rate of technical failure [7]. Similar to epidural analgesia, intrathecal morphine has been demonstrated to improve postoperative pain scores and reduce postoperative rescue analgesia requirements compared to intravenous opioid analgesia [8]. As such, a growing number of hospitals worldwide have adopted ITM as a preferred choice for perioperative analgesia for major open hepato-pancreatic-biliary surgery [6]. However, the benefits of ITM compared to conventional multimodal analgesic strategies for major open liver surgery remain unclear. Therefore, we conducted a retrospective observational study to determine if patients undergoing open liver resection who receive ITM in additional to receiving a standardized ERAS protocol have better postoperative analgesia compared to patients receiving ERAS alone. We hypothesize that for patients undergoing open liver resection using a standardized enhanced recovery after surgery protocol with multimodal analgesia, the addition of ITM results in less postoperative opioid use and enhanced postoperative analgesia.

Methods

Following prospective ethics approval by the Austin Health Human Research Ethics Committee (HREC no: LNR/18/Austin/79), we conducted a retrospective analysis of adult patients who underwent major open liver resection between July 2010 and June 2017 using a standardized ERAS protocol. All patients underwent surgery at the Austin Hospital, a university hospital in Melbourne, Australia with a dedicated high volume hepato-pancreatic-biliary and liver transplant centre. Eligible patients were identified by International Statistical Classification of Diseases (ICD) codes that included the following surgical categories: i.) excision of lesion of liver, ii.) segmental resection of liver, iii.) lobectomy of liver, iv.) trisegmental resection of liver, and v.) segmental resection of liver for trauma. In order to ensure a homogeneous patient cohort, we excluded patients receiving epidural analgesia, patients undergoing laparoscopic liver resection, and patients undergoing deroofing of liver cyst or liver biopsy. We also excluded patients with a history of chronic opioid use (defined as near-daily use of > 60 mg oral morphine equivalent) for 8 weeks or longer. A team of experienced high-volume surgeons ($n = 5$) and anaesthetists ($n = 6$) provided perioperative care based on a standardized liver enhanced recovery after surgery programme. As part of this protocol, all patients received an opioid based patient-controlled analgesia device for postoperative analgesia.

Key outcomes

The primary outcome was cumulative oral morphine equivalent daily dose in milligrams (oMEDD) on POD 1, adjusted for the following priori chosen variables: major resection, patient age, Charlson Comorbidity Index (CCI), duration of surgery, intraoperative oMEDD use, adjunct intrathecal clonidine, adjunct intrathecal bupivacaine, intraoperative ketamine and postoperative ketamine. These factors were chosen due to their potential influence on total morphine requirements after surgery. Secondary outcomes included average and maximum pain at rest and on movement over the first 24 postoperative hours, oMEDD use and postoperative pain scores in the PACU and on postoperative days 0, 2 and 3. We measured opioid related side effects, length of hospital stay, and performed a costs analysis (including readmissions within 30 postoperative days) for both groups of patients.

Definitions

oMEDD amounts were calculated using the Opioid Dose Equivalence document endorsed by the Faculty of Pain Medicine, Australian and New Zealand College of Anaesthetists [9]. Length of hospital stay was determined by the period from completion of surgery to discharge. Time to full ward diet was defined as the period from completion of surgery to the first mention of tolerating full ward diet in the patient medical records. Time to first oral opioid use was defined as the period from completion of surgery to the first administration of oral opioid after surgery. Daily postoperative pain scores were measured and recorded by a dedicated Acute Pain

Service using the Numerical Rating Scale (NRS). The NRS is a single 11-point numeric scale in which a respondent selects a whole number (integers from 0 to 10) that best reflects the intensity of their pain. A score of 0 indicates no pain, whereas a score of 10 indicates extreme or the worst pain imaginable [10]. Duration of surgery was defined from skin incision until the final stitch for wound closure. Major resection was defined as 4 segments or greater; minor resection was defined as 3 segments or less.

Complications were defined as any deviation from the normal postoperative course, guided by the European Perioperative Clinical Outcome definitions [11]. Complications were recorded by two independent clinicians, and then graded using Clavien-Dindo Classification - a widely used and validated approach to surgical outcome assessment that assigns severity grades to surgical complications [12]. In case of disagreement on grading by the two assessors, the case was discussed with a third author.

Costs related to the index hospital admission and any consequent readmission within 30 postoperative days were included. Costs related to the preoperative and perioperative course were not considered. Allocation of costs was done based on service volume, and costs were calculated using an activity-based costing methodology. Raw costing data was obtained from the hospital's business intelligent unit, and then allocated into categories based on individual itemisation codes for costs incurred during admission. These categories included 'intensive care unit', 'medical' (for example medical consults, allied health, pathology, blood products, and radiology), 'pharmacy', and 'ward' costs. For detailed cost analysis of complication incidence and severity, cost centres were further separated into 'allied health' (for example physiotherapy, speech pathology, dietician), 'blood products' (for example albumin, packed red cells), 'intensive care unit', 'pathology' (for example tissue diagnosis, blood testing), 'pharmacy' (drug dispensing), 'radiology' (for example scans, radiological procedures), and 'ward' (for example hospital bed, nursing, catering). Only in-hospital costs were considered, with both direct and indirect costs assessed to produce a total cost for each patient. Costs are displayed as medians and interquartile ranges to more accurately reflect the economic burden placed upon healthcare providers by catering for outliers. Costs were inflated to 2018 dollars based upon the average Australian Consumer Price Index from 2010 to 2017 inclusive, as reported by the Reserve Bank of Australia [13]. The average Consumer Price Index was applied pro rata to each patient based on the number of days between the admission date and the 1st of January 2018, to ensure all costs were inflated as accurately as possible reducing error in comparison. Conversion to the United States Dollar was completed using the market rate on the 1st of January 2018.

Data collection

Data was extracted from the patient's electronic medical records and the Hospital's computerized laboratory results. Austin Health utilizes Cerner® electronic health records that allows comprehensive electronic data capture and access to patient health information in the perioperative setting.

Preoperative data collected included gender, age, body mass index, American Society of Anesthesiologists (ASA) class, principle diagnosis, surgical procedure, segments resected, and Charlson Comorbidity Index (CCI). The ASA score provides a simple categorisation of a patient's physiological status before surgery and is useful in predicting perioperative morbidity and mortality [14]. The CCI is a validated method for classifying comorbid conditions and subsequently estimating the risk of mortality from comorbid diseases [15]. We additionally collected information on whether the patient had smoked in the 1 year prior to the operation, preoperative biochemistry, liver function test and full blood examination results.

Intraoperative data collected included duration of surgery, type of resection, and whether the resection was "major" or "minor". We collected the dose of intrathecal morphine administered just prior to the commencement of the surgery, type and amount of intraoperative analgesia delivered, and types and amounts of fluids and blood products used intraoperatively.

Postoperative data collected included length of stay, duration of PCA use, time to full ward diet, time to first oral opioid use, and time in the intensive care unit (ICU). We also collected data on postoperative analgesia agents and anti-emetics administered in the post-anaesthesia care unit (PACU), on postoperative day 0 (day of surgery) and postoperative days 1 to 3. The number and severity of postoperative complications, worst sedation scores and pain scores at rest and on movement in the PACU and POD 0–3 were also collected from the patient's electronic medical records.

Statistical methodology

For the primary and the key secondary outcomes, we used quantile regression modelling adjusted for the following a-priori defined covariates: major resection, patient age, Charlson Comorbidity Index, duration of surgery, intraoperative oMEDD use, adjunct intrathecal clonidine, adjunct intrathecal bupivacaine, intraoperative ketamine and postoperative ketamine. Quantile regression models were used due to the violation of the normality of residuals assumption required for standard linear regression and lack of suitable transformations to satisfy these assumptions. Quantile regression models the association between a set of input variables and specific percentiles (or quantiles) of the outcome variable and estimates differences in the quantiles of the outcome variable between standard care and ITM groups. For example, a median (50th percentile) regression of cumulative oMEDD use at 24 h on ITM use estimates the difference in the median oMEDD use at 24 h between standard care and ITM groups adjusted for the selected covariates. For each outcome, we included three quantile regression models: the 25th percentile, the 50th percentile (median), and the 75th percentile. Standard assessment of collinearity was conducted using variance inflation factors (VIF) and condition number. For all other outcomes, continuous data was summarized as medians and interquartile range (IQR) and compared using the Mann-Whitney U test. Categorical variables were summarized as counts (proportions) and compared using the chi-squared test or Fisher's Exact test, as appropriate. Statistical analysis was performed using statistical software RStudio (Boston, MA, USA). Figures were constructed using Prism 6.0 GraphPad software (La Jolla, CA, USA).

Results

Three hundred thirty-five patients underwent liver resection at the Austin Hospital between July 2010 and June 2017. Two hundred sixteen patients satisfied the inclusion criteria. Of these, 91 patients received usual care (Usual care group) and 125 patients received ITM in addition to usual care (ITM group). Data collection was complete for 216 (100%) patients. Reason for patients not satisfying inclusion criteria included: epidural analgesia ($n = 4$), laparoscopic liver resection ($n = 106$), deroofing of a liver cyst ($n = 5$), and liver biopsy whilst staging pancreatic cancer without sufficient parenchymal resection ($n = 4$).

The median (IQR) patient age was 60 (51:67) years. There were 125 (58%) males and 91 (42%) females. Median (IQR) body mass index (BMI), ASA score and CCI were 26.15 (23.1:30.4) kg/m^2, 3 (2:3), and 7 (4:8) respectively. The principal diagnosis and indication for resection was benign in 33 (15%) patients and malignant in 183 (85%) patients. 32 (15%) patients received chemotherapy within 3 months before surgery. 153 (71%) patients underwent a 'minor' (defined as 3 segments or less) liver resection, and the remaining 63 (29%) patients underwent a 'major' (defined as 4 segments or more) liver resection. The range of procedures performed included 35 (16%) right hepatectomies, 17 (8%) left hepatectomies, 2 (1%) central hepatectomies, 137 (63%) segmental resections (3 segments or less), and 25 (12%) extended left or right hepatectomies (5 segments or more). Baseline patient characteristics between the ITM and usual care groups is summarized in Table 1.

Key outcomes

The median (IQR) cumulative oMEDD use on postoperative day 1 was 126.7 (53:268) mg in the ITM group vs. 176.3 (105:270) mg in the usual care group ($p = 0.04$). Whilst patients in the ITM group required less morphine compared to the control group, the effect size of this difference depended on their distribution quartile. Patients in the 25th percentile required 55.7 mg less morphine (95% CI: 25.6 to 88.4; $p = 0.00025$); 50th percentile 53.3 mg less morphine (95% CI:-22.1 to 98.0; $p = 0.058$), and 75th percentile 13.9 mg more morphine (95% CI: − 53.1 to 42.4; $p = 0.65$). A boxplot of the cumulative oMEDD consumptions on postoperative day 1 is presented in Fig. 1.

Patients in the ITM group reported lower pain scores at rest and on movement over the first 24 postoperative hours (see Table 2). Pain scores at rest and in the 25th percentile showed the most statistically significant benefit from ITM.

Intraoperative outcomes

For patients receiving ITM, the minimum, median (IQR), and maximum dose of intrathecal morphine delivered were 150 μg, 300 μg (250:400), and 500 μg, respectively. To enhance or lengthen the duration of intrathecal analgesia, intrathecal bupivacaine and clonidine were administered with the ITM in 26 (21%) and 13 (10%) patients respectively. The median (IQR) doses of intrathecal clonidine and bupivacaine were 50 μg (30:15) and 10 mg (2:15), respectively. All patients received additional intraoperative systemic opioids (Table 3). The median (IQR) IV morphine equivalent of intraoperative opioid received was 29.8 mg (20.0:38.0). No statistically significant difference between the ITM group and the usual care group in total operative time or perioperative fluid use and blood product administration were identified. Patients in the ITM group received less intraoperative opioid compared to patients in the usual care group: median (IQR) 26.7 mg (20.0:33.3) vs. 33.3 mg (20.0:46.7) IV morphine equivalent, $p = 0.001$. The ITM group received less intraoperative ketamine: median (IQR) 36 mg (20:62.5) vs. 62.5 mg (38.8: 89.5) in the usual care group, $p = 0.003$. A higher number of patients in the ITM group required intraoperative ondansetron (51% vs. 32%, $p = 0.005$).

Postoperative opioid requirements

In the post anaesthesia care unit, the median (IQR) cumulative oMEDD requirement was lower in the ITM group: 0 mg (0:10.5) compared to the usual care group 6 mg (0:21), $p = 0.001$. Postoperative opioid requirements were lower in the ITM group on postoperative Days 0 to 1. No statistically significant differences were observed in cumulative oMEDD requirements between the ITM group and the usual group on postoperative days 2 and 3. For patients receiving ITM, there were no significant differences observed between the dose of ITM administered and the incidence of nausea and vomiting

Table 1 Baseline characteristics of patients receiving intrathecal morphine (ITM) or Usual care. Data presented as median (interquartile range) or number of patients (proportion)

	ITM (***n*** = 125)	Usual care (***n*** = 91)	***P***-value
Age (years)	61 (52.5:68.5)	59 (49:66)	0.26
Gender (male: female)	81 (65%): 44 (35%)	45 (49%): 46 (51%)	0.03
Body mass index (kg/m^2)	25.9 (22.8:30.6)	26.2 (23.4:30.1)	0.71
Charlson comorbidity index	6.5 (4.0:8.0)	7.0 (4.0:8.0)i	0.99
Preoperative chemotherapy within 3 months	21 (16.8%)	11 (12.1%)	0.44
AMERICAN SOCIETY OF ANAESTHESIOLOGISTS SCORE			
1	1 (0.8%)	2 (2.2%)	0.72
2	44 (35.2%)	35 (38.5%)	
3	77 (61.6%)	51 (56%)	
4	3 (2.4%)	3 (3.3%)	
BASELINE BIOCHEMISTRY			
Haemoglobin (g/L)	143 (129.5:150.5)	131 (122:146)	0.005
White cell count (× 10^9/L)	7 (5:8)	6 (5:8)	0.05
Platelet count (× 10^9/L)	220 (158:273.3)	222 (173.5:280)	0.52
Urea (mg/dL)	6 (4.5:7)	6 (4:7)	0.53
Creatinine (μmol/L)	76.5 (63.25:87)	71.5 (61.25:88)	0.34
Estimated glomerular filtration rate (mL/min/1.73m^2)	86 (75:90)	90 (74.5:90)	0.6
Alanine transaminase (U/L)	49 (33.5:97)	57.5 (41.5:88.25)	0.67
Aspartate transaminase (U/L)	53 (47:85.5)	68 (64:113)	0.24
Alkaline phosphatase (U/L)	147 (94:201.5)	176 (19.3:246.5)	0.33
Gamma-glutamyltransferase (U/L)	109 (65.75:157.5)	125 (72.5:220)	0.72
Albumin (g/L)	39 (35:42)	37.5 (34:39)	0.08
Bilirubin (μmol/L)	11.5 (6.25:16.75)	12 (7.5:21)	0.54
Activated partial thromboplastin time (s)	27 (24:29)	28 (25:30)	0.17
International normalized ratio	1 (1:1)	1 (1:1)	0.4
PATHOLOGY			
Benign	**13 (10.4%)**	**20 (21.9%)**	0.17
Adenoma	8 (6.4%)	8 (8.8%)	
Haemangioma	1 (0.8%)	2 (2.2%)	
Other liver pathology	4 (3.2%)	10 (11.0%)	
Malignant	**112 (89.6%)**	**71 (78.1%)**	
Hepatocellular carcinoma	36 (28.8%)	29 (31.9%)	
Cholangiocarcinoma	14 (11.2%)	5 (5.5%)	
Gallbladder tumor	4 (3.2%)	2 (2.2%)	
Metastatic colorectal	58 (46.4%)	35 (38.5%)	
COMPLEXITY OF RESECTION			
Minor resection (≤ 3 sections)	85 (68.0%)	68 (74.7%)	0.29
Major resection (≥ 4 sections)	40 (32.0%)	23 (25.3%)	
TYPE OF SURGERY			
Right hepatectomy	23 (18.4%)	12 (13.2%)	0.53
Left hepatectomy	9 (7.2%)	8 (8.8%)	
Central hepatectomy	2 (1.6%)	0 (0%)	
Segmental resection (< 3 segments)	76 (60.8%)	61 (67.0%)	
Extended left or right hepatectomy (> 5+ segments)	15 (12%)	10 (11.0%)	

requiring anti-emetics (150-200 μg vs. 300 μg, $p = 0.611$; 300 μg vs. 400-500 μg, $p = 0.272$; 150-200 μg vs. 400-500 μg, $p = 0.098$). Further, there were no significant differences observed in oMEDD use on postoperative day 1 in ITM patients who were administered other analgesic adjuncts compared to those who received ITM alone.

The median (IQR) postoperative ketamine requirement was lower in the ITM group on postoperative day 0: 30 mg (19.5:48) vs. 64 mg (35.8:96) in the usual care group, $p = 0.006$. No statistically significant differences in postoperative ketamine requirements were identified at other timepoints. A detailed overview of intraoperative outcomes and postoperative opioid and ketamine requirements is presented in Table 3.

Postoperative analgesia

In the PACU, the median (IQR) pain score at rest was 1 (0:3) in the ITM group compared to 4 (0:7) in the usual care group, $p = 0.001$. On postoperative day 0, median (IQR) pain scores at rest in the ITM group were 3 (0:5) vs. 5 (3:7) in the usual care group, $p = 0.003$. No statistically significant difference in pain scores at rest on postoperative days 1–3 were observed. Median (IQR) pain scores on movement on postoperative day 0 was 3 (1:5) in the ITM group vs. 4 (3:6) in the usual care group, $p = 0.007$. No statistically significant differences in pain scores on postoperative days 2 and 3 between the groups were identified. For patients receiving ITM, there were no significant differences in pain scores on movement or at rest between patients receiving 150-200 μg, 300 μg or 400-500 μg of ITM.

Postoperative outcomes and complications

No statistically significant differences were identified between the ITM group and usual care group in time to full ward diet, time to first oral opioid use, complications, length of stay and 30-day readmission. Patients in the ITM group had a longer median (IQR) stay in the ICU: 17 h (12:21.5) vs. 10 h (0:18), $p = 0.0001$. Patients in the usual care group had a greater incidence of severe sedation on postoperative day 0 (42.4% vs 28.8%, $p = 0.04$). A detailed overview of postoperative and complication outcomes for each study group is presented in Table 4. For patients receiving ITM, there were no significant differences observed in the severity or number of complications between patients receiving 150-200 μg, 300 μg or 400-500 μg of ITM. No significant changes were observed in the length of hospital stay over time period 2011 to 2017 ($P = 0.153$ Kruskal-Wallis).

Postoperative cost analysis

Median (IQR) total hospital costs for all patients were US$11,183 (8458:17,331). Costs relating to blood products, medical complications, MET calls, pharmacy,

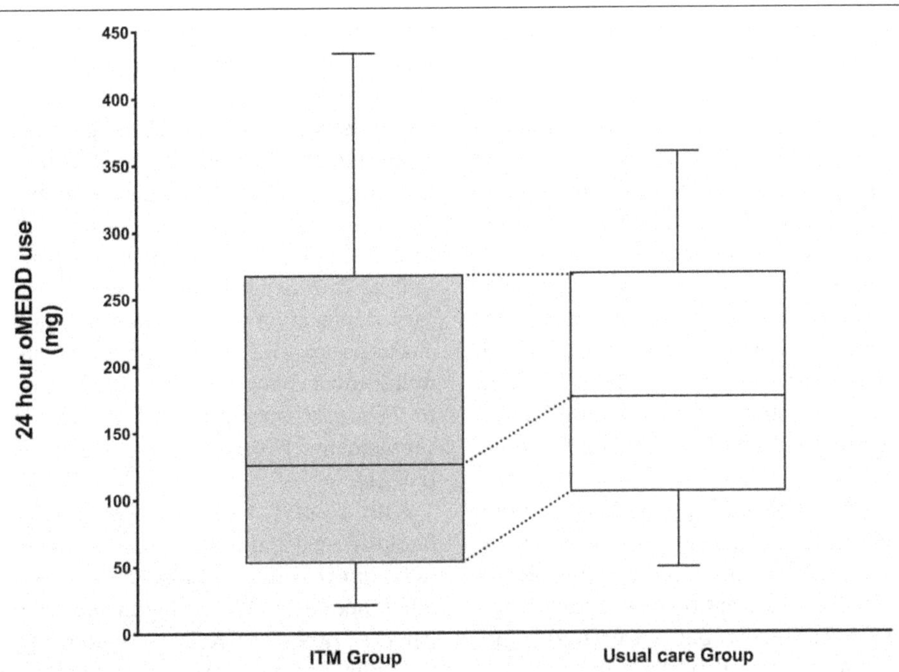

Fig. 1 Boxplots of oral morphine equivalent daily dose (oMEDD) use at 24-h post-surgery in patients of patients receiving intrathecal morphine (ITM) or Usual care

Table 2 Differences in morphine consumption and pain scores 24-h after surgery. Data presented as quartile differences (95% confidence interval) for the outcome variables between patients receiving receiving intrathecal morphine and Usual care. Adjustments for major resection, patient age, Charlton Comorbidity Index, duration of surgery, intraoperative oMEDD use, adjunct intrathecal clonidine, adjunct intrathecal bupivacaine, intraoperative ketamine and postoperative ketamine

		25th percentile		50th percentile		75th percentile	
		Adjusted	Unadjusted	Adjusted	Unadjusted	Adjusted	Unadjusted
Cumulative oMEDD use at 24 h (mg)	Difference	55.7 mg	52.3 mg	53.3 mg	50.7 mg	−13.9 mg	2.9 mg
	95% CI	25.6 to 88.4	35.3 to 77.9	− 22.1 to 98.0	13.4 to 87.8	−53.1 to 42.4	− 62.0 to 47.7
	p-value	0.00025	0.00015	0.058	0.03	0.65	0.94
Average pain at rest over 24 h	Difference	0.99	1	0.38	0	0.009	0
	95% CI	0.3 to 1.2	−0.6 to 1.0	0.04 to 1.1	0.0 to 3.9	−0.8 to 0.5	−2.1 to 1.8
	p-value	0.0005	0.48	0.37	1.0	0.98	1.0
Average pain on movement over 24 h	Difference	0.9	1	0.4	1	0.2	1
	95% CI	0.1 to 1.5	1.0 to 2.1	− 0.01 to 1.4	− 0.9 to 1.0	− 0.3 to 1.1	− 1.6 to 2.1
	p-value	0.09	1.0	0.33	0.37	0.58	0.48
Maximum pain on movement over 24 h	Difference	0.9	2	0.37	1	0.4	0
	95% CI	− 0.08 to 2.3	−1.6 to 2.0	− 0.4 to 2.1	−0.9 to 4.9	− 0.1 to 1.0	0.0 to 3.6
	p-value	0.18	0.15	0.35	0.37	0.26	1.0

radiology and ward were similar between the ITM and the usual care group. Costs relating to allied health, ICU and pathology were higher in the ITM group. The median (IQR) costs for allied health in US$ were $454 (362.7:933.8) in the ITM group vs. $366.6 (116.5:907.8) in the usual care group, $p = 0.002$; Median (IQR) total hospital costs (US$) were higher in the ITM group: $11, 640 (9106:17,247) vs. $10,338 (7419:18,664), $p = 0.05$. A detailed overview of postoperative costs for each study group is presented in Table 5.

Discussion

Key findings

We performed a single-centre observational study evaluating the opioid sparing and analgesic effects of ITM on adult patients undergoing open liver. As hypothesized, for patients undergoing open liver resection using a standardized enhanced recovery after surgery protocol with multimodal analgesia, the addition of ITM resulted in less postoperative opioid use and enhanced postoperative analgesia. Further, we found no statistically significant differences in opioid-related complications, time to mobilisation, and length of hospital stay. Hospital costs were significantly higher in patients receiving ITM, reflective of a longer mandatory stay in ICU. Our findings support the use of single shot intrathecal morphine as an efficacious analgesic technique in patients undergoing open hepatic resection.

Our findings of reduced oMEDD use at 24 h after surgery in the ITM group are congruent with other studies reporting that ITM reduces postoperative opioid requirements compared to conventional analgesia strategies for up to 24 h after surgery, but not beyond [8, 16, 17]. Thus ITM use provided statistically significant opioid sparing and analgesic benefits without any increase in opioid related side effects such as sedation and delayed respiratory depression, findings previously reported with high-doses of systematically administered opioids [18]. Interestingly, our findings revealed that ITM use significantly reduced postoperative opioid consumption at 24 h postoperatively in the 25th and 50th quartiles, implying the greatest benefit in this cohort of patients. Identifying these patients preoperatively remains challenging in the present time, however with modern computational functional genomics being rapidly developed, it may be possible to exploit genetic information from increasingly available data sets for patients with complex diseases, such as pain and liver cancer patients, that in turn may offer a new insight into which patients may benefit most from ITM therapy as part of complementary patient and surgery centric approaches.

Interestingly, postoperative pain scores shared the same temporal pattern as oMEDD use at 24 h after surgery, and pain was significantly reduced by ITM up to 24 h after surgery, but not beyond. The medical literature evaluating ITM analgesia in open liver resection, as well as in other procedures including thoracotomy and caesarian section, mirror our findings of ITM enhancing analgesia up to 24 h post operation [8, 16, 17, 19]. It is well-known that the analgesic effect of ITM can last up to 24 h post operation with a concomitant decrease in supplementary opioid requirement during this period [20, 21].

With respect to other postoperative outcomes, our findings reflect the array of studies which have universally reported that ITM causes no statistically significant difference in length of stay in open liver resection compared to other analgesic modalities [8, 16, 17, 19]. Similarly our findings were congruent with others reporting no differences in complication rate and complication severity between ITM and other analgesic modalities [8,

Table 3 Perioperative analgesia use and postoperative morphine consumption of patients receiving intrathecal morphine (ITM) or Usual care. Data presented as median (interquartile range) or number of patients (proportion)

	ITM (***n*** = 125)	Usual care (***n*** = 91)	***P***-value
Total operative time (minutes)	250 (196.5:338)	232 (180:310)	0.08
INTRAOPERATIVE ANALGESIA			
Patients receiving opioid	125 (100%)	91 (100%)	> 0.99
IV morphine equivalent (mg)	26.7 (20:33.3)	33.3 (20:46.7)	0.001
Patients receiving paracetamol	44 (35.2%)	27 (29.7%)	0.46
Median amount (mg)	1 (1:1)	1 (1:1)	0.15
Patients receiving ketamine	50 (40%)	26 (28.6%)	0.09
Median amount (mg)	36 (20:62.5)	62.5 (38.75:89.5)	0.003
Patients receiving clonidine	10 (8%)	8 (8.8%)	> 0.99
Median amount (mg)	75 (45:150)	75 (75:97.5)	0.61
Patients receiving IV lignocaine	7 (5.6%)	4 (4.4%)	0.76
Median amount (mg)	220 (150:660)	389 (364.5:467.5)	0.32
Patients receiving ondansetron	64 (51.2%)	29 (31.9%)	0.005
Median amount (mg)	4 (4:4)	4 (4:4)	0.31
Patients receiving metoclopramide	5 (4%)	2 (2.2%)	0.70
Median amount (mg)	20 (15:20)	20 (20:20)	> 0.99
Patients receiving naloxone	2 (1.6%)	3 (3.3%)	0.65
Median amount (µg)	110 (20:200)	100 (80:200)	> 0.99
POSTOPERATIVE oMEDD (mg)			
PACU	0 (0:10.5)	6 (0:21)	0.001
POD 0	25.9 (4:60)	46 (15:82)	0.007
POD 1	91.2 (39.6:204.7)	128.6 (79.0:187.3)	0.12
POD 1 (cumulative including POD 0)	125.7 (52.5:268.1)	176.3 (105:269.5)	0.04
POD 2	95.7 (44.7:164.5)	90 (51.1:165.7)	0.71
POD 2 (cumulative including POD 0–1)	231.1 (116.3:420.2)	255 (177:432.8)	0.14
POD 3	57 (30:104)	67.5 (30:116)	0.57
POD 3 (cumulative including POD 0–2)	283.6 (164.1:526.3)	343.5 (223.4:498)	0.13
POSTOPERATIVE KETAMINE			
Patients receiving ketamine in the PACU	6 (4.8%)	3 (3.3%)	0.74
Median amount (mg)	10 (8.75:21)	19.8 (10:30)	0.45
Patients receiving ketamine on POD 0	57 (45.6%)	27 (29.7%)	0.02
Median amount (mg)	30 (19.5:48)	64 (35.8:96)	0.006
Patients receiving ketamine on POD 1	59 (47.2%)	36 (39.6%)	0.27
Median amount (mg)	0 (0:96)	0 (0:130)	0.78
Patients receiving ketamine on POD 2	42 (33.6%)	27 (29.7%)	0.56
Median amount (mg)	0 (0:48)	0 (0:54)	0.71
Patients receiving ketamine on POD 3	19 (15.2%)	15 (16.5%)	0.85
Median amount (mg)	0 (0:0)	0 (0:0)	0.67
Patient controlled analgesia use (hours)	47.5 (40:71)	63.5 (42.25:71.5)	0.33

16, 17, 19]. No neurological sequelae of intrathecal administration were observed in our study. Concerns that intrathecal opioid use is associated with a higher incidence of opioid-related side effects such as sedation and respiratory depression were unfounded by our results. Among these side effects, respiratory depression is the most feared. Our findings are further supported by a meta-analysis of 28 studies for a range of surgical

Table 4 Postoperative outcomes of patients receiving intrathecal morphine (ITM) or Usual care. Data presented as median (interquartile range) or number of patients (proportion)

	ITM (***n*** = 125)	Usual care (***n*** = 91)	***P***-value
Time in the intensive care unit (hours)	17 (12:21.5)	10 (0:18)	0.0001
Time to full ward diet (hours)	79 (54.5:116.8)	73.75 (50.75:102.8)	0.41
Time to first oral opioid use (days)	2 (2:3)	2 (1:3)	0.98
Patients with at least one complication	88 (70.4%)	67 (73.6%)	0.65
NUMBER OF COMPLICATIONS			
0	37 (29.6%)	24 (27.0%)	0.90
1	31 (24.8%)	25 (28.1%)	
2	16 (12.8%)	11 (12.4%)	
3	9 (7.2%)	9 (10.1%)	
≥4	32 (25.6%)	20 (22.5%)	
WORST CLAVIEN-DINDO GRADE OF COMPLICATIONS			
I	26 (29.5%)	22 (33.8%)	0.13
II	51 (58.0%)	28 (43.1%)	
III	5 (5.7%)	8 (12.3%)	
IV	4 (4.5%)	7 (10.8%)	
V	2 (2.3%)	0 (0%)	
Respiratory depression requiring naloxone	1 (0.8%)	1 (1.1%)	> 0.99
Nausea or vomiting requiring anti-emetics	101 (80.8%)	72 (79.1%)	0.86
Pruritis requiring treatment with antihistamine, 5-hydroxytryptamine or dopamine receptor antagonist, or opiate-antagonist	17 (13.6%)	9 (9.9%)	0.53
SEVERE SEDATION			
POD 0	36/125 (28.8%)	38/90 (42.2%)	0.04
POD 1	19/122 (15.6%)	13/87 (14.9%)	0.99
POD 2	5/107 (4.7%)	9/75 (12.0%)	0.09
POD 3	1/25 (4%)	3/55 (5.5%)	0.99
Length of stay (days)	6 (5:10)	7 (5:10)	0.69
30-day readmission	11 (8.8%)	9 (9.9%)	0.82
Time in the intensive care unit (hours)	17 (12:21.5)	10 (0:18)	0.0001
Time to full ward diet (hours)	79 (54.5:116.8)	73.75 (50.75:102.8)	0.41
Time to first oral opioid use (days)	2 (2:3)	2 (1:3)	0.98
Patients with at least one complication	88 (70.4%)	67 (73.6%)	0.65

procedures, which found that there was no increased risk of respiratory depression with low-dose ITM (≤400 μg) compared to systemic opioids [22]. Nonetheless, ITM does need to be used with caution in elderly patients (> 80 years of age), patients with chronic respiratory and renal impairment, and patients with obstructive sleep apnoea [23]. As an additional safety precaution against delayed-onset respiratory depression, our hospital protocol mandates a 24-h stay in the ICU following surgery involving ITM analgesia to monitor for respiratory depression via the $ETCO_2$, PaO_2, $PaCO_2$, respiratory rate and oxygen saturation measurements [17, 23]. Reflective of this mandatory ICU stay, we showed that total postoperative hospital costs were increased in the ITM group.

Strengths and limitations

There are several strengths and limitations of this study. To date this is the largest review of ITM use in the context of open hepatic resection. A previous study assessing ITM in open liver resection was conducted by Sakowska et al. and involved 161 participants - less than half the size of our study [6]. Furthermore, our study collected comprehensive data detailing intraoperative and postoperative analgesia requirements, postoperative pain scores, and postoperative complications. Previous

Table 5 Postoperative costs in US dollars of patients receiving intrathecal morphine (ITM) or Usual care. Data presented as median (interquartile range)

Cost centre	ITM (**n** = 125)	Usual care (**n** = 91)	**P**-value
Allied health	\$454 (362.7:933.8)	\$366.6 (116.5:907.8)	0.002
Blood products	\$171.4 (120.3:1012)	\$1258 (92.46:3107)	0.21
Intensive care unit	\$2385 (1692:3355)	\$1600 (0:3375)	0.001
Medical	\$1470 (1047:1945)	\$1638 (1205:2318)	0.06
Medical emergency team	\$216.8 (201.8:403.6)	\$433.5 (263.5:605.4)	0.11
Pathology	\$1227 (795.7:1804)	\$898.4 (521:1440)	0.003
Pharmacy	\$359.6 (280.1:518.5)	\$344.1 (232.1:443)	0.08
Radiology	\$312.6 (142:1016)	\$231.6 (101.3:953.3)	0.65
Ward	\$4516 (3605:6935)	\$4824 (3781:6653)	0.35
Grand total	\$11,640 (9106:17,247)	\$10,338 (7419:18,664)	0.05

studies have been limited by failing to comprehensively report major outcomes, rather focusing on minor postoperative complications such as nausea, vomiting and sedation [8, 16, 23, 24]. In comparison, we have also detailed the incidence of all major systemic complications. Finally, to our knowledge, no other study has examined the costs of ITM in open liver resection compared to conventional analgesic modalities.

This is a single-centre study performed in a high-volume hepatobiliary unit within a tertiary healthcare centre, partly limiting the external validity of our findings. However, our hospital has all the typical characteristics of many tertiary institutions' hepatobiliary units, and the surgical and anaesthesia perioperative protocols adopted by our centre are aligned with those in many other tertiary centres. All patients were adults who underwent open hepatic resection, which also limits the generalisability of our findings to paediatric liver resections, and to adult patients undergoing other types of surgeries. Given the retrospective nature of the study, we cannot establish a causal relationship between ITM and the change in the perioperative variables we assessed.

Another significant limitation of our findings is that given the retrospective nature of our study, the collection of data may have been subject to human error in the interpretation and recording of data. However, we consider this an unlikely source of error given the comprehensive cross-checks required for data entry at our institution and the use of electronic medical records. Additionally, the data collection was conducted by a clinician not involved in postoperative patient care, thereby minimising the likelihood of detection bias. Being a retrospective observational study with no possibility of randomisation or subject blinding, our study lacks in validity compared to a randomized controlled trial. Nonetheless the large sample size, in addition to the congruence of our results with the existing medical literature, lends significant strength to our study. Our findings are hypothesis generating and may provide valuable data for power calculations for future studies on evaluating the effects of ITM on perioperative oMEDD use, analgesia, and various adverse outcomes. Finally, validation of our findings with a large multi-centre RCT, similar in design to the Multicenter Australian Study of Epidural Anesthesia Trial which involved 25 hospitals in Australia and South-East Asia, can be justified [4].

Conclusion

In patients undergoing open liver resection, ITM in addition to conventional multimodal analgesic strategies reduced postoperative opioid requirements and improved analgesia for 24 h after surgery, without any statistically significant differences in opioid-related complications, time to mobilisation, and length of hospital stay. Hospital costs were significantly higher in patients receiving ITM, reflective of a longer mandatory stay in ICU. Our findings support the use of single shot intrathecal morphine as an efficacious analgesic technique in patients undergoing open hepatic resection. A RCT evaluating the effects of ITM in addition to conventional multimodal analgesic is justified.

Abbreviations

ANZCTR: Australian New Zealand Clinical Trials Registry; ASA: American Society of Anesthesiologists; BMI: Body mass index; CCI: Charlson Comorbidity Index; ERAS: Enhanced recovery after surgery; $ETCO_2$: End tidal carbon dioxide; HREC: Health Human Research Ethics Committee; ICD: International Statistical Classification of Diseases; ICU: Intensive care unit; IQR: Interquartile range; ITM: Intrathecal morphine; NRS: Numerical Rating Scale; oMEDD: Oral morphine equivalent daily dose; PACU: Post-anaesthesia care unit; PaO_2: Partial pressure of oxygen; $PaCO_2$: Partial pressure of carbon dioxide; POD: Postoperative day; RCT: Randomized controlled trial

Acknowledgements

None.

Authors' contributions

LW: study conception and coordination, study design, data acquisition, analysis and interpretation, manuscript drafting and editing. LC, JT: statistical analysis, manuscript drafting and editing. CT, RH BP, LK, CH, JT: data acquisition, manuscript drafting and editing. All authors read and approved the final manuscript.

Author details

[1]Department of Anaesthesia, Austin Health, Heidelberg, Victoria, Australia. [2] Melbourne Medical School, University of Melbourne, Heidelberg, Victoria, Australia. [3]Department of Surgery, University of Melbourne, Austin Health, Heidelberg, Victoria, Australia.

References

1. Borromeo CJ, Stix MS, Lally A, Pomfret EA. Epidural catheter and increased prothrombin time after right lobe hepatectomy for living donor transplantation. Anesth Analg. 2000;91(5):1139–41 PMID: 11049898.
2. Moraca RJ, Sheldon DG, Thirlby RC. The role of epidural anesthesia and analgesia in surgical practice. Ann Surg. 2003;238(5):663–73 PMID: 14578727.
3. Rawal N. Epidural technique for postoperative pain-gold standard no more? Reg Anesth Pain Med. 2012;37(3):310–7 PMID: 22531384.
4. Rigg JR, Jamrozik K, Myles PS, Silbert BS, Peyton PJ, Parsons RW, et al. Epidural anaesthesia and analgesia and outcome of major surgery: a randomised trial. Lancet. 2002;359(9314):1276–82 PMID: 11965272.
5. Melloul E, Hubner M, Scott M, Snowden C, Prentis J, Dejong CH, et al. Guidelines for perioperative Care for Liver Surgery: enhanced recovery after surgery (ERAS) Society recommendations. World J Surg. 2016;40(10):2425–40 PMID: 27549599.
6. Sakowska M, Docherty E, Linscott D, Connor S. A change in practice from epidural to intrathecal morphine analgesia for hepato-pancreato-biliary surgery. World J Surg. 2009;33(9):1802–8 PMID: 19548026.
7. Mugabure B. A clinical approach to neuraxial morphine for the treatment of postoperative pain. Pain Res Treat. 2012;2012:612145 PMID: 23002426.
8. Dichtwald S, Ben-Haim M, Papismedov L, Hazan S, Cattan A, Matot I. Intrathecal morphine versus intravenous opioid administration to impact postoperative analgesia in hepato-pancreatic surgery: a randomized controlled trial. J Anesth. 2017;31(2):237–45 PMID: 27885425.
9. The Australian and New Zealand College of Anaesthetists. Opioid Dose Equivalence. From https://fpm.anzca.edu.au/documents/opioid-dose-equivalence.pdf. Accessed October 2018.
10. Hawker GA, Mian S, Kendzerska T, French M. Measures of adult pain: visual analog scale for pain (VAS pain), numeric rating scale for pain (NRS pain), McGill pain questionnaire (MPQ), short-form McGill pain questionnaire (SF-MPQ), chronic pain Grade scale (CPGS), short Form-36 bodily pain scale (SF-36 BPS), and measure of intermittent and constant osteoarthritis pain (ICOAP). Arthritis Care Res. 2011;63(Suppl 11):S240–52 PMID: 22588748.
11. Jammer I, Wickboldt N, Sander M, Smith A, Schultz MJ, Pelosi P, et al. Standards for definitions and use of outcome measures for clinical effectiveness research in perioperative medicine: European perioperative clinical outcome (EPCO) definitions: a statement from the ESA-ESICM joint taskforce on perioperative outcome measures. Eur J Anaesthesiol. 2015; 32(2):88–105 PMID: 25058504.
12. Dindo D, Demartines N, Clavien PA. Classification of surgical complications: a new proposal with evaluation in a cohort of 6336 patients and results of a survey. Ann Surg. 2004;240(2):205–13 PMID: 15273542.
13. Reserve Bank of Australia, Measures of Consumer Price Inflation. From https://www.rba.gov.au/inflation/measures-cpi.html. Accessed April 2018.
14. Irlbeck T, Zwissler B, Bauer A. ASA classification : transition in the course of time and depiction in the literature. Anaesthesist. 2017;66(1):5–10 PMID: 27995282.
15. Charlson ME, Pompei P, Ales KL, MacKenzie CR. A new method of classifying prognostic comorbidity in longitudinal studies: development and validation. J Chronic Dis. 1987;40(5):373–83 PMID: 3558716.
16. Devys J, Mora A, Plaud B, Jayr C, Laplanche A, Raynard B, et al. Intrathecal + PCA morphine improves analgesia during the first 24 hr after major abdominal surgery compared to PCA alone. Can J Anaesth. 2003;50(4):355–61 PMID: 12670812.
17. Ko JS, Choi SJ, Gwak MS, Kim GS, Ahn HJ, Kim JA, et al. Intrathecal morphine combined with intravenous patient-controlled analgesia is an effective and safe method for immediate postoperative pain control in live liver donors. Liver Transpl. 2009;15(4):381–9 PMID: 19326422.
18. Rathmell JP, Lair TR, Nauman B. The role of intrathecal drugs in the treatment of acute pain. Anesth Analg. 2005;101(5 Suppl):S30–43 PMID: 16334491.
19. Lee SH, Gwak MS, Choi SJ, Park HG, Kim GS, Kim MH, et al. Prospective, randomized study of ropivacaine wound infusion versus intrathecal morphine with intravenous fentanyl for analgesia in living donors for liver transplantation. Liver Transpl. 2013;19(9):1036–45 PMID: 23788468.
20. Jacobson L, Chabal C, Brody MC. A dose-response study of intrathecal morphine: efficacy, duration, optimal dose, and side effects. Anesth Analg. 1988;67(11):1082–8 PMID: 3189898.
21. Gwirtz KH, Young JV, Byers RS, Alley C, Levin K, Walker SG, et al. The safety and efficacy of intrathecal opioid analgesia for acute postoperative pain: seven years' experience with 5969 surgical patients at Indiana University Hospital. Anesth Analg. 1999;88(3):599–604 PMID: 10072014.
22. Gehling M, Tryba M. Risks and side-effects of intrathecal morphine combined with spinal anaesthesia: a meta-analysis. Anaesthesia. 2009;64(6): 643–51 PMID: 19462494.
23. Roy JD, Massicotte L, Sassine MP, Seal RF, Roy A. A comparison of intrathecal morphine/fentanyl and patient-controlled analgesia with patient-controlled analgesia alone for analgesia after liver resection. Anesth Analg. 2006;103(4):990–4 PMID: 17000818.
24. De Pietri L, Siniscalchi A, Reggiani A, Masetti M, Begliomini B, Gazzi M, et al. The use of intrathecal morphine for postoperative pain relief after liver resection: a comparison with epidural analgesia. Anesth Analg. 2006;102(4): 1157–63 PMID: 16551916.

22

Enhanced preoperative education about continuous femoral nerve block with patient-controlled analgesia improves the analgesic effect for patients undergoing total knee arthroplasty and reduces the workload for ward nurses

Xiaona Lin[1†], Yang Zhou[1†], Hongcai Zheng[1], Jing Zhang[1], Xiaoxiao Wang[2], Kaixi Liu[1], Jun Wang[1], Xiangyang Guo[1], Zhengqian Li[1*] and Bin Han[1*]

Abstract

Background: Total knee arthroplasty (TKA) is the most common treatment for end-stage knee osteoarthritis and continuous femoral nerve block (CFNB) has become the gold standard for analgesia. But the lack of knowledge about CFNB and patient-controlled analgesia (PCA) often leads to inappropriate dose of medications and increased workload for ward nurses.

Methods: After retrospectively registering to http://www.chictr.org.cn (ChiCTR1800018957), 60 patients undergoing unilateral TKA were randomly divided into groups A and B ($n = 30$ each). Patients in group B and their families received a nurse-led preoperative visit the day before surgery focusing on PCA educational pamphlets for postoperative pain management. Before returning to the ward, patients and their families in both groups received face-to-face PCA pump operation training. The usual postoperative follow-up was performed by nurse anesthetists for 2 consecutive days. Visual Analogue Scale (VAS) scores at rest and during movement, knowledge of the PCA evaluated by a ten-question questionnaire, knee flexion angles, and the number of PCA-related nurse calls were recorded.

Results: The VAS scores at rest and during movement of the patients in group B were both significantly lower than in group A on postoperative days 1 and 2. The questionnaire scores of the patients in group B were much higher than those in group A on postoperative day 1, but not on day 2. Patients in the 2 groups had similar knee flexion on postoperative days 1 and 2. Patients in group B asked for assistance from the ward nurses with the PCA fewer times than those in group A, and the ward nurses were more satisfied with the analgesic protocol in group B.

Conclusions: Enhanced preoperative education for CFNB with PCA can provide patients with a better grasp of postoperative pain management, improve the postoperative analgesic effect after TKA, and reduce the PCA-related workload for ward nurses.

Keywords: Total knee arthroplasty, Patient-controlled analgesia, Preoperative education, Nursing workload

* Correspondence: lizhengqianmazui@126.com; friendbinbin@163.com
†Xiaona Lin and Yang Zhou contributed equally to this work.
[1]Department of Anesthesiology, Peking University Third Hospital, No. 49, North Garden Rd, Haidian District, Beijing 100191, China

Background

Total knee arthroplasty (TKA) is the most common treatment for end-stage knee osteoarthritis [1, 2]. While the number of patients undergoing TKA is increasing annually with the aging global population, the management of postoperative pain has attracted much recent attention. It has been found that postoperative pain can directly affect early functional exercise and reduce the effectiveness of surgical treatment [3]. In recent years, continuous femoral nerve block (CFNB) has become the gold standard for analgesia after TKA [4]. However, the lack of knowledge by patients and their families about CFNB and patient-controlled analgesia (PCA) often leads to under-dosing or over-dosing of medications, a decrease in general analgesic efficacy, an increased workload for ward nurses, and an increased risk of falls [5]. While the importance of preoperative patient education has been emphasized, its role in improving postoperative analgesia and outcomes remains unclear. In this study, we explored whether preoperative CFNB education could improve postoperative analgesic efficacy; also, we evaluated whether preoperative CFNB education could reduce the PCA-related workload for ward nurses after TKA.

Accordingly, a prospective randomized clinical study was undertaken with the primary aim of evaluating the VAS on motion on POD1, and secondarily, to investigate the PCA-related workload for ward nurses postoperatively.

Subjects and methods

This study was approved by the Ethics Committee of Peking University Third Hospital and recorded on October 18, 2018 to chictr.org.cn (ChiCTR1800018957).

In total, 60 patients undergoing unilateral TKA in our hospital at 08:00–12:00 between November 2016 and March 2018 were enrolled and randomly divided into 2 groups (group A and group B; $n = 30$ each) using a random number table. The inclusion criteria included: a) being American Society of Anesthesiologists (ASA) grade I - II; b) undergoing unilateral TKA (left or right); c) receiving combined spinal-epidural anesthesia. The exclusion criteria were: a) inability to complete VAS scoring; b) lower-extremity muscle strength below grade V; c) intraoperative intraarticular injection of analgesic drugs; d) history of previous TKA; e) contraindications to spinal manipulation or patient insisting on general anesthesia. Before returning to the ward after surgery, patients in group A and their families received unified face-to-face PCA pump operation training by a nurse anesthetist. In contrast, patients in group B and their families received a nurse-led preoperative visit the day before surgery focusing on a PCA educational pamphlet (see the Additional file 1) about postoperative pain management. After surgery, they watched the PCA demonstration with group A patients/families before returning to the ward.

CFNB was performed by the same anesthesiologist in the post anesthesia care unit (PACU) or operating room before or after TKA. Under ultrasound guidance combined with nerve stimulation, the femoral nerve catheter was placed, and a single dose of 0.5% ropivacaine (20 ml) was administered. All of the patients received combined spinal-epidural anesthesia by the same anesthesiologist, along with subarachnoid administration of 2–3 ml of 0.5% bupivacaine. The epidural catheter was routinely placed 4 cm ahead. During the operation, 1% lidocaine was added to maintain the anesthesia via the epidural catheter according to the operative time (3 ml 1% lidocaine for test doses and 5 ml added each time according to the effect to maintain the block level at about T10). The same TKA procedure was performed, during which the lower-extremity tourniquet was routinely applied. After the operation, the femoral nerve tube was connected to the PCA pump (500 ml of 0.2% ropivacaine, with background infusion rate 5 ml·h^{-1}, lockout interval 15 min, and the patient controlled bolus 2 ml). In addition to the continuous femoral nerve PCA, all of the patients were intravenously administered 40 mg of parecoxib sodium twice daily for two consecutive days.

Data collection

After the patients returned to the ward, the ward surgeon routinely recorded the knee flexion angle, and the ward nurses recorded the number of PCA-related nurse calls. An appointed nurse anesthetist followed up the 2 groups for postoperative analgesia on the first and second days after the operation and carried out bedside education according to the specific PCA conditions. Meanwhile, the following data were collected: a) age, height, weight, ASA grade, timing and location of CFNB, time of operation, dosage of epidural drug, and level of postoperative anesthesia; b) VAS scores at rest and during movement on the first and second days after the operation; c) a ten-question questionnaire form (see the Additional file 1) on the first and second days after the operation, used to evaluate the patients' knowledge about CFNB and PCA - the results of which both the nurse anesthetist and patients were blinded to before the end of the two surveys; and d) the satisfaction (satisfied, not satisfied, and indifferent) of the ward nurses to the PCA mode of CFNB.

Statistical analysis

Power analysis was based on results of preliminary data comparing VAS score on motion on POD 1 between groups. In our preliminary study, 8 patients were recruited in each group. The medians and quartiles of VAS scores during movement were 4.5 ± 1 and 3 ± 1.75

in group A and B, respectively. Sample-size calculations showed that a Wilcoxon and Mann–Whitney U test with a type I error (two-sided) of $\alpha = 0.05$ would have 95% power to detect the aforementioned difference in VAS scores on motion between the two groups if the sample size in each group was 24. To account for possible loss in the follow-up period, we enrolled 30 cases per group. All statistical analysis was performed with SPSS for Windows (version 14.0, SPSS, Chicago, IL). Data were tested for normal distribution using the Kolmogorov–Smirnov test. Continuous variables were presented using means and standard deviations (SD) or median and interquartile values, and analyzed using Student's t test or the Wilcoxon-Mann-Whitney test, respectively. In the case of categorical variables, frequencies were used, and the count data were compared with a χ^2 test. A p value of < 0.05 was regarded as statistically significant.

Results

Follow-up and data collection were completed in all 60 patients. There were no significant differences in age, height, weight, and body mass index between the 2 groups (all $p > 0.05$). In both groups, 23 patients received CFNB in the PACU and 7 patients received it in the operating room ($p > 0.05$), and there was no significant difference between the groups in the timing of the CFNB. During intraoperative anesthesia management, 1 of 30 patients in Group A and 4 of 30 in Group B received additional epidural administration of 1% lidocaine (3.3% vs 13.3%, $\chi^2 = 0.873$, $p = 0.350$), the dosage of epidural lidocaine in Group A was 8 ml and the dosage in Group B was 5.5 (3, 8) ml. The anesthesia level immediate after surgery was maintained at about T10 in both groups, and there was no significant difference between the 2 groups (Table 1).

A 10-question questionnaire form was used to survey the patients on the first and the second postoperative days (Additional file 1). The results showed that the scores were significantly higher in group B than in group A on the first day ($p = 0.01$) (Table 2); however, the difference was not statistically significant on the second day ($p = 0.24$).

The VAS scores at rest and during movement in group B were significantly lower than those in group A on both the first and the second day after surgery ($p < 0.05$). There was no significant difference in knee flexion angle between the groups 2 days after the operation (Table 3). In addition, no adverse events such as falls occurred in either group.

The number of PCA-related nurse calls was significantly greater in group A than in group B ($p < 0.05$). The survey about the satisfaction of ward nurses with regard to the PCA showed that 60% of the nurses responsible for patients in group A were satisfied, 6.7% were not satisfied, and 33% were indifferent. For group B, 93.3% of the nurses were satisfied and 6.7% were indifferent. The difference between the groups was statistically significant ($p = 0.003$) (Table 4).

Discussion

TKA is commonly performed to relieve joint pain, and to improve quality of life in patients who have end-stage osteoarthritis, but is also associated with severe pain after surgery and a high incidence of chronic pain [6]. CFNB is the most commonly used postoperative analgesic method for TKA, not only could provide effective postoperative analgesia but also could improve joint function and quality of life even at 1 month postoperatively [7]. However, how to operate the device and how to cope with postoperative pain by self-administering analgesic is a problem and the efficacy of PCA highly depends on the patients' and their families' knowledge and skills [8]. If patients receiving PCA correctly maintain their appropriate concentration, the effect could be good and should lead to the decrease in demand for drugs and ward nurses; however, this assumption related to the patient's training has not been confirmed.

In the real-world clinical setting, the traditional preoperative oral education about PCA is often poorly understood by patients and their families, or quickly forgotten. Hekmatpou et al. found that about 80% of the information given to patients by their doctors was forgotten, and nearly half of the information remembered by patients was incorrect [9]. In our study, we developed a PCA educational pamphlet that focused on the knowledge of CFNB, PCA, and pain relief following TKA, with an attempt to intensify and improve preoperative PCA education. Our results suggested that the intensified education significantly improved the level of PCA-related knowledge in patients. However, in Yankova et al.'s study, although preoperative PCA education improved the use of the PCA device in patients, it showed no positive effect on postoperative analgesic efficacy (i.e., the VAS score) [10]. In contrast, our modified education model significantly lowered the VAS scores of patients at rest and during movement 2 days after surgery. Since the upper thoracic sensory block level immediately after surgery showed no significant differences between the groups, we followed up the patients on POD1 was 24 h postoperatively and no residual effect of central nerve blocks existed. Thus, we believe that the difference in postoperative analgesic efficacy might be explained by the preoperative education mode.

Since the VAS scores at rest and during movement on POD1 and POD2 in this research are quite similar, we doubt that the statistical significance may not make clinical difference. Actually, in the real-world clinical practice, no additional analgesics are provided when the VAS score is below 3. We hoped that readers could view these data objectively and carefully. From the perspective

Table 1 Anthropometric subject characteristics

Variable	Group A (*n* = 30)	Group B (*n* = 30)	*P*-Values
Age	66.6 ± 6.5	66.5 ± 8.1	0.986
Gender (female/male)	22/8	27/3	0.095
Height (cm)	158.8 ± 7.5	159.0 ± 7.7	0.919
Weight (kg)	66.3 ± 8.8	67.6 ± 11.2	0.601
BMI (kg/m^2)	26.4 ± 4.1	26.7 ± 4.0	0.756
ASA physical status (class I/II)	12/18	15/15	0.436
CFNB performance			
Side (left/right)	14/16	10/20	0.292
in PACU (pre–/post-op)	11/12	12/11	0.768
in OR (pre–/post-op)	6/1	7/0	1.000
Dosage of spinal bupivacaine (mg)	12.5 (12.5, 12.5)	12.5 (12.5, 12.5)	0.729
Upper thoracic sensory block level before surgery	10 (8, 10)	10 (8, 10)	0.629
Upper thoracic sensory block level immediately after surgery	10 (10, 10)	10 (10, 11)	0.564
Tourniquet application time (min)	62.1 ± 13.8	69.0 ± 14.7	0.349
Intraoperative blood loss (ml)	5 (5, 15)	10 (5, 20)	0.769
Duration of surgery (min)	74.3 ± 18.4	74.1 ± 18.1	0.972

Values are reported as mean ± SD or number of subjects. Non-normal data are expressed as median and interquartile values. *ASA* American Society of Anesthesiologists, *BMI* Body mass index, *CFNB* Continuous femoral nerve block

of clinical application, enhanced preoperative education about continuous femoral nerve block with PCA is still relatively limited in improving the postoperative analgesic effects.

PCA provides patients with a definite analgesic efficacy, allowing tailored self-management. However, while providing an analgesic effect, CFNB also remarkably weakens quadriceps femoris muscle strength, affects the early movement, and increases the risk of falls [11, 12]. Thacher et al. found that the first fall occurred 21 h (mean) after surgery [13]. In our study, fall precautions were highlighted in the pamphlet to improve postoperative safety. It was found that there were still 2 patients in group A that left the bed by themselves with walkers. One of them was a patient who was at high risk of falling less than 6 h after extubation. In group B, one patient became ambulatory with the assistance of his family members and medical staff 6 h after the catheter was removed. No falls occurred in our study, suggesting that the concentration and dosage of the analgesic drugs met the actual clinical needs.

Postoperative pain management is an ongoing challenge in surgical care and the nurses are very important participants [14]. The patients' inadequate knowledge and erroneous beliefs may hamper the appropriate use of analgesics and increase the workload of ward nurses [15]. However, the impact of PCA on the workload of ward nurses remains unclear. King et al. found that patients would call ward nurses due to problems with the PCA pump and the analgesic effect, which may be sources of workload for ward nurses [16]. Our data showed that intensified preoperative education significantly decreased the number of nurse calls within 2 days after the operation and thus effectively reduced the workload for ward nurses. As a result, the satisfaction of ward nurses with regard to the PCA in these patients

Table 2 Questionnaire scores for patients in two groups

Questionnaire scores	Group A (*n* = 30)	Group B (*n* = 30)	*P*-Values
POD 1	8.0 ± 1.4	9.4 ± 1.2	0.001
POD 2	9.8 ± 0.4	9.9 ± 0.3	0.235

Values are reported as mean ± SD. *POD* Postoperative day

Table 3 Analgesic effect of CFNB in two groups

	Group A (*n* = 30)	Group B (*n* = 30)	*P*-Values
VAS at rest			
POD 1	1 (1,2)	0 (0,1)	<0.001
POD 2	0 (0,1)	0 (0,0)	0.005
VAS on motion			
POD 1	4 (4,5)	3 (2,5)	<0.001
POD 2	3 (3,4)	2 (2,2)	<0.001
Knee flexion			
POD 1	100 (90, 120)	100 (90, 120)	0.916
POD 2	108 (98, 120)	110 (99, 120)	0.811

Non-normal data are expressed as median and interquartile values. *CFNB* Continuous femoral nerve block, *VAS* Visual Analogue Scale

Table 4 Nursing workload relief and satisfaction in the ward

	Group A ($n = 30$)	Group B ($n = 30$)	*P*-Values
Patients using PCA-related nurse call	15/15	7/23	0.032
Nursing satisfaction			
1	18 (60%)	28 (93.3%)	0.003
2	2 (6.7%)	0 (0%)	
3	10 (33%)	2 (6.7%)	

Values are reported as *n* and (percentages). *PCA* Patient-controlled analgesia

dramatically increased. Thus, the lower analgesia-related workload of ward nurses was associated with improved patient knowledge and skills about the PCA after the intensified education.

In summary, intensified preoperative analgesia education could be strengthened by the distribution of PCA educational materials, which allows patients and their families to have better knowledge and skills for pain relief after TKA, enhances their participation in postoperative rehabilitation, statistically improves the efficacy of postoperative analgesia, and definitely reduces workloads for ward nurses. Thus, preoperative PCA education can play an active role in pain management after TKA.

Abbreviations
ASA: American Society of Anesthesiologists; CFNB: Continuous femoral nerve block; PACU: Post anesthesia care unit; PCA: Patient-controlled analgesia; TKA: Total knee arthroplasty; VAS: Visual Analogue Scale

Acknowledgements
Not applicable.

Authors' contributions
XNL and YZ were the co-first authors of this article, responsible for the design and implementation of this project, data collection, data statistics, and article writing. HCZ, JZ and KXL were also responsible for the patient data collection. XXW participated in the analysis and interpretation of data. ZQL and BH were the corresponding authors of this article in charge of the project, responsible for the expenses, and were involved in the design of the project and modified the manuscript. JW and XYG modified the manuscript. All authors read and approved the final manuscript.

Author details
[1]Department of Anesthesiology, Peking University Third Hospital, No. 49, North Garden Rd, Haidian District, Beijing 100191, China. [2]Research Center of Clinical Epidemiology, Peking University Third Hospital, Beijing 100191, China.

References
1. Hofmann S, Seitlinger G, Djahani O, Pietsch M. The painful knee after TKA: a diagnostic algorithm for failure analysis. Knee Surg Sports Traumatol Arthrosc. 2011;19(9):1442–52.
2. Elmallah RK, Cherian JJ, Pierce TP, Jauregui JJ, Harwin SF, Mont MA. New and common perioperative pain management techniques in total knee arthroplasty. J Knee Surg. 2016;29(2):169–78.
3. Werner BC, Evans CL, Carothers JT, Browne JA. Primary total knee arthroplasty in super-obese patients: dramatically higher postoperative complication rates even compared to revision surgery. J Arthroplast. 2015;30(5):849–53.
4. Bauer MC, Pogatzki-Zahn EM, Zahn PK. Regional analgesia techniques for total knee replacement. Curr Opin Anaesthesiol. 2014;27(5):501–6.
5. Stevens JE, Mizner RL, Snyder-Mackler L. Quadriceps strength and volitional activation before and after total knee arthroplasty for osteoarthritis. J Orthop Res. 2003;21(5):775–9.
6. McCartney CJ, Nelligan K. Postoperative pain management after total knee arthroplasty in elderly patients: treatment options. Drugs Aging. 2014;31(2):83–91.
7. Wang F, Zhou Y, Sun J, Yang C. Influences of continuous femoral nerve block on knee function and quality of life in patients following total knee arthroplasty. Int J Clin Exp Med. 2015;8(10):19120–5.
8. Kissin I. Patient-controlled-analgesia analgesimetry and its problems. Anesth Analg. 2009;108(6):1945–9.
9. Hekmatpou D, Anoosheh M, Alhani F. Pathology of patient education: a qualitative study. Iran J Nurs. 2007;20:51–60.
10. Yankova Z. Patients' knowledge of patient controlled analgesia (PCA) and their experience of postoperative pain relief: a review of theimpact of structured preoperative education. J Adv Perioperative Care. 2008;3(3):91–99.
11. Elkassabany NM, Antosh S, Ahmed M, Nelson C, Israelite C, Badiola I, Cai LF, Williams R, Hughes C, Mariano ER, et al. The risk of falls after Total knee arthroplasty with the use of a femoral nerve block versus an Adductor Canal block: a double-blinded randomized controlled study. Anesth Analg. 2016;122(5):1696–703.
12. Kim DH, Lin Y, Goytizolo EA, Kahn RL, Maalouf DB, Manohar A, Patt ML, Goon AK, Lee YY, Ma Y, et al. Adductor canal block versus femoral nerve block for total knee arthroplasty: a prospective, randomized, controlled trial. Anesthesiology. 2014;120(3):540–50.
13. Thacher RR, Hickernell TR, Grosso MJ, Shah R, Cooper HJ, Maniker R, Brown AR, Geller J. Decreased risk of knee buckling with adductor canal block versus femoral nerve block in total knee arthroplasty: a retrospective cohort study. Arthroplast Today. 2017;3(4):281–5.
14. Bach AM, Forman A, Seibaek L. Postoperative pain management: a bedside perspective. Pain Manag Nurs. 2018;19(6):608–18.
15. van Dijk JF, Schuurmans MJ, Alblas EE, Kalkman CJ, van Wijck AJ. Postoperative pain: knowledge and beliefs of patients and nurses. J Clin Nurs. 2017;26(21–22):3500–10.
16. King S, Walsh K. I think PCA is great, but . . . '-surgical nurses' perceptions of patient-controlled analgesia. Int J Nurs Pract. 2007;13(5):276–83.

23

The effects of different doses of dexmedetomidine on the requirements for propofol for loss of consciousness in patients monitored via the bispectral index

Yang Gu[1,2†], Fan Yang[3†], Yonghai Zhang[3], Junwei Zheng[1], Jie Wang[1], Bin Li[1], Tao Ma[1], Xiang Cui[3], Kaimei Lu[1] and Hanxiang Ma[3*]

Abstract

Background: The α_2-adrenergic agonist dexmedetomidine (DEX) is a sedative and can be used as an adjunct to hypnotics. The study sought to evaluate the effects of different doses of DEX on the requirements for propofol for loss of consciousness (LOC) in patients monitored via the bispectral index (BIS).

Methods: In this randomized, double-blind, three arm parallel group design and placebo-controlled trial, 73 patients aged between 18 and ~ 65 years with a BMI range of 18.0–24.5 kg·m^{-2} and an American Society of Anesthesiologists (ASA) grade I or II who were scheduled for general anesthesia at the General Hospital of Ningxia Medical University were included in this study. Anesthesiologists and patients were blinded to the syringe contents. All patients were randomly assigned in a 1:1:1 ratio to receive a 0.5 μg·kg^{-1} DEX infusion (0.5 μg·kg^{-1} DEX group; $n = 24$), a 1.0 μg·kg^{-1} DEX infusion (1.0 μg·kg^{-1} DEX group; $n = 25$) or a saline infusion (control group; $n = 24$) for 10 min. Propofol at a concentration of 20 mg·kg^{-1}·h^{-1} was then infused at the end of the DEX or saline infusion. The propofol infusion was stopped when the patient being infused lost consciousness. The primary endpoint were propofol requirements for LOC and BIS value at LOC.

(Continued on next page)

* Correspondence: mahanxiang@hotmail.com
†Yang Gu and Fan Yang contributed equally to this work.
[3]Department of Anesthesiology, General Hospital of Ningxia Medical University, Yinchuan 750004, China

(Continued from previous page)

Results: The data from 73 patients were analyzed. The propofol requirements for LOC was reduced in the DEX groups compared with the control group (1.12 ± 0.33 mg·kg^{-1} for the 0.5 μg·kg^{-1} DEX group vs. 1.79 ± 0.39 mg·kg^{-1} for the control group; difference, 0.68 mg·kg^{-1} [95% CI, 0.49 to 0.87]; P = 0.0001) (0.77 ± 0.27 mg·kg^{-1} for the 1.0 μg·kg^{-1} DEX group vs. 1.79 ± 0.39 mg·kg^{-1} for the control group; difference, 1.02 mg·kg^{-1} [95% CI, 0.84 to 1.21]; P = 0.0001). The propofol requirements for LOC was lower in the 1.0 μg·kg^{-1} DEX group than the 0.5 μg·kg^{-1} DEX group (0.77 ± 0.27 mg·kg^{-1} vs. 1.12 ± 0.33 mg·kg^{-1}, respectively; difference, 0.34 mg·kg^{-1} [95% CI, 0.16 to 0.54]; P = 0.003). At the time of LOC, the BIS value was higher in the DEX groups than in the control group (67.5 ± 3.5 for group 0.5 μg·kg^{-1} DEX vs. 60.5 ± 3.8 for the control group; difference, 7.04 [95% CI, 4.85 to 9.23]; P = 0.0001) (68.4 ± 4.1 for group 1.0 μg·kg^{-1} DEX vs. 60.5 ± 3.8 for the control group; difference, 7.58 [95% CI, 5.41 to 9.75]; P = 0.0001).

Conclusion: The study showed that DEX (both 0.5 and 1.0 μg·kg^{-1} DEX) reduced the propofol requirements for LOC. DEX pre-administration increased the BIS value for LOC induced by propofol.

Keywords: Propofol, Dexmedetomidine, Bispectral index, Loss of consciousness

Background

A variety of sedatives, such as propofol combined with midazolam, are commonly used in induction of anesthesia. Dexmedetomidine (DEX) is now commonly used in anesthesia induction because of its sympatholytic effect and it can attenuate the cardiovascular response during intubation [1, 2]. However, there is still a lack of clinical experience in the combined use of these two drugs in the induction of anesthesia, and sedative overdose may occur during induction of anesthesia.

Along with other drugs, propofol is frequently used as a sedative-hypnotic drug to induce anesthesia. Unfortunately, propofol at the recommended induction dose (2.0–2.5 mg·kg^{-1}) often causes cardiovascular depression during anesthesia induction [3]. Theoretically, decreasing propofol dose is associated with a low incidence of hypotension during anesthesia induction [4]. The techniques decreasing propofol dose for anesthesia induction as guided by bispectral index [5] may reduce the incidence of hypotension induced by recommended propofol dose.

DEX is a widely used drug in anesthesia for its sympatholytic, sedative and analgesic effects [6]. It has been reported that DEX decreased the propofol requirements by bispectral index-guided closed-loop anesthesia [7]. Many studies have observed the opioid-free effect of DEX when combined with other drugs during anesthesia [8, 9]. But few study has focused on the effect of DEX on propofol requirements for loss of consciousness (LOC) during anesthesia induction. Indeed, anesthesia induction is an important phase in the perioperative period; thus, it is urgent to separately evaluate the effect of DEX on the propofol requirements for LOC during this phase. Considering the anesthetic-free effect of DEX, we hypothesized that DEX can decrease the propofol requirements for LOC during anesthesia induction. Therefore, the first purpose of this study was to verify that DEX decreases the propofol requirements for LOC during anesthesia induction.

The bispectral index (BIS) is a common tool to determine the depth of the sedative state. The BIS value is constantly maintained ranged from 40 to 60 during general anesthesia through the titration of anesthetic agents [10]. It had been demonstrated that there was a good relationship between the BIS values and the blood concentration of propofol at LOC [11]. However, the BIS value at LOC varies when different sedatives are used [12]. It has been proven that the BIS value was different at the loss of response to voice commands when fentanyl, nitrous oxide, or alfentanil was added to the propofol anesthesia [13]. DEX produced resembling stage 2 NREM sleep in the EEG and characteristic arousal sedation [14, 15], and these makes it distinguishes from propofol. Therefore, we hypothesized that the BIS value at LOC was different between propofol alone and propofol combined with DEX administration. Thus, the second goal of this study was to evaluate the effect of DEX on the BIS value at LOC induced by propofol.

Methods

The study was approved by the ethics committee of the General Hospital of Ningxia Medical University (2016167). The study was registered at ClinicalTrials.gov (NCT02783846). The study was conducted in accordance with applicable CONSORT guidelines. This was a prospective, double blind, single center randomized study with a three arm parallel group design. No changes were made regarding important changes to methods after trial commencement. Written informed consent was obtained from 87 patients with an American Society of Anesthesiologists (ASA) score I or II, an age of 18–65 years, and a body mass index (BMI) of 18.0–24.5 kg·m^{-2} who were scheduled for elective surgeries under general anesthesia. Exclusion criteria included an allergy to α_2-adrenergic agonists, bradycardia, atrioventricular block, neurologic disorders and the recent use of psychoactive medications, hearing impairment, or alcohol abuse.

Sample size estimation was performed using NCSS-PASS software (version 11.0.7, Update time 2013-01-22). In a one-way ANOVA study, we estimated that the sample sizes of 0.5 μg·kg^{-1} DEX group, 1 μg·kg^{-1} DEX group and control group were 22, 23, and 22, which means were to be compared. The total sample of 67 subjects achieves 90% power to detect differences among the means versus the alternative of equal means using an F test with a 0.05 significance level. The data of the pilot study were not included in data analysis in the current study. Given an anticipated dropout rate of 10%, a total of 73 patients ($n = 73$) were incorporated in the study and distributed randomly with a 1:1:1 ratio into three groups: the 0.5 μg·kg^{-1} DEX group ($n = 24$), the 1.0 μg·kg^{-1} DEX group ($n = 25$) and the control group ($n = 24$), respectively. No interim analysis were made.

A computer-generated randomization table was used to assign each patient to one of the three groups. Study drugs (DEX or normal saline) in the identical 50-ml syringes were prepared by a pharmacist, and the syringes were consecutively numbered according to the randomization schedule. The details were as follows: the solution administered to the 1.0 μg·kg^{-1} DEX group was prepared by dissolving one ampoule of DEX (containing 200 μg in a concentration of 100 μg·ml^{-1}) in normal saline to make a 50 ml solution, yielding a final concentration of 4 μg·ml^{-1}; the solution administered to the 0.5 μg·kg^{-1} DEX group was prepared by dissolving one-half of an ampoule of DEX in normal saline to make a 50 ml solution, yielding a final concentration of 2 μg·ml^{-1}; for the solution administered to the patients of the control group, only 50 ml of 0.9% saline was prepared. Each patient was assigned an order number and received the different drugs, and the anesthesiologists were blinded to the syringe contents. No changes were made regarding blinding. DEX (100 μg·ml^{-1}) and propofol (10 mg·ml^{-1}) were supplied by Sichuan Guorui Medicine Co. Ltd. (Sichuan, China) in identical 2-ml ampules and AstraZeneca Corporation (London, England) in identical 50-ml ampules, respectively.

Patients were admitted to the operating room with no pre-medication. An 18G catheter was inserted into the large forearm vein for fluid and drug administration. Lactated Ringer's solution was infused at a rate of 15 ml·kg^{-1}·h^{-1} before the study. Non-invasive arterial pressure, electrocardiogram, and peripheral oxygen saturation (SpO_2) were continuously measured throughout the study period. The BIS was derived from the frontal electroencephalogram and calculated by an Aspect Vista monitor (version 3.2, Aspect Medical System, Inc.) using BIS sensor electrodes. Four cutaneous electrodes (Zip-Prep; Aspect) were positioned: At_1 and At_2 (one each above the outer malar bones) with Fp (4 cm above the nasion) as the reference and Fp_2 (left forehead) as the ground. Impedance was kept at < 2000 Ω. The BIS (100 = awake, 0 = burse suppression) and its trend were displayed continuously. The time delay of the BIS should be addressed; therefore, the BIS data were recorded after the propofol infusion reached 61 s [16].

All groups were infused with a loading dose of DEX or normal saline via a Graseby syringe pump model 3500 at a speed of 1.5 ml·kg^{-1}·h^{-1} for 10 min. After the loading doses of DEX or normal saline, the propofol was not stopped with a continuous intravenous infusion by micro-pump at 20 mg·kg^{-1}·h^{-1} until the patient lost consciousness. The state of consciousness was evaluated once the propofol was initiated, with an interval of 10 s, until the patients lost consciousness. The endpoint of LOC was determined by loss of the eyelash reflex and not responded to their own name called loudly and repeatedly.

The primary outcomes were the propofol requirements for LOC and the BIS value at LOC. The secondary outcomes was the time to LOC. The mean arterial pressure (MAP), heart rate (HR) and the BIS value were recorded before infusion of the study drug, with an interval of 5 min throughout the study period. No changes were made regarding trial outcomes after the trial commenced.

If the systolic arterial blood pressure increased or decreased by 20% from the baseline or the systolic pressure was less than 90 mmHg, the urapidil or phenylephrine was administered immediately to adjust the blood pressure within a normal range. The atropine was used to maintain the HR above 50 beats·min^{-1}. Respiratory depression was treated with assisted ventilation via facemask.

The data were recorded using Microsoft Excel 2007 and analyzed with various statistical tests using SPSS 17.0 (SPSS Inc., Chicago, IL, USA). Sex distribution was analyzed using the chi-square (X^2) test. The propofol requirements for LOC, the BIS values at LOC, the time to LOC, and the patients' characteristics (age, height, and weight) were analyzed using analysis of variance (ANOVA) and LSD multiple comparisons. Statistical significance was defined as a P value of less than 0.05.

Results

The trial was conducted from June 16, 2016 to August 17, 2016 at the General Hospital of Ningxia Medical University. A total of 73 patients were ultimately enrolled. Twenty-four patients were randomly assigned to the control group, 24 patients received 0.5 μg·kg^{-1} DEX, and 25 patients received 1.0 μg·kg^{-1} DEX (Fig. 1). The

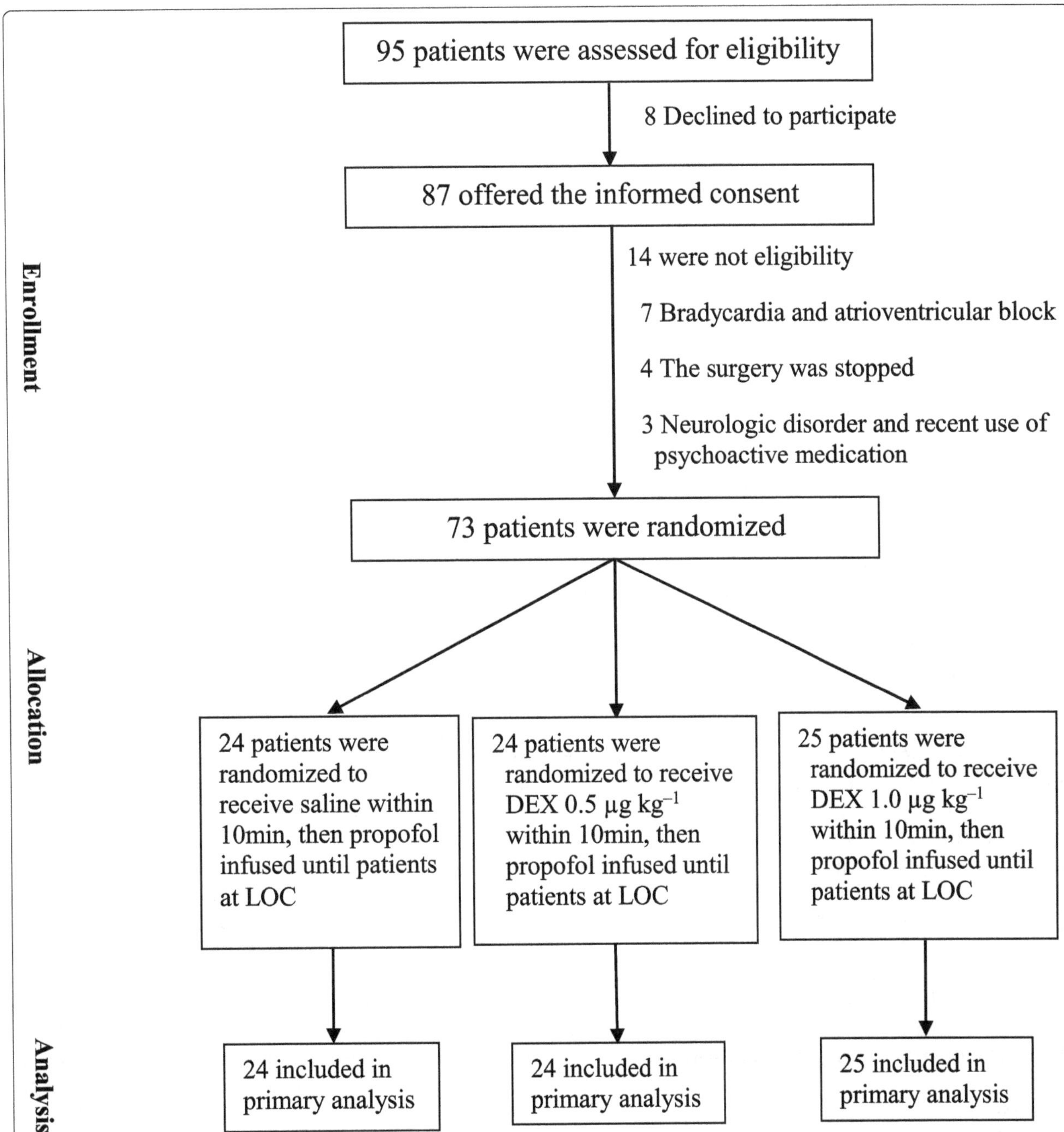

Fig. 1 Patient-flow diagram

Table 1 Patient characteristics and preoperative data before receiving drugs in the operating room

	Control group (***n*** = 24)	0.5 μg·kg^{-1} DEX group (***n*** = 24)	1.0 μg·kg^{-1} DEX group(***n*** = 25)	***P***
Weight (kg)	62.5 ± 9.0	61.0 ± 9.8	62.2 ± 9.0	0.805
Height (cm)	166.9 ± 6.9	166.3 ± 7.4	166.9 ± 6.4	0.932
Age (yr)	40.9 ± 7.4	40.0 ± 11.4	42.9 ± 11.8	0.748
Sex (female)	13 (54.1%)	12 (50.0%)	12 (48.0%)	0.912
BIS	96.7 ± 1.4	96.3 ± 1.6	97.0 ± 1.7	0.095

Data are presented as the means ± SD or numbers (%). Statistical significance was defined as $P < 0.05$

primary analysis was intention-to-treat (ITT) and involved all patients who were randomly assigned. The loading dose of DEX was not fully administered to one patient because bradycardia occurred in the 1.0 μg·kg^{-1} DEX group. There were no significant differences among the baseline and preoperative data (Table 1).

The propofol requirements for LOC decreased significantly in the DEX groups compared with the control group (ANOVA and LSD multiple comparisons, 1.12 ± 0.33 mg·kg^{-1} for the 0.5 μg·kg^{-1} DEX group vs. 1.79 ± 0.39 mg·kg^{-1} for the control group; difference, 0.68 mg·kg^{-1} [95% CI, 0.49 to 0.87]; $P = 0.0001$) (0.77 ± 0.27 mg·kg^{-1} for the 1.0 μg·kg^{-1} DEX group vs. 1.79 ± 0.39 mg·kg^{-1} for the control group; difference, 1.02 mg·kg^{-1} [95% CI, 0.84 to 1.21]; $P = 0.0001$), and the propofol requirements for LOC was lower in the 1.0 μg·kg^{-1} DEX group than that in the 0.5 μg·kg^{-1} DEX group (ANOVA and LSD multiple comparisons, 0.77 ± 0.27 mg·kg^{-1} vs. 1.12 ± 0.33 mg·kg^{-1}; difference, 0.34 mg·kg^{-1} [95% CI, 0.16 to 0.54]; $P = 0.0001$). At the time of LOC, the BIS value was higher in the DEX groups compared with the control group (ANOVA and LSD multiple comparisons, 67.5 ± 3.5 for the DEX 0.5 μg·kg^{-1} group vs. 60.5 ± 3.8 for the control group; difference, 7.04 [95% CI, 4.85 to 9.23]; $P = 0.0001$) (68.0 ± 4.1 for the 1.0 μg·kg^{-1} DEX group vs. 60.5 ± 3.8 for the control group; difference, 7.58 [95% CI, 5.41 to 9.75]; $P = 0.0001$). However, there was no difference between the two DEX groups (ANOVA, LSD multiple comparisons, $P = 0.621$). The time to LOC induced by propofol in both the 0.5 μg·kg^{-1} and 1.0 μg·kg^{-1} DEX groups was significantly shorter than that in the control group (ANOVA and LSD multiple comparisons, both $P = 0.0001$), and the time to LOC induced by propofol in the 1.0 μg·kg^{-1} DEX group was significantly shorter than that in the 0.5 μg·kg^{-1} DEX group (ANOVA and LSD multiple comparisons, $P = 0.0001$) (Tables 2 and 3). No patients in any of the groups developed hypoxia ($SpO_2 < 90\%$), hypotension or abnormal movements during the study period.

Discussion

In this study, we administered a loading dose of DEX before the infusion of propofol for anesthesia induction. The propofol requirements for LOC and the BIS value at LOC were measured. Our study showed that DEX facilitated LOC induced by propofol but increased the BIS value at LOC. The propofol requirements for LOC both decreased in the 0.5 μg·kg^{-1} and 1.0 μg·kg^{-1} DEX groups when compared with the control group. The result was similar to some early studies in which DEX was considered to decrease the propofol dose during anesthesia [5, 17]. The results indicated that synergistic effect existed between propofol and DEX when they were co-used for sedation. Norepinephrine release in the preoptic area of hypothalamus decreased by DEX makes the disinhibition of the GABAergic and galanergic inhibitory projections to the major arousal nuclei in the midbrain and pons and decreased noradrenergic signaling by DEX acted at the thalamus and cortex both can induce sedation and LOC [18]. Propofol produces sedation by potentiating the activity of $GABA_A$ receptors and inhibiting the NMDA-mediated excitatory neurotransmission [19, 20]. Thus, LOC induced by DEX combined with propofol displays a synergistic effect.

In the study, both BIS and clinical evaluation were used to measure the sedative depth. BIS is generally considered a reliable method to detect the level of sedation induced by some hypnotics, especially in propofol anesthesia. However, it had been reported that the BIS values can be influenced by different hypnotic drugs or their combinations [21, 22]. Our results showed the BIS value at LOC was higher when adding DEX to propofol than propofol administration alone. The former study demonstrated that the BIS values was less in DEX sedation than propofol sedation [22]. However, BIS values were higher at LOC when opioid combined with propofol [23]. One possible explanation is that the BIS value was dependent on the dose of propofol, and the BIS value is also larger when small dosage of propofol was administered. Other reasons may include that propofol mainly produces a delta to beta-frequency band in EEG [24], which was quite different from the delta, alpha, range activity induced by DEX [25]. What's more, the action site of DEX is different from that of propofol [18], which has been considered one factor that influences the BIS value. Furthermore, it should be noted that the BIS value has a time delay between 24 (7) and 122 (23) s [16, 26], which may influence the precision of the measurement of BIS values.

It is quite common that the circulatory and respiratory system were inhibited by propofol infusion. However, there were no episodes of hypotension or hypoxemia in

Table 2 ANOVA of the main results at LOC induced by propofol

	Control group(***n*** = 24)	0.5 μg·kg^{-1} DEX group (***n*** = 24)	1.0 μg·kg^{-1} DEX group (***n*** = 25)	***P***
Propofol requirements (mg·kg^{-1})	1.79 ± 0.39	1.12 ± 0.33	0.77 ± 0.27	0.0001
BIS	60.5 ± 3.8	67.5 ± 3.5	68.0 ± 4.1	0.0001
Time to LOC (s)	309 ± 28	209 ± 53	131 ± 40	0.0001

Data are presented as the means ± SD. Statistical significance was defined as $P < 0.05$

Table 3 LSD multiple comparison tests of the main results at LOC induced by propofol

	Propofol requirements ($mg{\cdot}kg^{-1}$)	BIS values	Time to LOC (s)
	Difference (95% CI) *P*	Difference (95% CI) *P*	Difference (95% CI) *P*
Control group vs. 0.5 μg· kg^{-1} DEX group	0.68 (0.49 to 0.87) 0.0001	−7.04 (− 9.23 to − 4.85) 0.0001	99.91 (76.20 to 123.63) 0.0001
Control group vs. 1.0 μg·kg^{-1} DEX group	1.02 (0.84 to 1.21) 0.0001	−7.58 (−9.75 to −5.41) 0.0001	177.56 (154.08 to 201.03) 0.0001
0.5 μg·kg^{-1} DEX group vs. 1.0 μg·kg^{-1} DEX group	0.34 (0.16 to 0.54) 0.0001	−0.54 (− 2.71 to1.63) 0.621	77.64 (54.17 to 101.12) 0.0001

Statistical significance was defined as $P < 0.05$

the control group, which might have been due to either the small dosages of propofol than the recommended dosage used in this study or the small number of participants in our study. During the infusion of DEX, one patient exhibited adverse events of severe bradycardia with an HR of 43 beats·min^{-1}. The reason for these events was most likely due to the sympatholytic effect of DEX, a common side effect of α_2-adrenergic agonists, especially administered with the infusion of loading doses of DEX. However, it could be easily prevented and treated after the administration of receptor-M antagonists. The patient was treated by 0.01 mg·kg^{-1} atropine, and then the patient's heart rate rose to over 50 beats·min^{-1} in a minute. Although the number of participants was small, the sample size was calculated by a statistical tool.

Conclusions

In conclusion, the pre-administration of 0.5 μg·kg^{-1} or 1.0 μg·kg^{-1} DEX could reduce the requirements of propofol for LOC. DEX pre-administration increased the BIS value at LOC induced by propofol.

Abbreviations

DEX: Dexmedetomidine; LOC: Loss of consciousness; BIS: Bispectral index; ASA: American society of anesthesiologists; BMI: Body mass index; MAP: Mean arterial pressure; HR: Heart rate; SpO_2: Peripheral oxygen saturation; ITT: intention-to-treat

Acknowledgments

Not applicable.

Authors' contributions

Conceived and designed the experiments: YG, FY, JWZ, XC and HXM. Performed the experiments: YG, FY, TM and YHZ. Analyzed the data: FY, JWZ, JW, BL, HXM, and KML. Wrote the paper: YG, FY and HXM. All authors have read and approval the final manuscript.

Author details

[1]Department of Anesthesiology, Ningxia Medical University, Yinchuan 750004, China. [2]Department of Anesthesiology, People's Hospital of Ningxia Hui Autonomous Region, Yinchuan 750002, China. [3]Department of Anesthesiology, General Hospital of Ningxia Medical University, Yinchuan 750004, China.

References

1. Wei L, Deng X, Sui J, Wang L, Liu J. Dexmedetomidine improves intubating conditions without muscle relaxants in children after induction with Propofol and Remifentanil. Anesth Analg. 2015;121(3):785–90.
2. Kakkar A, Tyagi A, Nabi N, Sethi AK, Verma UC. Comparision of clonidine and dexmedetomidine for attenuation of laryngoscopy and intubation response - a randomized controlled trial. J Clin Anesth. 2016;33:283–8.
3. Win NN, Kohase H, Yoshikawa F, Wakita R, Takahashi M, Kondo N, et al. Haemodynamic changes and heart rate variability during midazolam-propofol co-induction. Anaesthesia. 2007;62(6):561–8.
4. Upton RN, Martinez AM, Grant C. Comparison of the sedative properties of CNS 7056, midazolam, and propofol in sheep. Br J Anaesth. 2009;103(6): 848–57.
5. El-Shmaa NS, El-Baradey GF. The efficacy of labetalol vs dexmedetomidine for attenuation of hemodynamic stress response to laryngoscopy and endotracheal intubation. J Clin Anesth. 2016;31:267–73.
6. Weerink MAS, Struys MMRF, Hannivoort LN, Barends CRM, Absalom AR, Colin P. Clinical pharmacokinetics and pharmacodynamics of Dexmedetomidine. Clin Pharmacokinet. 2017;56(8):893–913.
7. Dutta A, Sethi N, Sood J, Panday BC, Gupta M, Choudhary P, et al. The effect of Dexmedetomidine on Propofol requirements during anesthesia administered by Bispectral index-guided closed-loop anesthesia delivery system: a randomized controlled study. Anesth Analg. 2019;129(1):84–91.
8. Le Guen M, Liu N, Tounou F, Augé M, Tuil O, Chazot T, et al. Dexmedetomidine reduces propofol and remifentanil requirements during bispectral index-guided closed-loop anesthesia: a double-blind, placebo-controlled trial. Anesth Analg. 2014;118(5):946–55.
9. Feld JM, Hoffman WE, Stechert MM, Hoffman IW, Ananda RC. Fentanyl or dexmedetomidine combined with desflurane for bariatric surgery. J Clin Anesth. 2006;18(1):24–8.
10. Punjasawadwong Y, Phongchiewboon A, Bunchungmongkol N. Bispectral index for improving anaesthetic delivery and postoperative recovery. Cochrane Database Syst Rev. 2014;6:CD003843.
11. Glass PS, Bloom M, Kearse L, Rosow C, Sebel P, Manberg P. Bispectral analysis measures sedation and memory effects of propofol, midazolam, isoflurane, and alfentanil in healthy volunteers. Anesthesiology. 1997;86(4): 836–47.
12. Ibrahim AE, Taraday JK, Kharasch ED. Bispectral index monitoring during sedation with sevoflurane, midazolam, and propofol. Anesthesiology. 2001; 95(5):1151–9.
13. Lysakowski C, Dumont L, Pellegrini M, Clergue F, Tassonyi E. Effects of fentanyl, alfentanil, remifentanil and sufentanil on loss of consciousness and bispectral index during propofol induction of anaesthesia. Br J Anaesth. 2001;86(4):523–7.
14. Shehabi Y, Howe BD, Bellomo R, Arabi YM, Bailey M, Bass FE, et al. Early sedation with Dexmedetomidine in critically ill patients. N Engl J Med. 2019; 380(26):2506–17.
15. Yu X, Franks NP, Wisden W. Sleep and sedative states induced by targeting the histamine and noradrenergic systems. Front Neural Circuits. 2018;12:4.
16. Musizza B, Ribaric S. Monitoring the depth of anaesthesia. Sensors (Basel). 2010;10(12):10896–935.
17. Ali AR, El Ghoneimy MN. Dexmedetomidine versus fentanyl as adjuvant to propofol: comparative study in children undergoing extracorporeal shock wave lithotripsy. Eur J Anaesthesiol. 2010;27(12):1058–64.
18. Brown EN, Pavone KJ, Naranjo M. Multimodal general anesthesia: theory and practice. Anesth Analg. 2018;127(5):1246–58.
19. Brotherton AL, Hamilton EP, Kloss HG, Hammond DA. Propofol for treatment of refractory alcohol withdrawal syndrome: a review of the literature. Pharmacotherapy. 2016;36(4):433–42.
20. Orser BA, Bertlik M, Wang LY, MacDonald JF. Inhibition by propofol (2,6 di-isopropylphenol) of the N-methyl-D-aspartate subtype of glutamate receptor in cultured hippocampal neurones. Br J Pharmacol. 1995;116(2): 1761–8.
21. de Valence T, Elia N, Czarnetzki C, Dumont L, Tramèr MR, Lysakowski C. Effect of sufentanil on bispectral index in the elderly. Anaesthesia. 2018; 73(2):216–22.

22. Kasuya Y, Govinda R, Rauch S, Mascha EJ, Sessler DI, Turan A. The correlation between bispectral index and observational sedation scale in volunteers sedated with dexmedetomidine and propofol. Anesth Analg. 2009;109(6): 1811–5.
23. Lysakowski, C. Effects of fentanyl, alfentanil, remifentanil and sufentanil on loss of consciousness and bispectral index during propofol induction of anaesthesia. Br J Anaesth.86(4):523–7.
24. Verdonck O, Reed SJ, Hall J, Gotman J, Plourde G. The sensory thalamus and cerebral motor cortex are affected concurrently during induction of anesthesia with propofol: a case series with intracranial electroencephalogram recordings. Can J Anaesth. 2014;61(3):254–62.
25. Sleigh JW, Vacas S, Flexman AM, Talke PO. Electroencephalographic arousal patterns under Dexmedetomidine sedation. Anesth Analg. 2018;127(4):951–9.
26. Zanner R, Pilge S, Kochs EF, Kreuzer M, Schneider G. Time delay of electroencephalogram index calculation: analysis of cerebral state, bispectral, and Narcotrend indices using perioperatively recorded electroencephalographic signals. Br J Anaesth. 2009;103(3):394–9.

The analgesic efficacy of ultrasound-guided transversus abdominis plane block for retroperitoneoscopic renal surgery

Xue Li[1], Zhen-Zhen Xu[1], Xue-Ying Li[2], Ting-Ting Jiang[1], Zeng-Mao Lin[1*] and Dong-Xin Wang[1]

Abstract

Background: Ultrasound-guided lateral transversus abdominis plane (TAP) block can provide definite analgesia to the anterior abdominal wall. However, whether this method is useful in renal surgery through the lateral abdominal wall pathway remains unknown. The study aimed to evaluate the analgesic efficacy of lateral TAP block for retroperitoneoscopic partial or radical nephrectomy.

Method: In this prospective, randomized, double-blind, placebo-controlled trial, eligible patients were randomized into two groups. After anaesthesia induction, ultrasound-guided lateral TAP block was performed with either 30 ml of 0.4% ropivacaine (Group T) or an equivalent volume of normal saline (Group C). The primary outcomes were opioid consumption during surgery and in the first 24 h after surgery. Secondary outcomes included postsurgical pain intensity immediately awakening from anaesthesia and at 0.5, 1, 2, 6, 12, and 24 h after surgery, as well as recovery variables including the incidence of postoperative nausea and vomiting (PONV), sleep quality, time to first ambulation, drainage and length of hospital stay.

Results: A total of 104 patients were enrolled and randomized (53 in Group T and 51 in Group C). Laparoscopic surgery was converted to open surgery in one patient of Group T; this patient was excluded from the outcome analysis. The opioid consumption during surgery (intravenous morphine equivalent dose: median 35.0 mg [interquartile range 18.0, 49.6] in Group C vs. 40.3 mg [20.9, 59.0] in Group T, $P = 0.281$) and in the first 24 h after surgery (10.8 mg [7.8, 21.7] in Group C vs. 13.2 mg [8.0, 26.6] in Group T, $P = 0.311$) did not differ significantly between groups. There were no significant differences between groups regarding the pain intensity at all time points after surgery and the recovery variables (all $P > 0.05$).

Conclusions: Our results showed that, in patients undergoing retroperitoneoscopic renal surgery, preoperative lateral TAP did not decrease intra- and postoperative opioid consumption, nor did it relieve pain intensity or promote postoperative recovery in the first 24 h after surgery. However, the trial might be underpowered.

Keywords: Transversus abdominis plane block, Analgesia, Retroperitoneoscopic renal surgery, Postsurgical recovery

* Correspondence: linzengmao@163.com
[1]Department of Anesthesiology, Peking University First Hospital, No. 7 Xishiku Street, Xicheng District, Beijing 100034, China

Background

For laparoscopic renal surgery, the retroperitoneal approach is an alternative pathway of the transperitoneal approach. The overall outcomes of both approaches, such as the rates of perioperative complications, positive surgical margin and postoperative recurrence, are similar; whereas the retroperitoneoscopic approach is advantageous in terms of easier hilar control and shorter total operative time, especially in patients with a past history of intraperitoneal procedures or with a posteriorly located renal tumour [1–3]. Therefore, the retroperitoneoscopic approach is the most popular approach for radical or partial nephrectomy in Peking University First Hospital. Multimodal analgesia including nerve block is advocated to improve early recovery after renal surgery [4, 5].

Transversus abdominis plane (TAP) block is an effective regional anaesthetic technique that blocks neural afferents of the T6-L1 spinal nerves innervating the anterolateral abdominal wall [6]. Since the original report by Rafi [7], there have been a plethora of studies on this block and variations of the original approach, among which lateral TAP is the most commonly used approach in abdominal surgery, with its dermatomal sensory block covering T10 to L1 [8]. A recent systematic review demonstrated that TAP block had definite analgesic efficiency for some kinds of lower abdominal surgeries, such as gynaecological surgery, caesarean section and hernia repair, but not urologic surgery [9]. However, it was worth noting that there was a high heterogeneity among the urologic studies included in that review. In addition, some studies focusing on renal surgery were missed.

To our knowledge, only three randomized controlled trials compared the effect of lateral TAP block with placebo in laparoscopic live-donor nephrectomy [10–12]. All of these found that TAP block surely reduced postoperative pain severity and opioid requirements. However, this conclusion can't be extrapolated to retroperitoneal laparoscopic renal surgery (RLRS) of which the main incision is completely different from those of live-donor nephrectomy. Theoretically, the dermatomes of lateral TAP block can only partially cover the incision in RLRS. Therefore, whether it could reduce opioid consumption and subjective pain intensity, and ultimately promote postoperative recovery in patients undergoing RLRS remains unknown. The purpose of this study was to determine whether lateral TAP block could provide effective analgesia and improve recovery in patients undergoing RLRS.

Methods

Study design

This prospective, randomized, double-blinded trial was approved by the Biomedical Research Ethics Committee of Peking University First Hospital (2017–1398). It was registered at http://www.chictr.org.cn with an identification number of ChiCTR-INR-17013244. Written informed consent was obtained from each patient. The study adhered to the CONSORT guidelines.

Participants

Potential participants were screened the day before surgery. Patients aged between 18 and 70 years and scheduled to undergo elective laparoscopic radical or partial nephrectomy through the retroperitoneal approach were included. Patients who met any of the following criteria were excluded: (1) chronic opioid addiction and/or use of other kinds of analgesic drugs for more than 3 months; (2) inability to communicate due to severe dementia, language barrier, or end-stage disease; (3) allergic to local anaesthetics; (4) nerve block contraindication such as an infection in the puncture site or severe coagulation dysfunction; and (5) refusal to participate in the study. Patients who were enrolled for this trial were taught how to evaluate pain intensity by using the numeric rating scale (NRS, an 11-point scale where 0 indicates no pain and 10 indicates the worst pain) and how to use a patient-controlled analgesia (PCA) device.

Anaesthesia management and surgical technique

All patients were managed according to a standardized anaesthetic protocol. Anaesthesia was induced with sufentanil, propofol and etomidate. Endotracheal intubation was facilitated with cisatracurium or rocuronium. Anaesthesia was maintained with continuous infusion of propofol, remifentanil (and intermittent sufentanil) or sufentanil, with or without dexmedetomidine; the aim was to maintain the BIS values between 40 and 60, and the mean arterial pressure and heart rate within 20% of the preoperative values. At 30 min before the end of surgery, 50 mg of flurbiprofen axetil and 5 mg of tropisetron were administered intravenously. After emergence from anaesthesia, all patients were monitored in the post-anaesthesia care unit (PACU) for at least 1 h before transferred to the general ward.

The retroperitoneal laparoscopic procedure was usually performed through three ports. The primary port was invariably placed through the incision made for the creation of the working space, which was just below the tip of the 12th rib on the posterior axillary line. The secondary port was placed 2 cm above the iliac crest on the midaxillary line. The third port was placed under the costal margin on the anterior axillary line. In case of radical nephrectomy, the initial incision was extended ventrally for kidney removal. The pneumoperitoneum was maintained at approximately 12–14 mmHg throughout the procedure (Fig. 1).

For all patients, a standard postoperative pain management was provided, i.e., a PCA pump, which was

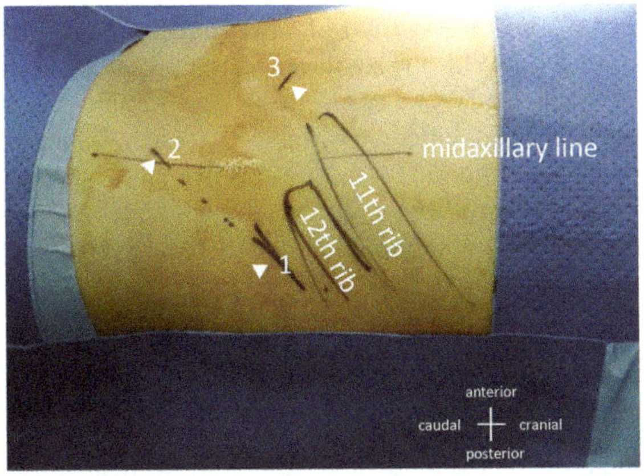

Fig. 1 The three trocar sites for retroperitoneoscopic renal surgery

established with 1.25 μg/ml sufentanil and programmed to administer a background rate of 0.5 ml/h and an on-demand bolus of 4 ml every 10 min, together with a rigorous rescue analgesia plan. The target was to maintain the NRS pain score below 4. In the PACU, regular pain evaluation was performed every 30 min. If the NRS score was higher than 4, a PCA bolus of 4 ml was administered first, and pain was evaluated 5 min later. If the NRS score remained higher than 4, another 3–5 μg sufentanil was administered intravenously according to the patient's body weight. No more rescue analgesics were administered if the NRS score decreased to 4 or less. In the general ward, pain evaluation was performed at 2, 6, 12, and 24 h after surgery; in addition, patients were instructed to request additional analgesia in case of breakthrough pain. Pain control measures were similar to those in the PACU, except that morphine (3–5 mg) was administered instead of sufentanil. NSAIDS or other analgesics could also be administered according to the surgeons' prescription.

Randomization and intervention

Stratified randomization with a block size of 4 was performed using the SAS statistical package version 9.3 (SAS Institute, Cary, NC, USA) by a biostatistician (XLN) who was not involved in the data management and statistical analyses. Stratification was performed according to the planned type of surgery, i.e., radical or partial nephrectomy. The randomization results were then sealed in sequentially numbered envelopes, transferred to a study coordinator (TTJ) with the Good Clinical Practice (GCP) certification and stored at the site of the investigation until the end of the study.

The day before surgery, an investigator (ZML) screened potential participants and recruited patients after obtaining written informed consents. On the day of surgery, the study coordinator opened the envelopes consecutively according to the recruitment sequence and prepared the study drugs for each patient, but did not participate in the rest of the trial. All study drugs were provided as clear aqueous solutions in the same 20 ml syringes for TAP block. In this way patients were randomly assigned into two groups: patients in Group T received 30 ml of 0.4% ropivacaine, while those in Group C received an equivalent amount of normal saline. Apart from the study drugs used for TAP block, other perioperative management was identical in both groups. All health-care team members, investigators, and patients themselves were fully blinded to the group assignments throughout the study period.

Ultrasound-guided TAP block was performed by two experienced anaesthetists (DH and HK) immediately after the induction of anaesthesia and approximately 15 min before skin incision. With the patient in the supine position, the ultrasound probe was placed at the midaxillary line between the lower costal margin and the iliac crest. At this point, the plane between the internal oblique and transverse abdominal muscles was identified (Fig. 2a). A special needle used for nerve block (80 mm or 100 mm, Stimuplex D, Germany) was inserted using an in-plane technique in the anteroposterior direction. After aspiration, to avoid inadvertent intravascular injection and abdominal paracentesis, an injection with 2 ml of normal saline was used to ensure correct positioning of the needle. The prepared study drug was then injected into this plane. Successful study drug injection was defined as the appearance of a hypoechoic ellipsoid with well-defined margins on ultrasonic imaging (Fig. 2b).

Follow-up schedule and outcomes

Investigators (XL, ZZX, and ZML) who were blinded to the study group assignment were in charge of the perioperative data collection. Patients were followed-up at several time points in the first 24 h after surgery. In addition, the electronic medical record was reviewed to obtain necessary data.

The primary outcomes were opioid consumption (intravenous morphine equivalent dose) during surgery and within the first 24 h after surgery. The secondary outcomes included the following: (1) the NRS pain scores both at rest and with coughing immediately awakening from anaesthesia and at 0.5, 1, 2, 6, 12 and 24 h after surgery; (2) time to the first bolus demand in the PCA system, as well as the numbers of required and administered bolus; (3) time to the first rescue analgesic, as well as its use and frequency in addition to the PCA system; (4) the incidence of postoperative nausea and vomiting (PONV) within 24 h after surgery and the use of antiemetics; (5) subjective sleep quality on the night of surgery evaluated by the NRS (an 11-point scale where 0 indicates the best sleep quality and 10 indicates the worst sleep experience); (6) time to the first

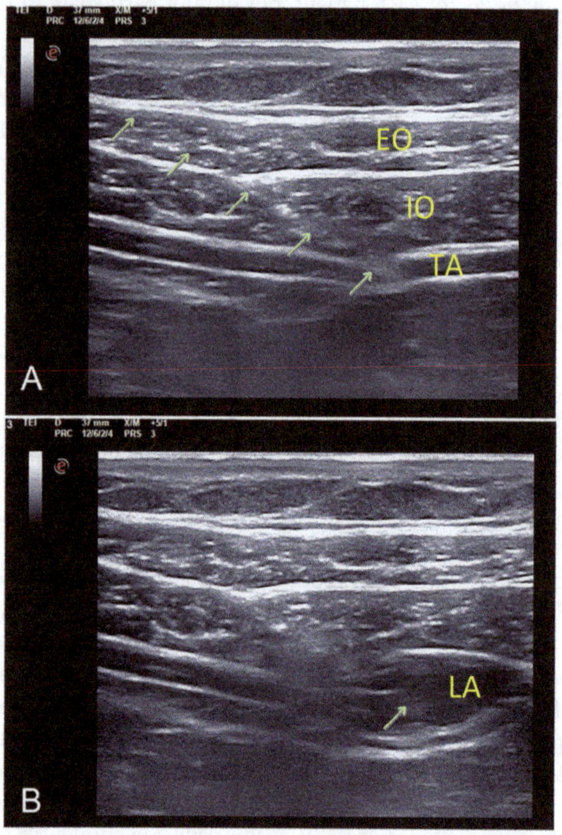

Fig. 2 Sonography of the lateral TAP block, indicating the ultrasound anatomical structure (**a**) and the spread of local anaesthetic (**b**). The green arrow indicates the needle trajectory; EO: external oblique; IO: internal oblique; TA: transversus abdominis; LA: local anaesthetic

ambulation after surgery; (7) drainage during the first 24 h after surgery; and (8) the length of hospital stay after surgery.

Safety outcomes were monitored from the beginning of anaesthesia until 24 h after surgery. The adverse events associated with TAP block included but not limited to the following: numbness in the lower extremities, haematoma and bleeding in the needle trajectory, visceral organ injury, anaphylaxis, local anaesthetic toxicity. Other perioperative adverse events were also documented.

Statistical analysis

Sample size estimation

According to previous studies [10, 12, 13], the use of TAP block decreased opioid consumption by 13.5–45.3% compared with the placebo during the first 24 h after surgery. We conservatively assumed that opioid consumption would be reduced by 10% in the TAP block group. Sample size calculation was performed based on the previous data obtained from our clinical follow-up system, which showed that the total consumption of sufentanil (within 24 h after surgery) in patients who underwent RLRS without TAP block was 36.5 ± 5.4 μg. With the significance and power set at 0.05 (two-sided) and 90%, respectively, the sample size required to detect differences was 94 patients. Taking into account a drop-out rate of approximately 10%, we planned to enrol 104 patients. Sample size calculation was performed with the PASS 11.0 software (Stata Corp. LP, College Station, TX).

Outcome analyses

Normally distributed continuous variables are expressed as the mean ± standard deviation and were compared using a two-tailed Student's t-test. Non-normally distributed continuous variables and ordinal data are expressed as medians (interquartile range) and were compared using the Mann-Whitney U test. Categorical variables are expressed as numbers (percentages) and were compared with Chi-squared analysis or Fischer's exact test. Time-to-event data were analysed by the Kaplan-Meier estimator, with the difference between groups compared by the log-rank test. Per-protocol analysis was performed. Two-sided P values of less than 0.05 were regarded as statistically significant. All statistical analyses were performed with the SPSS statistical package version 25.0 (IBM SPSS Inc., Chicago, IL, USA).

Results

From January 1, 2018, to March 20, 2018, 166 patients were screened for eligibility; of these, 130 met the inclusion/exclusion criteria, 104 gave consents and were randomized into the study, with 53 patients in Group T and 51 in Group C. During surgery, one patient developed major haemorrhage and was converted to open surgery. This patient was excluded from the per-protocol analysis. Flow diagram of the study was shown in Fig. 3 and original dataset was listed as Additional file 1.

No patient received opioid treatment before surgery. The two groups were comparable regarding the demographic or baseline characteristics except that the percentage with diabetes mellitus was higher in Group T ($P = 0.041$; Table 1). Intraoperative variables, including durations of anaesthesia and surgery, use and dose of dexmedetomidine, and estimated blood loss, did not differ significantly between groups (Table 2).

The opioid consumption during surgery (intravenous morphine equivalent dose: median 35.0 mg [interquartile range 18.0, 49.6] in Group C vs. 40.3 mg [20.9, 59.0] in Group T, $P = 0.281$) and in the first 24 h after surgery (10.8 mg [7.8, 21.7] in Group C vs. 13.2 mg [8.0, 26.6] in Group T, $P = 0.311$) did not differ significantly between groups. Stratified analysis did not find any significant differences regarding intraoperative and postoperative morphine equivalent dose between the two groups in

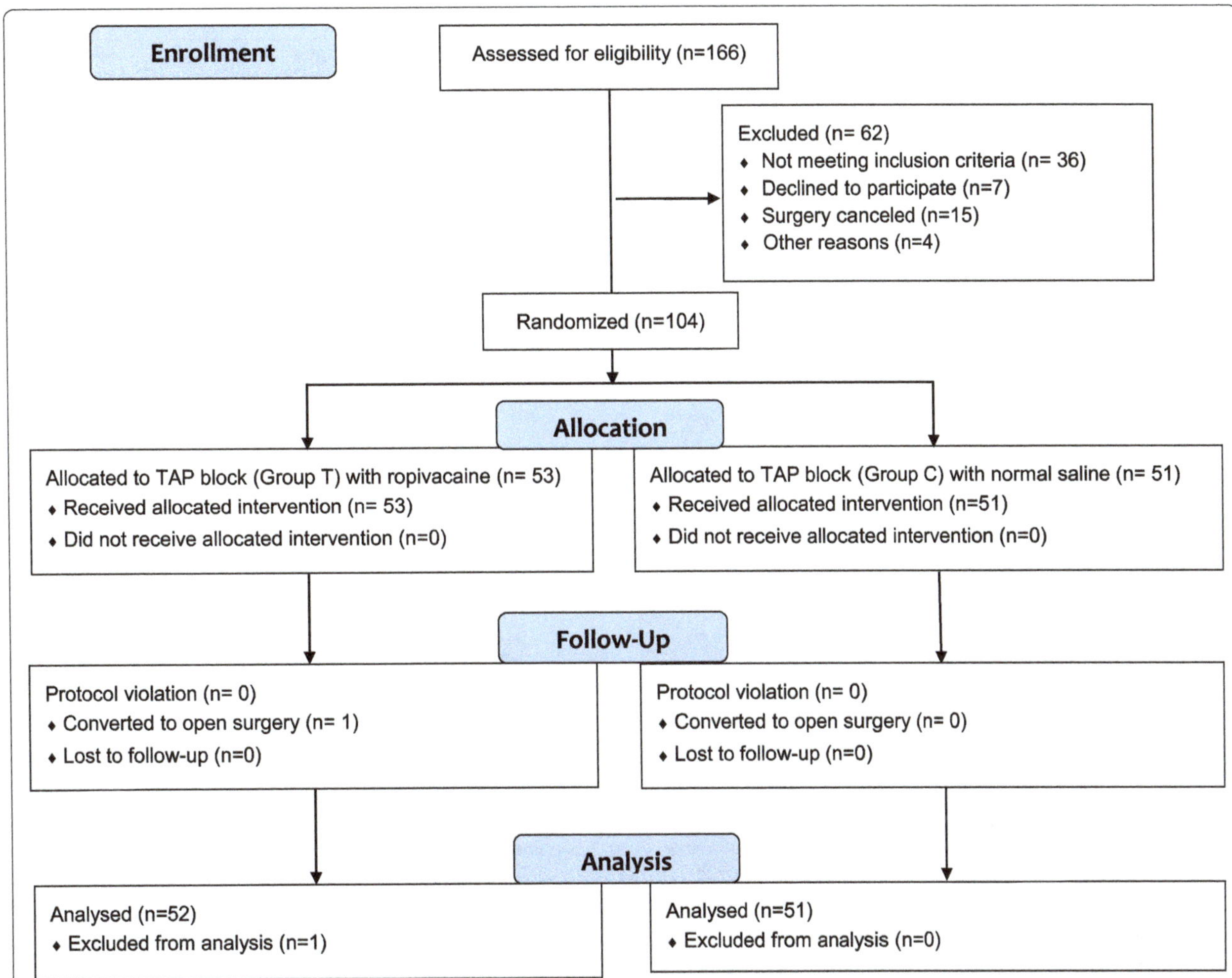

Fig. 3 Flow diagram of the study

patients receiving either the partial or radical nephrectomy (Table 3).

There were no significant differences between groups regarding the numbers of required and administered bolus, as well as the time to the first required bolus from the PCA system ($P = 0.335$, 0.338 and 0.088, respectively). There were no significant differences between groups regarding the percentage and frequency of rescue analgesics, as well as the time to first dose rescue analgesics in addition to the PCA system ($P = 0.153$, 0.306, and 0.843, respectively) (Table 3). Post-surgical pain scores at those abovementioned time points were similar between the two groups both at rest and with coughing (all $P > 0.05$) (Fig. 4a and b).

As for postoperative recovery in the first 24 h, the incidence of PONV, percentage of antiemetic therapy, subject sleep quality, time to the first ambulation, volume of drainage, and length of stay in hospital after surgery were not significantly different between the two groups (all $P > 0.05$) (Table 4).

No adverse events related to the TAP block technique were observed in either group. One patient in Group T developed major haemorrhage during surgery (estimated blood loss of 6500 ml), one patient in Group C developed emergence delirium. Perioperative management was uneventful in other patients.

Discussion

To our knowledge, this was the first study investigating the efficiency of lateral TAP block in patients undergoing RLRS. Our results showed that preoperative lateral TAP block did not decrease intra- and postoperative opioid consumption, nor did it relieve pain intensity or promote postoperative recovery early after surgery. Our study added new evidence to the current knowledge of analgesic measures for laparoscopic urological surgery.

Our results conflicted with those of previous studies. For example, both Parikh et al. and Guner et al. found that lateral TAP block performed at the end of laparoscopic donor nephrectomy significantly decreased pain

Table 1 Demographic and baseline characteristics

	Group C (*n* = 51)	Group T (*n* = 52)	*P* value
Age, year	51.1 ± 11.1	51.9 ± 10.3	0.717
Body mass index, kg/ m^2	24.8 ± 3.3	24.8 ± 3.8	0.929
Male	31 (60.8%)	32 (61.5%)	0.937
Type of surgery			
Radical nephrectomy	24 (47.1%)	24 (46.2%)	0.927
Partial nephrectomy	27 (52.9%)	28 (53.8%)	
ASA class			
I	27 (52.9%)	24 (46.2%)	0.421
II	24 (47.1%)	27 (51.9%)	
III	0 (0.0%)	1 (1.9%)	
NYHA class			
I	51 (100%)	50 (96.2%)	0.495
II	0 (0.0%)	2 (3.8%)	
Comorbidities			
Stoke	2 (3.9%)	4 (7.7%)	0.692
Hypertension	19 (37.3%)	16 (30.8%)	0.487
Coronary artery disease	1 (2.0%)	3 (5.8%)	0.624
Diabetes Mellitus	3 (5.9%)	10 (19.2%)	0.041
Asthma and/or COPD	2 (3.9%)	0 (0.0%)	0.243
Previous abdominal or back surgery	14 (27.5%)	10 (19.2%)	0.324

Data are presented as mean ± standard deviation or number (%)
ASA America Society of Anaesthesiologists, *NYHA* New York Heart Association, *COPD* chronic obstructive pulmonary disease

score and total opioid consumption in the first 24 h [11, 12]. Similarly, Hosgood et al. also claimed that TAP block reduced the early morphine requirement (within 6 h after surgery) in a similar patient population [10]. It should be noted that there were two important differences between our study and the above-mentioned others. First, the location of the main surgical incision for kidney retrieval and trocar sites in the present study was completely different from those in the previous studies [10, 11]. Second, we performed TAP block before surgery, whereas others performed TAP block after surgery [11, 12]. Thus, when comparing results among different trials, it is crucial to take the surgical technique, the block approach and the time of block into consideration. Full clarification of our negative findings requires detailed understanding of the innervation of the abdominal wall.

The anterolateral abdominal wall is mainly innervated by the anterior rami of thoracolumbar spinal nerves (T6-L1), which follow a curvilinear course from the back towards the midline of the body [6]. Generally, as they proceed, after giving off lateral cutaneous branches near the costal angle innervating the lateral areas of the abdominal wall [14], they enter into the TAP with a varied course and finally perforate the rectus abdominis and end as the anterior cutaneous branches innervating the anterior abdomen (area from the midline to the midclavicular line) [15]. Most of the lateral cutaneous branches arise before the main nerves enter the TAP, and only those of T11 and T12 have a short course within or through the TAP [15]. Thus, it is not surprising that lateral TAP block can reliably provide analgesia for the lower anterior abdomen but not the lateral abdomen

Table 2 Intraoperative data

	Group C (*n* = 51)	Group T (*n* = 52)	*P* value
Duration of anaesthesia, min	144 (122, 168)	140 (126, 165)	0.805
Duration of surgery, min	78 (59, 112)	79 (64, 102)	0.934
Use of dexmedetomidine	20 (39.2%)	13 (25.0%)	0.122
Dose of dexmedetomidine, μg	30 (23, 39) (*n* = 20)	30 (22, 50) (*n* = 13)	0.785
Estimated blood loss, ml	50 (50, 50)	50 (50, 50)	0.387

Data are presented as median (interquartile range) or number (%)

Table 3 Effectiveness outcomes

	Group C (*n* = 51)	Group T (*n* = 52)	Estimated effects (95% CI) [a]	*P* value
Opioid consumption during surgery				
Sufentanil, μg	20 (15, 38)	23 (20, 30)	Median D = 0 (−5, 5)	0.685
Remifentanil, μg	600 (502, 794) (*n* = 33)	607 (428, 818) (*n* = 39)	Median D = 0 (− 119, 120)	0.977
Morphine equivalent dose, mg	35.0 (18.0, 49.6)	40.3 (20.9, 59.0)	Median D = 4.4 (−3.6, 13.4)	0.281
Morphine equivalent dose, mg/kg	0.58 (0.29, 0.77)	0.59 (0.30, 0.87)	Median D = 0.05 (−0.06, 0.18)	0.326
Opioid consumption within 24 h after surgery				
Sufentanil, μg	33 (23, 65)	40 (24, 80)	Median D = 4 (−4, 14)	0.311
Morphine equivalent dose, mg	10.8 (7.8, 21.7)	13.2 (8.0, 26.6)	Median D = 1.2 (−1.3, 4.8)	0.311
Morphine equivalent dose, mg/kg	0.16 (0.12, 0.31)	0.19 (0.12, 0.39)	Median D = 0.02 (−0.02, 0.07)	0.252
Laparoscopic partial nephrectomy	(*n* = 27)	(*n* = 28)		
Intraoperative MED, mg	41.2 (14.0, 49.6)	38.0 (19.0, 60.4)	Median D = 4.4 (−10.6, 16.6)	0.480
Postoperative MED within 24 h, mg	10.1 (7.4, 19.8)	17.7 (8.4, 26.1)	Median D = 3.1 (−0.3, 10)	0.070
Laparoscopic radical nephrectomy	(*n* = 24)	(n = 24)		
Intraoperative MED, mg	30.0 (19.2, 52.7)	40.7 (26.9, 53.8)	Median D = 5.5 (−6.8, 18.7)	0.370
Postoperative MED within 24 h, mg	14.5 (8.2, 25.0)	10.6 (8.0, 27.8)	Median D = -0.9 (−6.0, 4.4)	0.773
Data from the PCA system				
Number of required bolus	4 (1, 10)	6 (1, 15)	Median D = 1 (−1, 4)	0.335
Number of administered bolus	3 (1, 10)	5 (1, 12)	Median D = 1 (−1, 3)	0.338
Time to first required bolus, hour [b]	1.7 (0.4, 3.0)	6.0 (2.8, 9.2)	HR = 1.46 (0.93, 2.30)	0.088
Data of rescue analgesia within 24 h after surgery				
Percentage of rescue analgesics	12 (23.5%)	19 (36.5%)	OR = 0.53 (0.23, 1.26)	0.153
Frequency of rescue analgesics	2 (1, 3)	1 (1, 4)	Median D = 0 (−1, 0)	0.306
Time to first rescue analgesics, hour [b]	21.0 (14.4, 27.6)	25.0 (19.3, 30.7)	HR = 1.08 (0.52, 2.24)	0.843

Data are presented as median (interquartile range) or number of patient (%), unless otherwise indicated
D difference, *MED* morphine equivalent dose, *PCA* patient controlled analgesia
[a]Calculated as Group T vs. or minus Group C
[b]Data were analysed by Kaplan-Meier analysis and compared by log-rank test; the results are presented as the median (95% confidence interval)

wall. Ma et al. further confirmed this by detecting the blocking dermatomes in 19 areas of the abdominal wall after lateral TAP block [16]. This might be an important reason for our negative results. The dermatomes of lateral TAP block we performed only covered part of the wounds in RLRS. For urological surgery, the posterior TAP approach [13, 17] or quadratus lumborum block [18] may be the better choice because they can block the lateral cutaneous branches of thoracolumbar spinal nerves and provide better lateral abdominal wall analgesia.

Regarding postoperative recovery, we observed no advantages in Group T in terms of the incidence of PONV. This was understandable since the perioperative opioid consumptions were comparable in the two groups. Similar findings were also reported in other studies [10, 19]. We found rather low sleep quality in both groups with no significant difference. We believed that not only pain intensity but also the surrounding environment in the ward affected sleep quality. Given that none of the above variables were different, it was no wonder that the length of hospital stay was similar in the two groups.

Our study has some limitations. First, we did not assess sensory dermatome blockage to confirm a successful TAP block because the block was performed after anaesthesia induction for blinding. Second, we only collected opioid consumption at a single time point (24 h after surgery) during the follow-up periods. Since we didn't record the opioid consumption at earlier postsurgical time-points, such as at 6 and 12 h after surgery, we could not analyse the early effect of TAP block. Third, the range of 95% confidence interval of the median difference in opioid consumption between the two groups were large, which indicated that the present trial might be underpowered.

Conclusions

Results of this prospective, randomized, double-blind trial showed that preoperative single-shot lateral TAP block did not decrease intra- and postoperative opioid

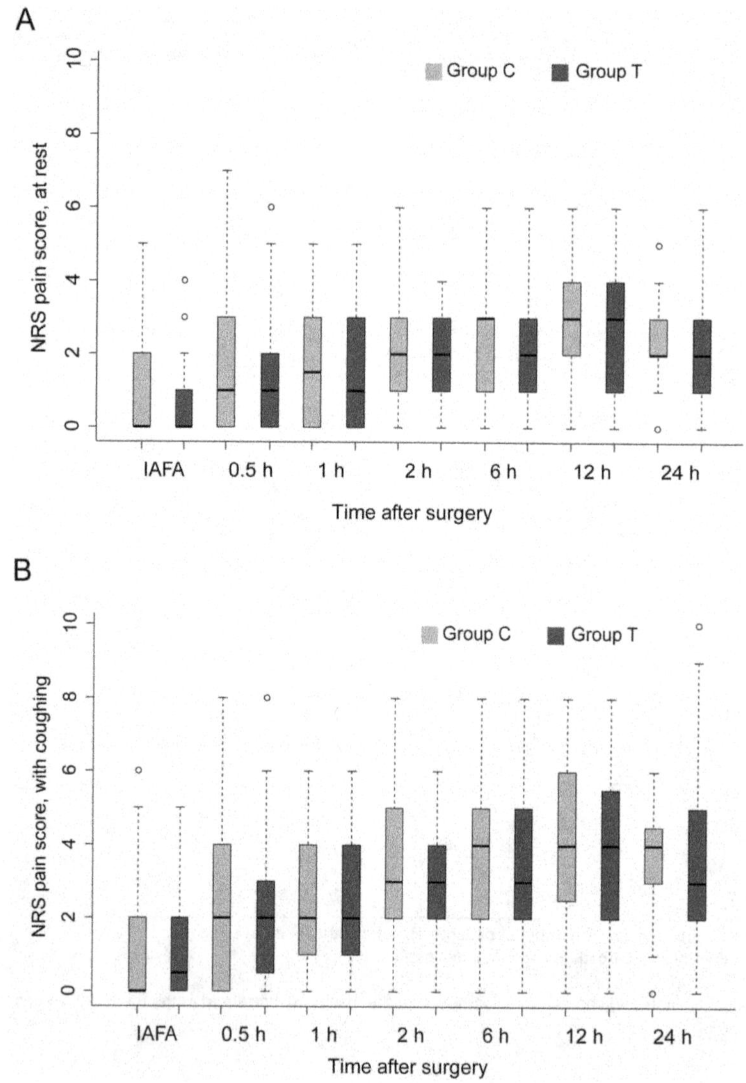

Fig. 4 NRS pain score at rest (**a**) or with coughing (**b**) within 24 h after surgery. There were no significant differences between the two groups. IAFA: immediate awakening from anaesthesia

Table 4 Comparisons of recovery variables

	Group C ($n = 51$)	Group T ($n = 52$)	*P* value
PONV within 24 h	15 (29.4%)	17 (32.7%)	0.719
Use of antiemetics within 24 h	10 (19.6%)	8 (15.4%)	0.573
NRS subject sleep quality, score [a]	5 (2, 7)	4 (2, 7)	0.717
Time to first ambulation, hour [b]	19.5 (17.8, 21.2)	20.0 (18.2, 21.8)	0.314
Volume of drainage within 24 h, ml	30 (0, 55)	35 (0, 90)	0.248
LOS in hospital after surgery, day [b]	4.0 (3.7, 4.3)	4.0 (3.6, 4.4)	0.754

Data are presented as number (%) or median (interquartile range)
PONV postoperative nausea and vomiting, *NRS* numeric rating scale, *LOS* length of stay
[a]Subjective sleep quality on the night of surgery
[b]Data were analyzed by Kaplan-Meier analysis and compared by log-rank test; the results are presented as median (95% confidence interval)

consumption, nor did it relieve pain intensity or promote postoperative recovery in the first 24 h after surgery for patients undergoing retroperitoneoscopic renal surgery. However, considering the wide range of confidence interval of median difference in opioid consumption between the two groups, the trial might be underpowered.

Abbreviations

ASA: America Society of Anaesthesiologists; BIS: Bispectral Index; BMI: Body mass index; COPD: Chronic obstructive pulmonary disease; NRS: Numeric rating scale; NSAIDs: Non-steroidal anti-inflammatory drugs; NYHA: New York Heart Association; PACU: Post-anaesthesia care unit; PCA: Patient-controlled analgesia; PONV: Postoperative nausea and vomiting; RLRS: Retroperitoneal laparoscopic renal surgery; TAP: Transversus abdominis plane

Acknowledgements

We thank Ms. Xiao-Lu Nie for creating the randomization sequence, making the opaque envelopes and giving statistical consultation. We appreciate the efforts of Drs. Da Huang and Hao Kong for performing the TAP block. We also acknowledge the team members of the Departments of Anaesthesiology and Urological Surgery in Peking University First Hospital for supporting the research.

Authors' contributions

XL: Study design, data collection and analysis, manuscript drafting. ZZX: Data collection, data analysis and interpretation. XYL: Sample size calculation. TTJ: Randomization implementation and drug preparation. ZML: Study design, data collection, manuscript revision. DXW: Data interpretation, and critical revision of the manuscript. All authors have read and approved the final manuscript.

Author details

[1]Department of Anesthesiology, Peking University First Hospital, No. 7 Xishiku Street, Xicheng District, Beijing 100034, China. [2]Department of Biostatics, Peking University First Hospital, No. 7 Xishiku Street, Xicheng District, Beijing 100034, China.

References

1. Liatsikos E, Kallidonis P, Do M, Dietel A, Al-Aown A, Constantinidis C, Stolzenburg JU. Laparoscopic radical and partial nephrectomy: technical issues and outcome. Word J Urol. 2013;31(4):785–91.
2. Ren T, Liu Y, Zhao X, Ni S, Zhang C, Guo C, Ren M. Transperitoneal approach versus retroperitoneal approach: a meta-analysis of laparoscopic partial nephrectomy for renal cell carcinoma. PLoS One. 2014;9(3):e91978.
3. Fan X, Xu K, Lin T, Liu H, Yin Z, Dong W, Huang H, Huang J. Comparison of transperitoneal and retroperitoneal laparoscopic nephrectomy for renal cell carcinoma: a systematic review and meta-analysis. BJU Int. 2013;111(4):611–21.
4. Tan M, Law LS, Gan TJ. Optimizing pain management to facilitate enhanced recovery after surgery pathways. Can J Anaesth. 2015;62(2):203–18.
5. Nasrallah G, Souki FG. Peri-anesthetic management of laparoscopic kidney surgery. Curr Urol Rep. 2018;19:1):1.
6. Tsai HC, Yoshida T, Chuang TY, Yang SF, Chang CC, Yao HY, Tai YT, Lin JA, Chen KY. Transversus abdominis plane block: an updated review of anatomy and techniques. Biomed Res Int. 2017;2017:8284363.
7. Rafi AN. Abdominal field block via the lumbar triangle revisited. Anaesthesia. 2012;67(12):1399–401.
8. Tran TM, Ivanusic JJ, Hebbard P, Barrington MJ. Determination of spread of injectate after ultrasound-guided transversus abdominis plane block: a cadaveric study. Br J Anaesth. 2009;102(1):123–7.
9. Brogi E, Kazan R, Cyr S, Giunta F, Hemmerling TM. Transversus abdominal plane block for postoperative analgesia: a systematic review and meta-analysis of randomized-controlled trials. Can J Anaesth. 2016;63(10):1184–96.
10. Hosgood SA, Thiyagarajan UM, Nicholson HF, Jeyapalan I, Nicholson ML. Randomized clinical trial of transversus abdominis plane block versus placebo control in live-donor nephrectomy. Transplantation. 2012;94(5):520–5.
11. Parikh BK, Waghmare VT, Shah VR, Mehta T, Butala BP, Parikh GP, Vora KS. The analgesic efficacy of ultrasound-guided transversus abdominis plane block for retroperitoneoscopic donor nephrectomy: a randomized controlled study. Saudi J Anaesth. 2013;7(1):43–7.
12. Guner CM, Goz R, Berber I, Kaspar C, Cakir U. Ultrasound/laparoscopic camera-guided transversus abdominis plane block for renal transplant donors: a randomized controlled trial. Ann Transplant. 2015;20:418–23.
13. Aniskevich S, Taner CB, Perry DK, Robards CB, Porter SB, Thomas CS, Logvinov II, Clendenen SR. Ultrasound-guided transversus abdominis plane blocks for patients undergoing laparoscopic hand-assisted nephrectomy: a randomized, placebo-controlled trial. Local Reg Anesth. 2014;7:11–6.
14. Sakamoto H, Akita K, Sato T. An anatomical analysis of the relationships between the intercostal nerves and the thoracic and abdominal muscles in man. I. Ramification of the intercostal nerves. Acta Anat (Basel). 1996;156(2):132–42.
15. Hebbard PD, Barrington MJ, Vasey C. Ultrasound-guided continuous oblique subcostal transversus abdominis plane blockade: description of anatomy and clinical technique. Reg Anesth Pain Med. 2010;35(5):436–41.
16. Ma J, Pan Y, Yang J, Xie Z, Li J. Efficacy of mid-axillary approach to transversus abdominis plane block in each abdominal and back region. Chin J Anesthesiol. 2016;10(01):1247–9 (in chinese).
17. Qu G, Cui XL, Liu HJ, Ji ZG, Huang YG. Ultrasound-guided transversus abdominis plane block improves postoperative analgesia and early recovery in patients undergoing Retroperitoneoscopic urologic surgeries: a randomized controlled double-blinded trial big up tri, open. Chin Med Sci J. 2016;31(3):137–41.
18. Elsharkawy H, Ahuja S, DeGrande S, Maheshwari K, Chan V. Subcostal approach to anterior quadratus lumborum block for pain control following open urological procedures. J Anesth. 2019;33(1):148–54.
19. Ma N, Duncan JK, Scarfe AJ, Schuhmann S, Cameron AL. Clinical safety and effectiveness of transversus abdominis plane (TAP) block in post-operative analgesia: a systematic review and meta-analysis. J Anesth. 2017;31(3):432–52.

The erector spinae plane block causes only cutaneous sensory loss on ipsilateral posterior thorax

Jingxiong Zhang[1], Yuting He[1], Shi Wang[1], Zhengjie Chen[1], Yu Zhang[1], Yuan Gao[1], Quanguang Wang[1], Yun Xia[2], Thomas J. Papadimos[1,2] and Riyong Zhou[1*]

Abstract

Background: Ultrasound-guided erector spine plane (ESP) block is widely used in perioperative analgesia for back, chest and abdominal surgery. The extent and distribution of this block remain controversial. This study was performed to assess the analgesia range of an ultrasound-guided ESP block.

Methods: This prospective observational volunteer study consisted of 12 healthy volunteers. All volunteers received an erector spinae plane block at the left T5 transverse process using real-time ultrasound guidance. Measured the cutaneous sensory loss area (CSLA) and cutaneous sensory declination area (CSDA) using cold stimulation at different time points after blockade until its disappearance. The CSLA and CSDA were mapped and then calculated. The block range was described by spinous process level and lateral extension. The effective block duration for each volunteer was determined and recorded.

Results: The cold sensory loss concentrates at T6-T9. The decline concentrates primarily at T4-T11. The lateral diffusion of block to the left side did not cross the posterior axillary line, and reached the posterior median line on the right. The area of cutaneous sensory loss was (172 ± 57) cm^2, and the area of cutaneous sensory decline was (414 ± 143) cm^2. The duration of cutaneous sensory decline was (586 ± 28) minutes.

Conclusion: Ultrasound-guided erector spine plane block with 20 mL of 0. 5% ropivacaine provided a widespread cutaneous sensory block in the posterior thorax, but did not reach the anterior chest, lateral chest, or abdominal walls. The range of the blockade suggested that the dorsal branch of spinal nerve was blocked.

Keywords: Ultrasound, Nerve block, Erector Spinae plane, Cutaneous sensory block area, Volunteer study

* Correspondence: riyongzhou@126.com
[1]Department of Anesthesiology, the First Affiliated Hospital of Wenzhou Medical University, Zhejiang, China

Backgroud

Forero et al. [1] first reported the use of an ultrasound-guided ESP block, an interfascial plane block that successfully treats severe thoracic neuropathic pain. In ESP blockade, local anesthetic drugs are injected into the superficial or deep portion of the erector spinae using ultrasound guidance, then through the costotransverse foramina into the region of the spinal nerves and the origins of the dorsal and ventral rami [1]. It is simple, safe, and suitable to perform with an indwelling catheter to prolong postoperative analgesia, it may also prove to have the potential to replace the paravertebral block (PVB) in many clinical situations [2, 3].

Increasing cases of ultrasound-guided erector spinae plane block appeared in clinical applications [4, 5]. At the same time, in order to demonstrate the effect of ultrasound-guided ESP block, many clinical randomized controlled trials (RCT) have been conducted [3, 6–11]. Tulgar et al. [6] confirmed that bilateral ultrasound guided ESP block leads to effective analgesia and reduce analgesia requirement in first 12 h in patients undergoing laparoscopic cholecystectomy (LC). However, Chen et al. [7] demonstrated that ultrasound-guided multiple-injection PVB provided superior analgesia to intercostal nerve blocks (ICNB) and single-injection ESP block, while ICNB and single-injection ESP block were equally effective in reducing pain after thoracoscopic surgery. It has been reported that single-injection ESP block require more morphine [7]. Recently, a cadaveric study conducted by Aponte et al. [12] indicated that the dye and contrast agents diffuse in a cephalad-to-caudal direction in the dorsal region of T1-T11, and laterally diffuse to the ribs, as demonstrated by CT scan and anatomical observation. Moreover, no dye or contrast agent was observed to spread to the paravertebral region. Based on the contradiction between clinical trials and cadaveric research reports, it was of importance to perform a volunteer study to determine the range of the ESP block, and to clarify the applicability of the technique.

In this study, ultrasound-guided ESP blocks were performed in healthy volunteers, and the area of blockade was determined by dermal stimulation of cold sensors using ice. The main outcome measured was the range of sensory loss and decline in cutaneous cold sensation, and the secondary outcome measurement was the area of blockade and the duration of decreased cold sensation.

Methods

Volunteers

This observational volunteer study was approved by the University's Institutional Review Board (IRB No.2017–22) and written informed consent was obtained from all subjects participating in the trial. The trial was registered prior to patient enrollment at Chinese Clinical Trial Registry (registration number: CHiCTR1800014438), Principal investigator: Jingxiong Zhang, Date of registration: December 11th, 2017. This study adheres to the applicable CONSORT guidelines.

All 12 volunteers that were enrolled provided written informed consent. The age of volunteers ranged from 25 to 50 years old, and the study was not gender limited. Volunteers required an American society of anesthesiologists (ASA) physical classification system status of I-II, a Body mass index (BMI) of 18.5–28.0 kg/m^2, the area of study for cutaneous sensation needed to be intact in order to be confirmed by the cold stimulation test. Exclusion criteria were as follows: allergy to Ropivacaine or other drugs used in this trial, and inability to communicate, ASA grade ≥ 3, BMI less than 18.5 kg/m^2 or greater than 28 kg/m^2, abnormal platelet function or other coagulopathy, infectious disease of the skin sensation, abnormal skin sensation, spinal deformity, neuropathy, spinal cord disease, torso scar in area studied, and/or a history of abdominal surgery.

Procedures

Intravenous access was established after the subject was admitted into the designated block ward, and routine monitoring was performed in all participants (noninvasive blood pressure, continuous electrocardiogram, and pulse oximetry). All participants were sedated with 1 to 2 mL of an intravenous mixture of 20 μg/mL fentanyl and 1 mg/mL midazolam.

The volunteer was placed in a sitting position (Fig. 1a). The operator prepared a 80 mm 22G needle (Stimuplex® D; B. Braun Melsungen AG, Melsungen, Germany) and used a 38 mm wide high frequency 6-15MHZ ultrasound probe for high frequency linear sensors (Sonosite X-Porte; Sonosite Inc., Bothell, WA, USA), for block placement.

The apex of the left T5 transverse process (TP) was determined by using a high-frequency ultrasonic probe to identify the fifth rib, and then moved slowly in a medial direction to locate the transverse process. The apex of the T5 TP was identified by using the probe to determine the horizontal and sagittal sections of the T5 TP. The probe was placed in the longitudinal sagittal aspect to find the ultrasound image of the apex of T5 TP, approximately 3 cm lateral to the posterior medial line (Fig. 1b), and then the site was marked.

For the ESP blocks the operative area was disinfected, and the ultrasonic probe was covered with a sterile protective cover, and placed longitudinally at the marked point. The probe was adjusted to identify the three important layers of muscles (from posterior to anterior), i.e., trapezius, rhomboid, and erector spinae, and the optimal point for injection was identified (the apex of the left T5 TP). Local anesthesia with 1% lidocaine was instilled at the site of injection, 1 cm from the probe on

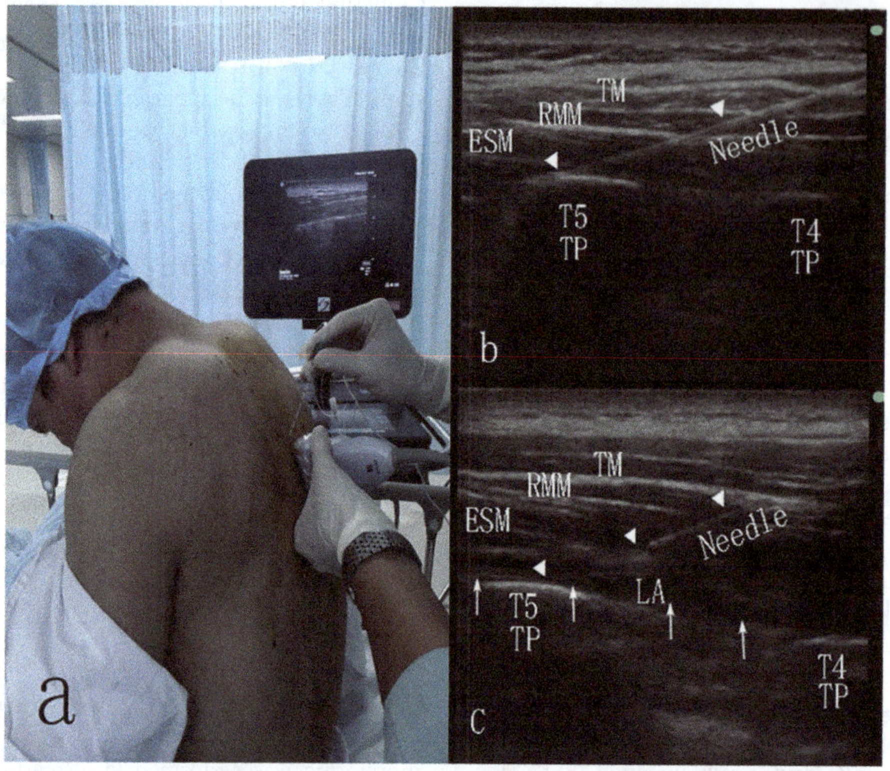

Fig. 1 **a**: Positioning and scanning during erector spinae plane (ESP) block. The needle is inserted in a cephalad-to-caudal direction; **b**: The needle (triangle indicates) is inserted through the trapezius muscle (TM), rhomboid major muscle (RMM) and Erector Spinae Muscle (ESM), to the transverse process; **c**: An injection at this point creates a linear pattern of local anesthetic spread (arrows) that displaces the ESM downward

the cephalad side. An 80 mm 22 G needle was inserted under ultrasound guidance (in plane), aiming towards the TP. Saline 1-2 ml was injected to determine the gap, and then 20 mL of 0. 5% ropivacaine (Naropin, AstraZeneca AB, Sweden) was injected. Another experienced anesthesiologist and the operator rechecked the needle tip and local anesthetic diffusion in the plane between the erector spinae and the TP with ultrasound (Fig. 1c).

Measurement and calculation

Important landmarks included: the posterior median line, the left scapular line, the left posterior line, the left 12th costal margin line, the left inferior angle of scapular, and the T1 to L4 spines (Fig. 2). For range of distribution measurements, the volunteers were kept in sitting position, and for the remaining time were in the supine position. The patients allowed to leave to urinate and to imbibe water as needed.

The determination of the cutaneous sensory block area was done using cold stimulation (ice cubes) by an attending physician (other than the operator) at 0.5 h, 1 h, and every hour after injection. According to previous experiments, the block lasts for 10 h. Thus, 9 h after the block, we measured every 15 min until cutaneous sensory returns to normal. The time from the end of injection to the last measurement was considered the blockade duration, and was recorded as such. Sensation was evaluated on a 3-point scale: 0 = loss of cold sensation, 1 = decreased cold sensation compared with the sensation at unaffected areas, 2 = normal sensation. The cold stimulus was moved laterally at approximately 2 cm/s from the opposite posterior axillary line at 1 cm intervals and measurements ceased at the left midaxillary line. During application of the cold stimulus, areas of sensory change were marked on the skin, and the marked dots were connected in order to map the blocked area. We marked block levels 1 and 0 with black and red dots, respectively. During the observation period, when the block range was no longer expanding, we connected the black and red dots to map the CSDA and CSLA. Then photos were taken (and saved) (Fig. 3). We covered the CSDA and CSLA with a 37 cm*52 cm transparent rectangular film, and then transferred all surface landmarks/lines to it.

Afterwards, the transferred transparency was converted into a transparent digital-based images with a fixed pixel value (1057*1485) (size: 37 cm*52 cm) using a scanner (Fujitsu FI-7460), and then saved as a JPG format (Fig. 3). After completing the trial, we used the magnetic lasso tool to select the target area that needed

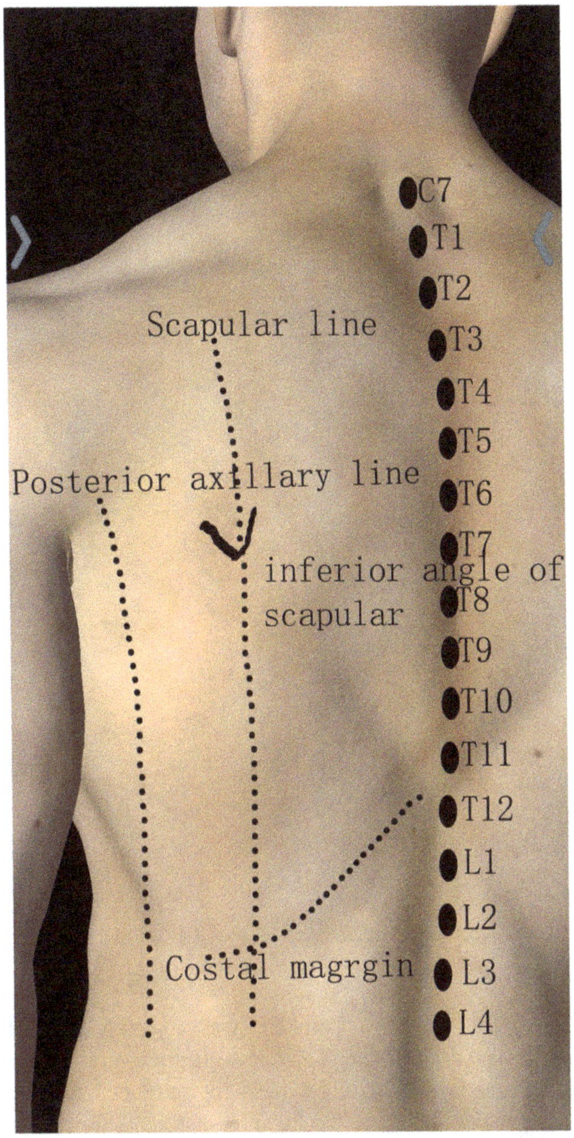

Fig. 2 Marked lines and points

to be calculated, and used the histogram toolbar to see/determine the pixel size of the selected area. The actual size of this digital picture was 1924 cm^2 [target area pixel / total pixel (fixed pixel)]. We were able to calculate the CSLA and CSDA. The highest and lowest level of spinous processes were observed and recorded.

Any systemic toxicity events regarding local anesthetics, nausea, and vomiting during the block were recorded.

Statistics analysis

Statistical analysis was performed with SPSS statistical software (version 21.0; SPSS, Chicago, Illinois) using the one-sample Kolmogorov-Smirnov normality test. The demographic data, cutaneous cold sensory area, and cutaneous sensory block duration, were expressed as mean ± SD.

Results

Demographic data

This study involved 12 volunteers, 8 were male. The ages ranged from 27 to 48 years, weight ranged from 62 kg to 79 kg, and height ranged from 158 cm to 177 cm. More details are in Table 1.

Block range of cold cutaneous sensation

The range of sensory loss was maximal at 1 h, with no further expansion. The cold sensory loss was from the T3 spinous process down to the T12 spinous process, and was most concentrated at T6-T9. Except for two volunteers, the lateral diffusion to the left side reached scapular line, did not cross the posterior axillary line; and to the right it reached 1 cm to the left of the posterior median line.

The cold sensory decline was from the T1 spinous process down to the L4 spinous process, and was concentrated at T4-T11. The lateral diffusion to the left side reached scapular line, did not cross the posterior axillary line, and to the right it reached the left of the posterior median line (Figs. 3 and 4).

Block area

The average cutaneous sensory block area in the left posterior thorax was (172 ± 57) cm^2, and the decline area was (414 ± 143) cm^2 at 1 h.

The duration of block

The ESP block retarded the cold cutaneous sensation in posterior thorax for 555--645 min, and the duration of sensory decline was (586 ± 28) minutes (Fig. 5).

Side effects and complications

During the operative/block process and subsequent measurement process, the general condition of the patients was very good, and there were no systemic toxicity events regarding local anesthetics, and there was no nausea and vomiting observed.

Discussion

This is a detailed volunteer study on the blockade range of the ultrasound-guided ESP block. The results of this study suggest that a 20 ml injection of 0.5% ropivacaine in the erector spinae plane administered to the left side of the T5 transverse process results in a significant block of the ipsilateral dorsal cutaneous sensory block. The cold sensory range of declination was from the T1 down to L4 spinous process, with a concentration at T4-T11, and a lateral effect extending between the posterior median and the posterior axillary line. The anterior chest wall, lateral chest wall and abdominal wall were not affected.

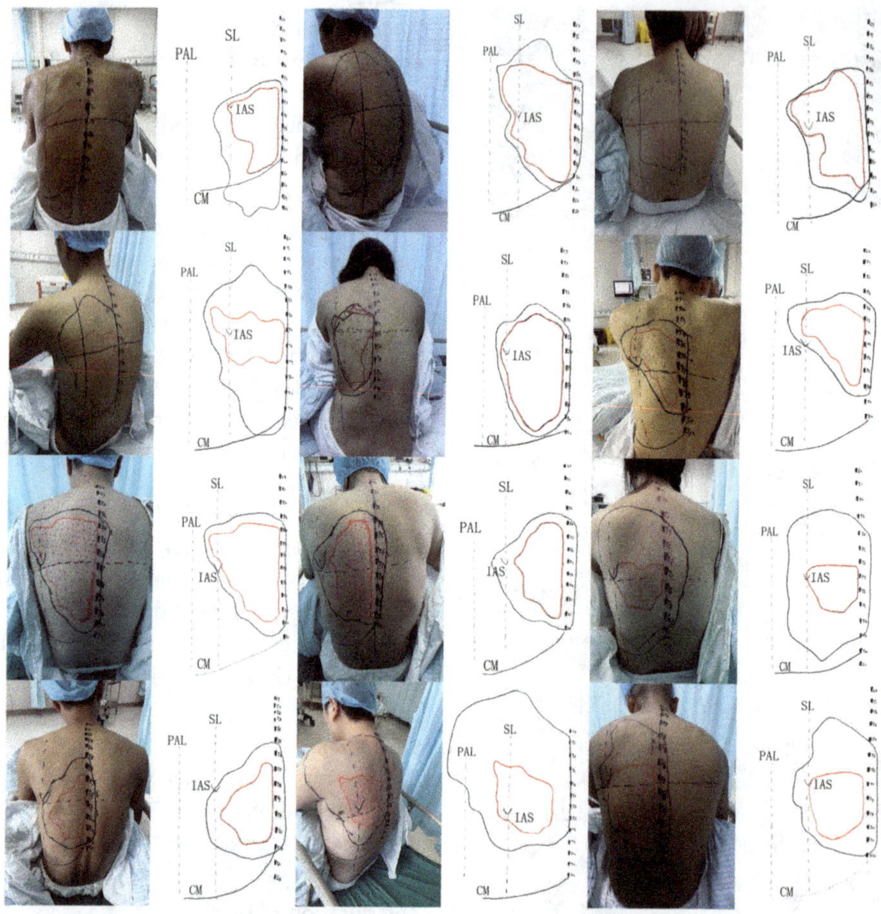

Fig. 3 Photos and scanned transparencies; scapular line (SL), posterior axillary line (PAL); costal margin (CM); inferior angle of scapula (IAS)

Table 1 Demographic data

Volunteer	Sex	Age (y)	Weight (kg)	Height (cm)	Body mass index (kg/m²)
#1	M	48	67	169	23.46
#2	F	47	62	158	24.84
#3	F	42	66	160	25.78
#4	M	27	73	180	22.53
#5	F	34	64	161	24.69
#6	M	38	60	169	21.01
#7	M	32	74	175	24.16
#8	M	30	73	176	23.57
#9	F	39	68	163	25.59
#10	M	31	72	173	24.06
#11	M	33	76	177	24.26
#12	M	35	79	175	25.80
Total	M:F(8:4)	36 ± 7	70 ± 6	170 ± 8	24.1 ± 1.4

The ESP block we applied, was injected the local anesthesia towards the TP, between transverse process and muscle layers. Actually, there are many clinical modifications to ESP block. Cosarcan SK et al. [13] advanced the needle over the intertransverse ligament, added the injection of local anesthetics above the superior costotransverse ligament (SCTL) to increase the spread into the paravertebral space. Tulgar S et al. [14] demonstrated different injection points of ESP block, costotransverse block (CTB),and mid-transverse process (MTP) block. It should be emphasized that our method of ESP block does not penetrate the intertransverse ligament. There are many problems with the modified ESP blocks mentioned in the article, such as their nomenclature problem, the problem of ligament recognition under ultrasound [14], which is contrary to the simplicity and safety of the traditional ESP block. Therefore, we insist on adopting traditional ESP block towards TP, while the modified ESP blocks are still controversial and out of our research scope.

Oksuz et al. [10] reported that bilateral ESP block after breast reduction is superior to local anesthesia in analgesic drug consumption and pain score. ESP blocks can be used

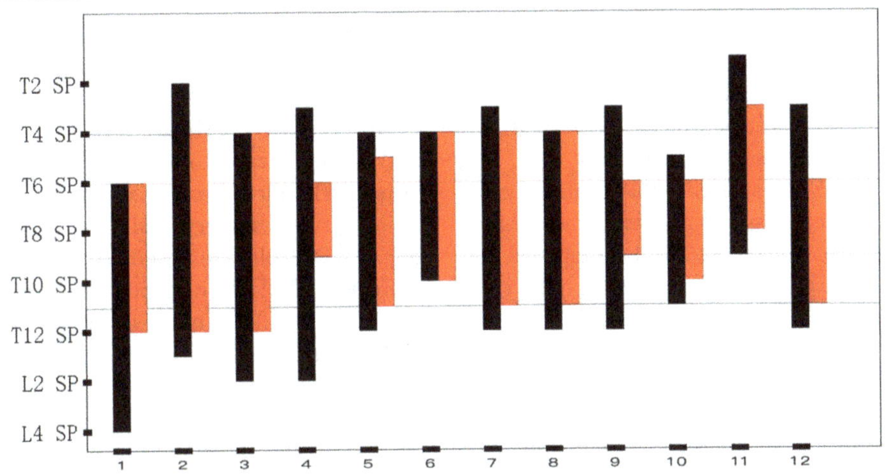

Fig. 4 The cold sensory block reached the spinous process (SP). The black bars represent the range of cold sensation declination, the red bars represent the range of cold sensation loss

as a suitable, effective and safe method of analgesia after mastectomy. However, Ueshima et al. [15] reported that an ESP block cannot effectively achieve the full analgesia of T2-T6 anterior branch, and cannot be assumed to provide complete analgesia for breast cancer surgery. Drennen et al. [16] questioned the pain scores of Oksuz et al. [10] in that they were higher when compared to previous reports, and questioned the efficacy and use of ESP block in breast reduction surgery without better evidence. Therefore, whether ESP block can produce reliable postoperative analgesia in breast surgery remains uncertain.

A single-center study [3] concluded that the ESP block and thoracic PVB have similar analgesic effects in patients undergoing open thoracic surgery. The advantage of ESP blocks is that they have a low incidence of adverse reactions. Taketa et al. [17] suggested that ESP blocks have the properties of a strong lateral cutaneous branch block that are similar to pectoral nerves (PECS) block, but not to PVB or ICNB. Whether ESP blocks can be effectively used in thoracoscopic surgery is still in dispute. Some reports have indicated [6, 11, 18] ESP blocks can be used for abdominal surgery.

Currently most clinical studies support the use of ESP blocks for postoperative analgesia in surgeries involving the posterior thorax, chest, and abdomen. The literature [1, 19, 20] indicates that the specific mechanism of the ESP block involves local anesthetic diffusion in a cephalad-to-caudal direction in the erector spinae plane. It may enter the paravertebral space through the connective tissue complex attached to the transverse process, and then on through the intervertebral foramen. Therein, the ventral and dorsal branches of the spinal nerve are blocked.

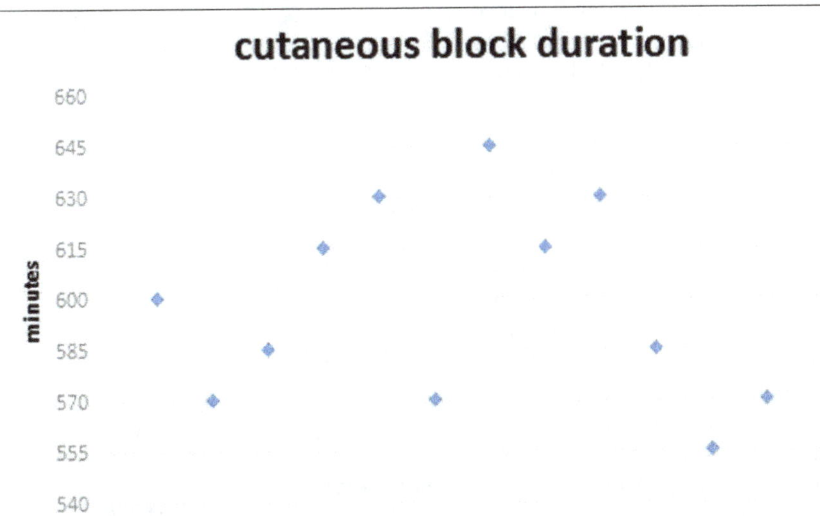

Fig. 5 The duration of cold sensory block

Gaweda et al. [9] conducted a RCT study that showed the addition of PECS block to ESP block improved postoperative pain control and increased patient satisfaction. If the mechanism of ESP block is diffusion to the paravertebral space, the results for both groups should be the same. Nuclear magnetic resonance studies by Adhikary et al. [21] and Schwartzmann et al. [20] suggested that contrast agents can enter the paravertebral space, and even the epidural space. Further cadaveric studies [22, 23] also suggested that dyes can enter the paravertebral area. However, other studies have raised concerns and objections. Otero PE et al. [24] according to inject dye in the erector spinae plane in a porcine living model, found there is no evidence of anterior spread of dye involving thoracic paravertebral or epidural spaces. The cadaver study by Ivanusic et al. [25] also demonstrated that there was no spread of dye anteriorly to the paravertebral space to involve the origins of the ventral and dorsal branches of the thoracic spinal nerves. Therefore, the theory of paravertebral diffusion and intercostal nerve block is not supported. They speculated that the lateral thoracic wall block may be related to the lateral diffusion of local anesthetic drugs affecting the lateral cutaneous branch of the intercostal nerve [25]. Taketa et al. [17] also confirmed the loss of cold sensation and the disappearance of acupuncture pain when measured at the anterior axillary line and the midclavicular line during an ESP block. Additionally, CT reconstruction by Forero et al. [1] and the use of nuclear magnetic resonance by Schwartzmann et al. [20] indicated that contrast media has limited diffusion to the lateral side. Adhikary et al. [21] made anatomical observations suggesting that in ESP blocks, the dye diffusion was within 10 cm from the posterior median line, thereby not supporting the theory of the lateral spread of local anesthetic drugs. There still remains contradictory evidence regarding paravertebral diffusion in ESP blocks between the different cadaveric studies and medical imaging studies.

Our volunteer trials suggested that ultrasound-guided ESP block only affects the dorsal branch of the ipsilateral spinal nerve. There was no evidence of the block affecting the paravertebral space, intercostal nerve, or lateral branch of the intercostal nerve. Nevertheless, we cannot exclude other anatomical mechanisms, independent of diffusion to the paravertebral space, which could result in the analgesic efficacy of the ESP block observed in clinical practice.

The thoracolumbar fascia, which is a complex structure of several layers that forms a girdle with a sustaining and stabilizing function, seems to contain a high density of nerves and sympathetic fibers [26]. The diffusion of local anesthetic drugs in the thoracolumbar fascia helps to modulate the somatic and visceral pain. Recently, Otero PE et al. [24] found that the thoracic lymph nodes were stained when exploring the mechanism of ESP block in a porcine model. They considered it might be that the local anesthesia entered the lymphatic reflux and desensitized the sensory nerve fibers connected to the lymphatic finger, contributing to clinical analgesic effects. Regardless of the mechanism, further clinical research is needed to apply ESP block to thoracoabdominal surgery.

However, the ESP block does produce a definite block in the dorsal branch of the spinal nerve, and can be used in pediatric oncological posterior thoracic [27] and posterior cervical surgery [28]. The future research directions of ESP block use should study the effect of high-thoracic ESP block in scapular surgery and cervical dorsal surgery, and the effect of middle and lower thoracic ESP blocks in thoracic vertebral surgery.

There are several limitations in our study: 1) this is a volunteer study and the sample size is small. There was not a large enough sample size to study drug concentration, capacity, and the effect of the patient's position on drug diffusion, 2) we only used cold stimulation to measure the cold sensation range. The pain sensitivity and tactile sensation were not measured, and the disappearance and decrease of the cold sensation were biased due to the subjective feelings of the volunteers.3) we didn't adopt modified ESP blocks, modified ESP blocks may lead to different results.

Conclusion

Ultrasound-guided ESP blocks using 20 mL of 0.5% ropivacaine can provide a widespread cutaneous sensory blockade of posterior chest wall, while sparing the anterior and lateral chest walls, and the abdominal wall. The range of blockade suggested only that the dorsal branch of spinal nerve was blocked.

Abbreviations

ESP: Erector spinae plane; CSLA: Cutaneous sensory loss area; CSDA: Cutaneous sensory declination area; PVB: Paravertebral block; RCT: Randomized controlled trial; LC: Laparoscopic cholecystectomy; ICNB: Intercostal nerve block; ASA: American Society of Anesthesiologists; BMI: Body mass index; TP: Transverse process; SCTL: Superior costotransverse ligament; CTB : Costotransverse block; MTP : Mid-transverse process; PECS: Pectoral nerves

Acknowledgements

Not applicable.

Authors' contributions

J.Z: this author helped study design, conduct of the study, data collection, data analysis and manuscript preparation. Y.H: this author helped conduct of the study. S.W: this author helped study design, conduct of the study and data collection. Z. C: this author helped data analysis. Y.Z: this author helped conduct of the study and data collection. Y.G: this author helped data collection. Q.W: this author helped data collection. Y.X: this author helped study design and data analysis. T.J.P: this author helped revising manuscript. R.Z: this author helped study design, conduct of the study, data analysis and manuscript preparation. All authors have read and approved the manuscript.

Author details

[1]Department of Anesthesiology, the First Affiliated Hospital of Wenzhou Medical University, Zhejiang, China. [2]Department of Anesthesiology, Ohio State University Wexner Medical Center, Columbus, OH, USA.

References

1. Forero M, Adhikary SD, Lopez H, Tsui C, Chin KJ. The erector Spinae plane block: a novel analgesic technique in thoracic neuropathic pain. Reg Anesth Pain Med. 2016;41(5):621–7.
2. Forero M, Rajarathinam M, Adhikary S, Chin KJ. Continuous erector Spinae plane block for rescue analgesia in thoracotomy after epidural failure: a case report. A A Case Rep. 2017;8(10):254–6.
3. Fang B, Wang Z, Huang X. Ultrasound-guided preoperative single-dose erector spinae plane block provides comparable analgesia to thoracic paravertebral block following thoracotomy: a single center randomized controlled double-blind study. Ann Transl Med. 2019;7(8):174.
4. Chin KJ, Malhas L, Perlas A. The erector Spinae plane block provides visceral abdominal analgesia in bariatric surgery: a report of 3 cases. Reg Anesth Pain Med. 2017;42(3):372–6.
5. Ueshima H, Otake H. Clinical experiences of ultrasound-guided erector spinae plane block for thoracic vertebra surgery. J Clin Anesth. 2017;38:137.
6. Tulgar S, Kapakli MS, Senturk O, Selvi O, Serifsoy TE, Ozer Z. Evaluation of ultrasound-guided erector spinae plane block for postoperative analgesia in laparoscopic cholecystectomy: a prospective, randomized, controlled clinical trial. J Clin Anesth. 2018;49:101–6.
7. Chen N, Qiao Q, Chen R, Xu Q, Zhang Y, Tian Y. The effect of ultrasound-guided intercostal nerve block, single-injection erector spinae plane block and multiple-injection paravertebral block on postoperative analgesia in thoracoscopic surgery: a randomized, double-blinded, clinical trial. J Clin Anesth. 2019;59:106–11.
8. Altiparmak B, Korkmaz Toker M, Uysal AI, Gumus Demirbilek S. Comparison of the efficacy of erector spinae plane block performed with different concentrations of bupivacaine on postoperative analgesia after mastectomy surgery: ramdomized, prospective, double blinded trial. BMC Anesthesiol. 2019;19(1):31.
9. Gaweda B, Borys M, Belina B, Bak J, Czuczwar M, Woloszczuk-Gebicka B, Kolowca M, Widenka K. Postoperative pain treatment with erector spinae plane block and pectoralis nerve blocks in patients undergoing mitral/tricuspid valve repair - a randomized controlled trial. BMC Anesthesiol. 2020; 20(1):51.
10. Oksuz G, Bilgen F, Arslan M, Duman Y, Urfalioglu A, Bilal B. Ultrasound-guided bilateral erector Spinae block versus tumescent anesthesia for postoperative analgesia in patients undergoing reduction mammoplasty: a randomized controlled study. Aesthet Plast Surg. 2019;43(2):291–6.
11. Abu Elyazed MM, Mostafa SF, Abdelghany MS, Eid GM. Ultrasound-guided erector Spinae plane block in patients undergoing open Epigastric hernia repair: a prospective randomized controlled study. Anesth Analg. 2019; 129(1):235–40.
12. Aponte A, Sala-Blanch X, Prats-Galino A, Masdeu J, Moreno LA, Sermeus LA. Anatomical evaluation of the extent of spread in the erector spinae plane block: a cadaveric study. Can J Anaesth. 2019;66(8):886–93.
13. Cosarcan SK, Dogan AT, Ercelen O, Gurkan Y. Superior costotransverse ligament is the main actor in permeability between the layers? Target-specific modification of erector spinae plane block. Reg Anesth Pain Med 2019.
14. Tulgar S, Ahiskalioglu A, Thomas DT, Gurkan Y. Should erector spinae plane block applications be standardized or should we revise nomenclature? Reg Anesth Pain Med. 2020;45(4):318–19.
15. Ueshima H, Otake H. Limitations of the erector Spinae plane (ESP) block for radical mastectomy. J Clin Anesth. 2018;51:97.
16. Drennen A. Erector spinae block to reduce pain after reduction mammoplasty: we need more evidence. Aesthetic Plast Surg. 2019;43(5): 1406–7.
17. Taketa Y, Irisawa Y, Fujitani T. Ultrasound-guided erector spinae plane block elicits sensory loss around the lateral, but not the parasternal, portion of the thorax. J Clin Anesth. 2018;47:84–5.
18. Restrepo-Garces CE, Chin KJ, Suarez P, Diaz A. Bilateral continuous erector Spinae plane block contributes to effective postoperative analgesia after major open abdominal surgery: a case report. A A Case Rep. 2017;9(11):319–21.
19. Chin KJ, Adhikary S, Sarwani N, Forero M. The analgesic efficacy of pre-operative bilateral erector spinae plane (ESP) blocks in patients having ventral hernia repair. Anaesthesia. 2017;72(4):452–60.
20. Schwartzmann A, Peng P, Maciel MA, Forero M. Mechanism of the erector spinae plane block: insights from a magnetic resonance imaging study. Can J Anaesth. 2018;65(10):1165–6.
21. Adhikary SD, Pruett A, Forero M, Thiruvenkatarajan V. Erector spinae plane block as an alternative to epidural analgesia for post-operative analgesia following video-assisted thoracoscopic surgery: a case study and a literature review on the spread of local anaesthetic in the erector spinae plane. Ind J Anaesth. 2018;62(1):75–8.
22. Vidal E, Giménez H, Forero M, Fajardo M. Erector spinae plane block: a cadaver study to determine its mechanism of action. Rev Esp Anestesiol Reanim. 2018;65(9):514–9.
23. Yang HM, Choi YJ, Kwon HJ, O J, Cho TH, Kim SH. Comparison of injectate spread and nerve involvement between retrolaminar and erector spinae plane blocks in the thoracic region: a cadaveric study. Anaesthesia. 2018; 73(10):1244–50.
24. Otero PE, Fuensalida SE, Russo PC, Verdier N, Blanco C, Portela DA. Mechanism of action of the erector spinae plane block: distribution of dye in a porcine model. Reg Anesth Pain Med. 2020;45(3):198–203.
25. Ivanusic J, Konishi Y, Barrington MJ. A cadaveric study investigating the mechanism of action of erector Spinae blockade. Reg Anesth Pain Med. 2018;43(6):567–71.
26. Willard FH, Vleeming A, Schuenke MD, Danneels L, Schleip R. The thoracolumbar fascia: anatomy, function and clinical considerations. J Anat. 2012;221(6):507–36.
27. Munoz F, Cubillos J, Bonilla AJ, Chin KJ. Erector spinae plane block for postoperative analgesia in pediatric oncological thoracic surgery. Can J Anaesth. 2017;64(8):880–2.
28. Evans HT, Leslie GJ, Rutka O, Keevil E, Burckett-St Laurent D. Bilateral erector Spinae plane block for surgery on the posterior aspect of the neck: a case report. A A Pract. 2019;12(10):356–8.

26

Effects of dexmedetomidine on stress hormones in patients undergoing cardiac valve replacement

Hanhua Wu[1†], Jinqing Tang[2†], Jiamei Pan[1], Ming Han[1], Huijun Cai[1] and Hong Zhang[1*]

Abstract

Background: Stress response always occurs in cardiac valve replacement patients undergoing cardiopulmonary bypass (CPB).

Methods: 60 patients undergoing cardiac valve replacement were recruited and randomized into control and Dex groups. Dex group received 1.0 µg·kg-1 of Dex for 10 min intravenously before anesthesia, followed by 0.5 µg·kg-1·h-1 of Dex, steadily administered throughout the procedure. And controlled group received the identical velocity of saline as Dex group. Plasma level of cortisol (Cor), epinephrine (E), norepinephrine (NE), and serotonin (5-HT) were evaluated at four timepoints: Before administration (T0), sawn sternum (T1), end of extracorporeal circulation (T2), and 24 h post operation (T3). General data of operation and recovery such as heart rate (HR), mean arterial pressure (MAP), intraoperative bispectral index (BIS), and hospitalization time in the intensive care unit (ICU) were also compared.

Results: Increase of Cor, E, NE, and 5-HT for the Dex group was significant lesser than that in the control group ($P < 0.05$), and ICU hospitalization time and ventilator support time was significantly shorter in the Dex group. The proportion of patients discharged from the hospital with better prognosis was significantly higher than that in the control group, while there were no significant differences in hospitalization costs and vasoactive drugs use between the two groups.

Conclusions: Dex reduces plasma Cor, E and NE elevations in patients after CPB, alleviates the stress reaction of the body, shortens the hospitalization time and ventilator support time in ICU, and plays a positive role in the rehabilitation of patients undergoing cardiac valve replacement.

Keywords: Dexmedetomidine, Cardiopulmonary bypass, Hormones

* Correspondence: zhzmcc@sina.com
Hanhua Wu and Jinqing Tang are Co-first author
[1]Department of Anesthesiology, Affiliated Hospital of Zunyi Medical University, No. 149 Dalian Road, Huichuan District, Zunyi 563003, Guizhou Province, China

Background

Cardiopulmonary bypass (CPB) immensely facilitated open heart surgical procedures such as cardiac valve replacement, benefitting patients for decades [1]. However, procedural exposure to a non-physiological condition, elicited a strong neuroendocrine stress response in patients due to several reasons such as cardiac arrest, blood dilution, and ischemia-reperfusion injury [2]. Generally, the serum hormones have a physiological circadian rhythm, with a peak in the morning between 8 and 9 a.m. Surgical stress response may be a major causative factor leading to physiological and biochemical disturbance of the homeostatic axes, primarily affecting the hypothalamic-pituitary-adrenal cortex (HPA) and locus coeruleus-sympathetic-adrenal medullary system [3]. Previously, changes in secretion of HPA related hormones such as corticotropin releasing hormone (CRH), adrenocorticotropic hormone (ACTH), glucocorticoid (GC) and Cortisol (Cor) were observed [4]. Similarly changes in the locus system related hormones such as noradrenaline (NE), epinephrine (E) and dopamine (DA) were observed [5, 6].

Increased secretion of surgical stress response associated hormones could cause tachycardia and elevate myocardial oxygen demand, peripheral vascular resistance, and oxygen consumption. Moreover, α-receptor activated sympathetic nerve stimulation may also lead to contraction of the coronary artery inducing myocardial ischemia [7]. Clinically, administration of anesthetic drugs to alleviate stress, could be effective in decreasing postoperative complications and mortality [8]. Dexmedetomidine hydrochloride (Dex) is a highly specific and selective α2 adrenergic receptor agonist (α2-AR), having the following physiological effects: sedation, analgesia, inhibition of sympathetic nerve, alleviation of inflammatory response, and reduction of stress response [9]. Moreover, Dex was effective for blunting the elevation in systolic blood pressure and stabilizing heart rate perioperatively. And it had little adverse effect [10].

We aimed to investigate if Dex can alleviate intraoperative stress response and accelerate patient recovery by observing its effects on Cor, E, NE, and 5-HT concentration in plasma of patients undergoing cardiac valve replacement.

Methods

Study design

This was a randomized controlled clinical trial to evaluate effects of Dex administration in order to control intraoperative stress response, by observing changes in hormone levels at different timepoints. The trial adheres to CONSORT guidelines and was approved by the Ethics Committee of the First Affiliated Hospital of Zunyi Medical University and registered in the China Clinical Trial Registry (Registration No. ChiCTR-IPR-17010954).

Participants

We selected patients who underwent cardiac valve replacement between 9:00 and 11:00 am, from March 2016 to April 2017, in the First Affiliated Hospital of Zunyi Medical University.

Inclusion criteria: (1) Age, 40–65 years; (2) American Society of Anesthesiologists (ASA) physical status classification of II or III; (3) expected operative time less than 5 h; (4) altitude of permanent residence less than 2500 m; (5) absence of symptoms of rheumatic fever (RF < 20).

Exclusion criteria: (1) Patients who discontinued anticoagulants for less than 3 days before operation; (2) Second cardiac surgery, (3) Hypertension (systolic blood pressure ≥ 180 mmHg or diastolic blood pressure ≥ 110 mmHg), anemia (hemoglobin less than 7.0 g/L), low blood volume or low protein (< 30 g/L); (4) Sinus node dysfunction with impaired conduction of impulses; (5) Severe liver dysfunction (AST > 120 U/L or ALT> 129 U/L), kidney dysfunction (SCR ≥ 150 μmol/L) and coagulation disorders (INR < 1.8 or INR > 2.0 for aortic valve replacement patients, INR < 2.0 or INR > 2.5 for mitral valve replacement patients, INR < 2.5 or INR > 3.0 for tricuspid valve replacement patients); (6) Severe pulmonary infections and diseases (imaging results of pulmonary inflammation or respiratory symptoms such as coughing); (7) Heparin resistance and allergy in patients.

Termination criteria: (1) Uncontrollable procedural emergencies; (2) If the patient's condition was serious and they could not be successfully rescued during or 24 h after surgery; (3) Re-cardiopulmonary bypass or surgery; (4) Difficulty in cardiac resuscitation (defibrillation > 4 beats) and cardiopulmonary bypass stopping; (5) Surgical procedures that could develop sever stress response such as intraaortic balloon pump, extracorporeal membrane oxygenation (ECMO), and deep hypothermic circulatory arrest.

The flow-diagram of participant selection is summarized in Fig. 1. Data of 60 patients were analyzed in this study.

Procedures and assessments

Participants received detailed information about this study and provided informed consent before baseline assessment, following which, study assistants opened a prepared sealed envelope containing group allocation information. Participants were randomly allocated to either a Dex group (0.2 mg Dex extracted to 50 mL normal saline) or control group (50 mL normal saline). In the Dex group (Group D), 1.0 μg·kg^{-1} Dex was infused intravenously for 10 min before inducing

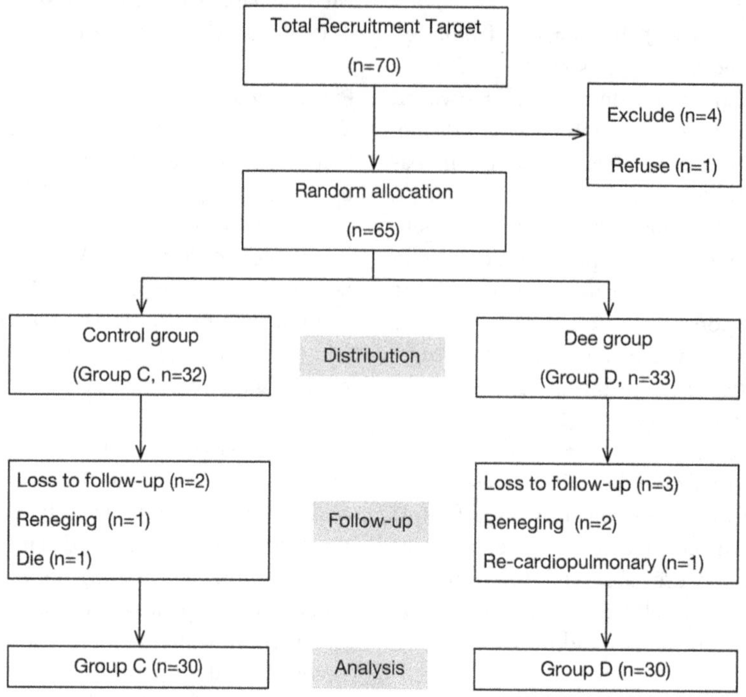

Fig. 1 Study flow chart

anesthesia. Subsequently, 0.5 μg·kg^{-1}·h^{-1} Dex was administered for maintenance until the end of operation. Participants in the control group (Group C) were administered saline at an infusion velocity identical to that of the Dex group, in the induction and maintenance phase of the procedure.

Demographic features such as gender, age, weight, ASA level and Euroscore were collected before the surgery. During the operation, the CPB transit time, ascending aorta occlusion time, operative time and condition of cardiac resuscitation (automatic cardiac resuscitation or cardiac resuscitation after defibrillation) were recorded. Moreover, four timepoints were chosen for testing the heart rate (HR), mean arterial pressure (MAP), bispectral index (BIS) and concentration of hormones in the blood as follows: before administration (T0), at sternum sawing (T1), at end of extracorporeal circulation (T2) and 24 h after operation (T3). Five milliliters of blood sample of each patients were tested for the level of Cor, E, NE and 5-HT. After the surgery, the hospitalization time in ICU, ventilator support time, condition of improvement and hospitalization expense were recorded and compared between two groups. The different vasoactive drugs use (during the operation and after the operation) was also recorded and compared between two groups of patients. Patients with improvement were defined as improvement of cardiac function, no abnormity of valve replacement, normal coagulation function and general condition. The primary outcome of this study were the plasma Cor, E, NE and 5-HT level at T3, while the concentration at other timepoints were considered as secondary outcomes. In addition, the secondary outcomes included HR, MAP and BIS at all follow-ups, the ICU hospitalization time, ventilator support time, proportion of patients with improvement and discharged from hospital, hospitalization costs and the intraoperative and postoperative vasoactive drug dosage.

Laboratory analysis

Cor in plasma was measured using an enzyme-linked immunosorbent assay (ELISA) kit (Shanghai Jianglai Biotechnology Co., Ltd. Shanghai). We evaluated E, NE, and 5-HT in plasma by High Performance Liquid Chromatography (HPLC) Using Agilent 1200 high performance liquid chromatography (Agilent Company, USA). The purity of E, NE, and 5-HT standard products was higher than 99%, purchased from Sigma Chemical Reagent Company. E was recovered by 100–117%. NE and 5-HT were successfully recovered by 100–110%, respectively, and relative standard deviation of less than 5%. The normal range for Cor was 20-250 ng/mL. Normal ranges were 0.30–3.00 pg/μL for E, 0.36–1.98 pg/μL for NE and 0.97–2.09 pg/μL for 5-HT.

Anesthesia induction and cardiopulmonary bypass management

Anesthesia induction was achieved with midazolam (0.06–0.1 mg·kg^{-1}), sufentanil (1–3 μg·kg^{-1}), etomidate fat emulsion (0.15–0.3 mg·kg^{-1}), and rocuronium (1 mg·kg^{-1}). Continuous propofol (4–12 mg·kg^{-1}·h^{-1}) and sufentanil (1–2 μg·kg^{-1}·h^{-1}) infusions were administered intraoperatively to maintain anesthesia and muscle relaxation, and inhalational anesthetics such as sevoflurane were also used in certain situation. To ensure the safety of our patients, we kept the hemodynamics and BIS in a safe range. In order to maintain effective visceral perfusion, the MAP was controlled between 50 and 80 mmHg, and the HR was maintained between 60 and 120 bpm. The BIS was maintained over 45 during anesthesia induction. Then the BIS was maintained between 40 and 60 during the surgery. Moreover, we also administered routine adjuvant drugs such as omeprazole, ulinastatin, and tranexamic acid.

Here, we used the cardiopulmonary bypass machine (C5, Sorin; Munich, Germany), hollow fiber super filter (0.8m^2, MicroPort, Dongguan, China), CPB pipeline (adult, TPRI; Tianjin, China), BIS monitoring module monitor (BeneViewT5, Mandary; Shenzhen, China) and membrane oxygenator (541,Medtronic, Memphis, United States). Crystal and colloid liquid ratio of CPB pre-filling fluid was approximately 1:1. Hematocrit (Hct) was maintained between 21 and 25%, and suspended red blood cells were administered as required. Pre-filling fluid volume was approximately 1700–2000 mL, and cardiopulmonary bypass was conducted during low body temperature and medium-high flow. After routine disinfection and laying the towel, skin incision, thoracotomy, 3 mg·kg^{-1} heparinization, and pericardiectomy were carried out through a median incision. CPB was established by connecting the superior and inferior vena cava and ascending aorta with the corresponding pipelines of the pre-filled artificial cardiopulmonary machine. We used a perfusion needle to fix the aortic root, followed by connecting a myocardial protective fluid perfusion device. We commenced CPB after activated prothrombin time (ACT) of > 480 s. During CPB, we maintained the nasopharyngeal temperature at 32–34 °C, Hct at 25–30%, perfusion flow between 50 and 100 mL·min^{-1}·kg^{-1}, and MAP at 50–80 mmHg. Furthermore, the ion-acid-base balance was maintained according to blood gas analysis. Both biological and artificial valves were used in this study.

Statistical analysis

For the sample size calculation, we considered a difference in E level of 1.0 pg/μL (δ) between the group treated with Dex and saline as clinically relevant and we specified such an effect to be detected with 90% power (0.9) and a significance level alpha of 0.05. For the population variance, our pilot study showed that in similar patients, the SD of E level was 1.3 pg/μL(σ). Then we used the formula $N = 2 \times [(\alpha + \beta)\ \sigma\ /\ \delta]^2$ to calculate the sample size, and the sample size was at least $N = 28$ patients in each group. The experimental data were analyzed by Statistical Package for the Social Sciences ver. 17.0 software (SPSS Inc., Chicago, IL). Measurement data were expressed by mean ± SD. Count variables were compared by the Chi squared test. Two independent sample t-test was used for inter-group comparison, and repeated measurement data variance analysis was used for intra-group comparison. We considered $P < 0.05$ as statistically significant.

Results

Initially 70 patients were recruited for the study, of which 5 were excluded (4 did not meet the criteria and 1 refused to participate). After randomized allocation, there were 32 cases in the control group and 33 cases in the Dex group. During the follow-up, 2 patients refused the test and quit halfway, 1 patient was re-operated and 1 patient expired. Finally, a total of 60 patients were included in the analysis, including 30 in Group C and 30 in Group D (Fig. 1).

Comparison of clinical data between the two groups

There were no significant differences in sex, age, weight, ASA category, Euroscore, CPB transit time, ascending aorta occlusion time, operative time, and cardiac resuscitation between the two groups ($P > 0.05$, Table 1).

Comparison of HR, MAP, and BIS in the two groups

There were no differences in BIS values at identical time points between the two groups ($P > 0.05$). MAP at T2 was lower than that at T0 in both the groups ($P < 0.05$), HR at T1 in the Dex group was the lowest, but within the normal clinical range. HR and MAP of both groups had no significant differences among other timepoints. At T1, HR in Group D was significantly lower than that in Group C ($P < 0.05$), with no significant change in MAP. Additionally, there were no significant differences in HR and MA*P* values between the two groups at other timepoints ($P > 0.05$, Table 2).

Comparison of plasma Cor, E, NE, and 5-HT levels in the two groups

In order to eliminate the influence of hemodilution after CPB on the results, Hct before CPB bypass was used as the standard reference. The formula was: correction value = measurement value * (Hct before bypass / Hct at the corresponding blood collection times).

Comparing the two groups at different times: Compared with T0, Cor, E and NE levels showed an increasing trend, while Cor and NE concentration in both groups at T1, T2, and T3 increased significantly ($P <$ 0.05). The plasma Cor concentration at T2 and T3 in Group C was significantly higher than that at T1 ($P <$

Table 1 Comparison of clinical data between the two groups

Clinical data	Group C ($n = 30$)	Group D ($n = 30$)	t(x^2)	*P*
Gender [M/F, n (%)]	19 (63)/11 (37)	16 (55)/14 (47)	0.617	0.432
Age (years)	51 ± 6	49 ± 4	1.420	0.161
Weight (kg)	55 ± 9	54 ± 8	0.015	0.988
ASA [II/III, n (%)]	5 (17)/25 (83)	9 (30)/21 (70)	1.491	0.222
Euroscore	2.03 ± 1.63	1.80 ± 1.58	0.562	0.576
CPB transit time (min)	115 ± 34	110.74 ± 37	0.502	0.618
Ascending aorta occlusion time (min)	73 ± 25	74 ± 36	0.150	0.881
Operative time (min)	247 ± 39	244 ± 49	0.261	0.795
Automatic cardiac resuscitation [YES/NO, n (%)]	2 (7)/28 (93)	3 (10)/27 (90)	0.218	0.640

0.05), while there were no significant differences for the same at T1, T2, and T3 in Group D. The plasma E concentration at T3 in Group C was significantly higher than that at T0 ($P < 0.05$), while there were no significant differences between the values at T1 and T2. There were no significant differences at T0, T1, T2, and T3 in group D. Plasma NE concentration at T0, T1, T2, and T3 in both groups, results showed a significantly increasing trend, while concentrations at each timepoint were significantly lower than the next timepoint ($P < 0.05$). The plasma 5-HT concentration at T2 and T3 was significantly higher than that at T0. When compared with T1, plasma 5-HT concentrations increased significantly at T2 and T3 ($P < 0.05$).

At T0, there was no significant difference in plasma E, NE, 5-HT, and Cor for both groups ($P > 0.05$). At T1, T2, and T3, the plasma E, NE, and Cor levels in Group D were lower than those in Group C ($P <$ 0.05). At T2 and T3, the plasma 5-HT levels in Group D were lower than those in Group C ($P < 0.05$, Figs. 2, 3, 4, and 5).

Postoperative follow-up

ICU hospitalization time ($P = 0.026$) and ventilator support time ($P = 0.042$) were significantly shortened in Group D than in Group C (Table 3). Proportion of patients with improvement and discharged from hospital was significantly increased ($P = 0.020$). There were no significant differences in hospitalization costs and the intraoperative and postoperative vasoactive drug dosage between the two groups ($P > 0.05$, Table 3 and Table 4).

Discussion

Our results showed plasma concentrations of Cor, E, NE, and 5-HT gradually increased with the prolongation of operation time. The plasma concentration of Cor, NE, and 5-HT at T2 was significantly higher than that at T0 and T1. Application of Dex preoperatively could significantly reduce plasma Cor, E, NE, and 5-HT concentrations than the control group, indicating that Dex could inhibit the stress response in patients undergoing valve replacement undergoing CPB. Moreover, 24-h follow-up showed that application of Dex could significantly improve ICU hospitalization time, ventilator support time, and rate of improvement and discharge, suggesting that it could be conducive to the recovery of patients who are undergoing CPB.

In our study, there was no difference between Dex and control group in terms of hemodynamics, and it might

Table 2 Comparison of HR, MAP and BIS in the two groups ($\overline{X}$ ±SD, $n = 30$)

Index	Group	T0	T1	T2	T3
HR (beats/min)	Group C	95 ± 23	98 ± 27	105 ± 20	103 ± 16
	Group D	94 ± 22	78 ± 14^{a*}	108 ± 18^{ab}	106 ± 16^{ab}
MAP (mmHg)	Group C	87 ± 13	83 ± 12	70 ± 10^{a}	78 ± 11^{a}
	Group D	91 ± 10	80 ± 14^{a}	74 ± 7^{a}	82 ± 9^{ac}
BIS	Group C	90.4 ± 1.7	37.9 ± 1.8	36.4 ± 1.7	–
	Group D	90.7 ± 1.8	38.3 ± 1.8	36.2 ± 1.7	–

T0 baseline; *T1* at sternum sawing; *T2* at shutdown; *T3* 24 h after operation
* $P < 0.05$ as compared with group C
[a] $P < 0.05$ as compared with T0
[b] $P < 0.05$ as compared with T1
[c] $P < 0.05$ as compared with T2

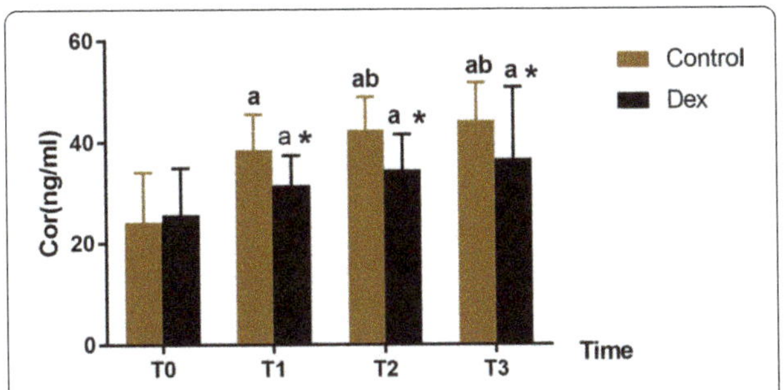

Fig. 2 Comparison of Cor concentration at different timepoints between the two groups

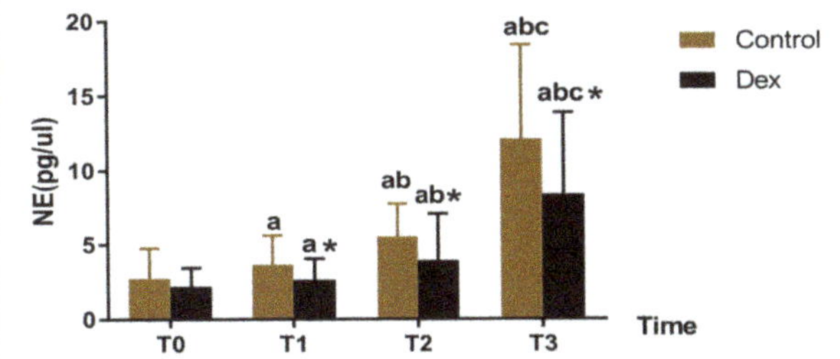

Fig. 4 Comparison of plasma NE concentration at different timepoints between the two groups

due to our study design. With regard to the MAP, Hashemian et al. found there was no difference between Dex and control group 0-2 h post CPB, and the difference of MAP was only found 1-2 h post operation [11]. Our study was partly in accordance with their results. However, the MAP of the control group was more than 80 mmHg 1-2 h post operation in their study, while we set our safe range of MAP between 50 and 80 mmHg. This unintentional control of HR and MAP might explain that we did not find any difference about HR and MAP between these two groups.

In healthy people, hormone secretion has a physiological circadian rhythm. For Cor, the peak of serum Cor concentration showed between 8 and 9 a.m. Then the concentration gradually decreased till 12–14 p.m. with a second peak during this period [12]. In our study, we chosen 9–11 a.m. to test the concentration of different hormones as for avoiding the impact of physiological circadian rhythm.

Recent study reported that the postoperative Cor levels did not show any difference between patients with and without CPB, which supported that CPB procedure did not specifically induce the stress response compared with other surgeries [13]. During the CPB procedure, an obvious increase of Cor and catecholamines level and presence of stress response have been reported in other studies [5, 13, 14], similar to our study. Cor is a stress response biomarker and is necessary in the defense reaction of the body [15]. Moreover, it has been reported that higher Cor levels are related to longer duration of stay, longer ventilator time, higher inotrope scores, and larger fluid requirement [16]. With regard to the effect of Dex on Cor released during operation, studies showed that it could inhibit Cor secretion [17]. However, there are studies which argue about the effects of short-term Dex usage in humans. Bekker et al. reported that Dex could have a negative impact on the plasma Cor levels [18]. However, Bulow et al. did not find any differences Cor levels while using Dex in the patients undergoing mini-CPB surgery [9]. In our study, we observed that patients in Dex group had a lower plasma Cor levels. Our study used etomidate for induction, which had been reported had negative effect on Cor level till 7 h postinduction [19]. However, both groups of patients received etomidate for induction, and we believed the difference on Cor level between Dex and control group could reflect the effect of Dex on plasma Cor level.

Considering plasma catecholamines levels, it has been reported that CPB is associated with the release of catecholamines. However, our results showed a slight increase in the E and significant change in the NE values after CPB, contrary to the result of a previous study, which indicated that the elevation of plasma E level was several times higher than the plasma NE level in patients after CPB [20]. This might be due to differences in the

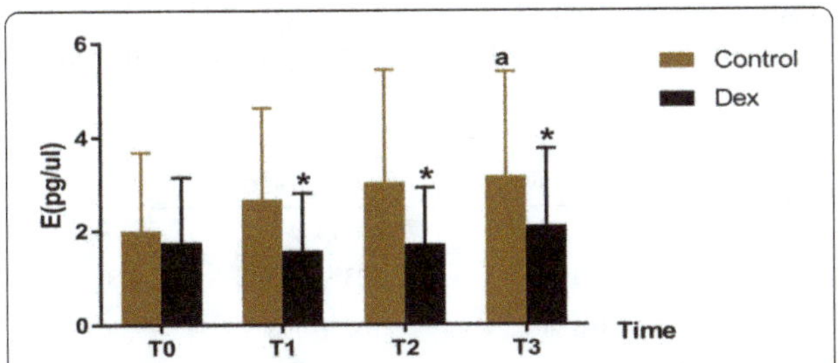

Fig. 3 Comparison of plasma E concentration at different timepoints between the two groups

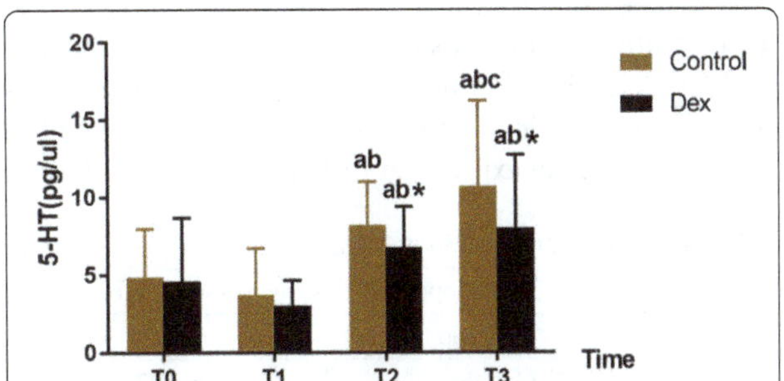

Fig. 5 Comparison of plasma 5-HT concentration at different timepoints between the two groups. Different timepoints as follows: T0: baseline; T1: at sternum sawing; T2: at end of extracorporeal circulation; T3: 24 h after operation

Table 3 Comparison of postoperative follow-up between the two groups ($\overline{X}$ ±SD, $n = 30$)

Postoperative follow-up	Group C	Group D	t(x^2)	P value
Hospitalization time in ICU (h)	90.4 ± 72.0	55.4 ± 41.9	2.30	0.026
Ventilator support time (h)	44.5 ± 40.20	19.3 ± 16.3	2.11	0.042
Patients with improvement^ [YES/NO, n (%)]	25 (83)/5 (17)	30 (100)/0 (0)	5.46	0.020
Hospitalization expenses (Ten thousand yuan)	12.5 ± 5.1	11.4 ± 4.4	0.57	0.572

^ Patients with improvement were defined as improvement of cardiac function, no abnormity of valve replacement, normal coagulation function and general condition

activation of the sympathetic nerve and adrenal medulla [21]. Plasma NE level is primarily affected by the activation of sympathetic system, which is particularly mediated by baroreceptor activation and physical issues. Additionally, hypothermia might significantly affect sympathetic nerve activation, resulting in increased plasma NE levels [20]. However, plasma E level is primarily associated with psychological stress and general and metabolic threat. Due to surgical intervention and the application of anesthetic drugs such as opioids, external nerve afferent impulse and neuroendocrine autonomic response might be blocked, resulting in an imbalances change of plasma E and NE levels [22].

Additionally, we observed that Dex had negatively affected both plasma E and NE levels than the control group, similar to a previous report, suggesting that the application of Dex could significantly lower the plasma Cor, E, NE, and blood glucose in pediatric cardiac surgery [23]. As the selective α2-AR agonist, Dex could specifically bind to presynaptic α2-AR and inhibit central sympathetic outflow trough a negative feedback mechanism. Due to the fact that these receptors are primarily located in the brain stem and locus coeruleus, Dex administration could significantly affect plasma NE levels [24]. Furthermore, a previous study also reported that Dex could suppress NE transporters by competitively inhibiting substrate transport [25]. With regard to the changes in the plasma E levels, it is our assumption that it might be due to the activation of both pre- and post-synaptic α ARs.

It has been reported that Dex could also inhibit the release of other neurotransmitters such as γ-aminobutyric acid, DA, and 5-HT in non-adrenergic neurons [26]. According to a previous animal study, 5-HT is involved in regulation of gene expression of hypothalamic hormones and the secretion of pituitary gland hormones. The study showed that 5-HT1A receptor activation promoted acetylcholine and NE release in brain and increased the blood concentration of CRH, ACTH, and Cor [27]. Dex administration could be significantly more beneficial in treating serotonin syndrome than the current treatment involving the use of benzodiazepines in rats [28]. There is also clinical evidence demonstrating that Dex could temporally stabilize the autonomic nervous system, improve agitation, and benefit successful extubation in three cases of severe serotonin syndrome [29]. Here, we also found Dex had a negative effect on the plasma 5-HT levels of patients who underwent CPB, which might indirectly contribute to decreased Cor and catecholamine levels. Moreover, it might have a direct effect on the central 5-HT system, resulting in improved recovery after the procedure.

In our study, we found that although Dex had an elimination half-life of 2-3 h, patients received Dex treatment showed lower plasma Cor, E, NE and 5-HT level 24 h after the surgery. It might due to the protective effect of Dex during the surgery, which lead to relatively low level of plasma hormone after surgery. Moreover, it might reduce the stress and inflammatory response, and prevent the cardiac complications among adults undergoing surgery [9, 24]. Chi et al. found that intraoperatively Dex use could attenuates myocardial injury in off-pump coronary artery bypass graft surgery, and it could stabilize the HR even 48 h after surgery [30]. In our study, we found patients in Dex group had shorter ventilator time and hospitalization time, and it might also due to the protective effect of Dex during the surgery. As an α2 adrenergic receptor agonist, Dex has minimal effects on respiration compared with other drugs [31]. Moreover, Dex could attenuate the lung injury and inflammation

Table 4 Comparison of dosage of vasoactive drugs used during and after the operation ($\overline{X}$ ±SD, mg)

Vasoactive drugs	Intraoperative dosage of vasoactive drugs (mg)			Postoperative dosage of vasoactive drugs (mg)		
	Group C	Group D	P value	Group C	Group D	P value
Adrenaline	0.55 ± 0.06	0.55 ± 0.07	0.798	0.97 ± 0.10	0.93 ± 0.17	0.272
Deoxyepinephrine	0.22 ± 0.18	0.22 ± 0.19	0.891	0.48 ± 0.34	0.47 ± 0.31	0.910
Dopamine	55.23 ± 7.10	55.00 ± 8.59	0.911	155.53 ± 18.42	155.44 ± 17.52	0.983
Glyceryl trinitrate	5.48 ± 0.74	5.46 ± 0.71	0.958	5.06 ± 0.68	4.99 ± 0.71	0.730

due to causes such as ischemia-reperfusion and ventilator, which might benefit respiratory function and reduce ventilator time [32, 33]. With regard to hospitalization time, study reported that intraoperative use of Dex was associated with faster recovery in patients who underwent major spinal surgery [18]. In addition, less postoperative complications might also lead to shorter hospitalization time.

There are certain limitations of our study. First, the sample size in our study is comparatively small, which might negatively influence our data. Second, we observed that a significant increase of plasma E level at T3, which might be correlated to the continued postoperative pumping of E and stimulus of intubation, misleading the real physical values of plasma E. Third, samples could only be collected from the blood plasma, which reflects the real situation from a single perspective. Fourthly, we conducted our surgeries between 9 and 11 am. Although this period is after the peak of the plasma Cor level, the circadian rhythm of Cor could still be a factor affecting the results. Lastly, after Dex administration, there may be a significant decrease in the heart rate, which may lead to the failure of the double blinded design for this clinical trial.

Conclusions

Patients underwent CPB developed elevation of Cor, E, NE and 5-HT during the surgery. Dexmedetomidine can reduce Cor, E, NE, and 5-HT elevation in plasma after CPB in patients undergoing cardiac valve replacement, which then alleviated the stress response of the body. Moreover, it could shorten the hospitalization time and ventilator support time in the ICU, and had a positive effect on patient rehabilitation.

Abbreviations

5-HT: Serotonin; ACT: Activated prothrombin time; ACTH: Adrenocorticotropic hormone; ASA: American Society of Anesthesiologists; BIS: Bispectral index; Cor: Cortisol; CPB: Cardiopulmonary bypass; CRH: Corticotropin releasing hormone; DA: Dopamine; Dex: Dexmedetomidine hydrochloride; E: Epinephrine; ECMO: Extracorporeal membrane oxygenation; ELISA: Enzyme-linked immunosorbent assay; GC: Glucocorticoid; Hct: Hematocrit; HPA: Hypothalamic-pituitary-adrenal cortex; HPLC: High Performance Liquid Chromatography; HR: Heart rate; ICU: Intensive care unit; MAP: Mean arterial pressure; NE: Norepinephrine; α2-AR: α2 adrenergic receptor agonist

Acknowledgements

Not applicable.

Authors' contributions

HHW and JQT developed the concept and drafted the manuscript; JMP and MH performed the experiments and data acquisition; HJC contributed to the literature research and data analysis; HZ revised the manuscript. All have read the final version of this paper and have agreed with this submission.

Author details

[1]Department of Anesthesiology, Affiliated Hospital of Zunyi Medical University, No. 149 Dalian Road, Huichuan District, Zunyi 563003, Guizhou Province, China. [2]Department of Anesthesiology, Third Affiliated Hospital of Zunyi Medical University, Zunyi 563003, Guizhou Province, China.

References

1. Featherstone PJ, Ball CM. The origins of cardiopulmonary bypass. Anaesth Intensive Care. 2018;46(4):351–3.
2. Zakkar M, Guida G, Suleiman MS, Angelini GD. Cardiopulmonary bypass and oxidative stress. Oxidative Med Cell Longev. 2015;2015:189863.
3. Mauricio Del Rio J, Nicoara A, Swaminathan M. Neuroendocrine stress response: implications for cardiac surgery-associated acute kidney injury. Rom J Anaesth Intensive Care. 2017;24(1):57–63.
4. Gajarski RJ, Stefanelli CB, Graziano JN, Kaciroti N, Charpie JR, Vazquez D. Adrenocortical response in infants undergoing cardiac surgery with cardiopulmonary bypass and circulatory arrest. Pediatr Crit Care Med. 2010; 11(1):44–51.
5. Winterhalter M, Brandl K, Rahe-Meyer N, Osthaus A, Hecker H, Hagl C, Adams HA, Piepenbrock S. Endocrine stress response and inflammatory activation during CABG surgery. A randomized trial comparing remifentanil infusion to intermittent fentanyl. Eur J Anaesthesiol. 2008;25(4):326–35.
6. Tan CK, Glisson SN, El-Etr AA, Ramakrishnaiah KB. Levels of circulating norepinephrine and epinephrine before, during, and after cardiopulmonary bypass in man. J Thorac Cardiovasc Surg. 1976;71(6):928–31.
7. Onk D, Akarsu Ayazoglu T, Onk OA, Aksut M, Gunay M, Turkmen K, Ozensoy A, Yazici Ersoy C, Coban A. Comparison of TIVA and Desflurane added to a Subanaesthetic dose of Propofol in patients undergoing coronary artery bypass surgery: evaluation of Haemodynamic and stress hormone changes. Biomed Res Int. 2016;2016:3272530.
8. Wijeysundera DN, Naik JS, Beattie WS. Alpha-2 adrenergic agonists to prevent perioperative cardiovascular complications: a meta-analysis. Am J Med. 2003;114(9):742–52.
9. Bulow NM, Colpo E, Pereira RP, Correa EF, Waczuk EP, Duarte MF, Rocha JB. Dexmedetomidine decreases the inflammatory response to myocardial surgery under mini-cardiopulmonary bypass. Braz J Med Biol Res. 2016;49(4): e4646.
10. Wang XW, Cao JB, Lv BS, Mi WD, Wang ZQ, Zhang C, Wang HL, Xu Z. Effect of perioperative dexmedetomidine on the endocrine modulators of stress response: a meta-analysis. Clin Exp Pharmacol Physiol. 2015;42(8):828–36.
11. Hashemian M, Ahmadinejad M, Mohajerani SA, Mirkheshti A. Impact of dexmedetomidine on hemodynamic changes during and after coronary artery bypass grafting. Ann Card Anaesth. 2017;20(2):152–7.
12. Debono M, Ghobadi C, Rostami-Hodjegan A, Huatan H, Campbell MJ, Newell-Price J, Darzy K, Merke DP, Arlt W, Ross RJ. Modified-release hydrocortisone to provide circadian cortisol profiles. J Clin Endocrinol Metab. 2009;94(5):1548–54.
13. Glumac S, Kardum G, Karanovic N. A prospective cohort evaluation of the cortisol response to cardiac surgery with occurrence of early postoperative cognitive decline. Med Sci Monit. 2018;24:977–86.
14. Bangalore H, Checchia PA, Ocampo EC, Heinle JS, Minard CG, Shekerdemian LS. Cortisol response in children after second cardiopulmonary bypass. Pediatr Cardiol. 2019;40(1):47–52.
15. Hoda MR, El-Achkar H, Schmitz E, Scheffold T, Vetter HO, De Simone R. Systemic stress hormone response in patients undergoing open heart surgery with or without cardiopulmonary bypass. Ann Thorac Surg. 2006; 82(6):2179–86.
16. Wald EL, Preze E, Eickhoff JC, Backer CL. The effect of cardiopulmonary bypass on the hypothalamic-pituitary-adrenal axis in children. Pediatr Crit Care Med. 2011;12(2):190–6.
17. Maze M, Virtanen R, Daunt D, Banks SJ, Stover EP, Feldman D. Effects of dexmedetomidine, a novel imidazole sedative-anesthetic agent, on adrenal steroidogenesis: in vivo and in vitro studies. Anesth Analg. 1991;73(2):204–8.
18. Bekker A, Haile M, Kline R, Didehvar S, Babu R, Martiniuk F, Urban M. The effect of intraoperative infusion of dexmedetomidine on the quality of recovery after major spinal surgery. J Neurosurg Anesthesiol. 2013;25(1):16–24.
19. Hohl CM, Kelly-Smith CH, Yeung TC, Sweet DD, Doyle-Waters MM, Schulzer M. The effect of a bolus dose of etomidate on cortisol levels, mortality, and health services utilization: a systematic review. Ann Emerg Med. 2010;56(2): 105–13 e105.
20. Corr L, Grounds RM, Brown MJ, Whitwam JG. Plasma catecholamine changes during cardiopulmonary bypass: a randomised double blind comparison of trimetaphan camsylate and sodium nitroprusside. Br Heart J. 1986;56(1):89–93.
21. Zamparelli R, De Paulis S, Martinelli L, Rossi M, Scapigliati A, Sciarra M, Meo F, Schiavello R. Pulsatile normothermic cardiopulmonary bypass and plasma catecholamine levels. Perfusion. 2000;15(3):217–23.
22. Okuyama K, Wada K, Sakurada S, Mizoguchi H, Komatsu H, Sora I, Tamura G,

Ohkawara Y, Takayanagi M, Ohno I. The involvement of micro-opioid receptors in the central nervous system in the worsening of allergic airway inflammation by psychological stress in mice. Int Arch Allergy Immunol. 2010;152(4):342–52.

23. Mukhtar AM, Obayah EM, Hassona AM. The use of dexmedetomidine in pediatric cardiac surgery. Anesth Analg. 2006;103(1):52–6.
24. Duncan D, Sankar A, Beattie WS, Wijeysundera DN. Alpha-2 adrenergic agonists for the prevention of cardiac complications among adults undergoing surgery. Cochrane Database Syst Rev. 2018;3:CD004126.
25. Park JW, Chung HW, Lee EJ, Jung KH, Paik JY, Lee KH. alpha2-adrenergic agonists including xylazine and dexmedetomidine inhibit norepinephrine transporter function in SK-N-SH cells. Neurosci Lett. 2013;541:184–9.
26. Kiski D, Malec E, Schmidt C. Use of dexmedetomidine in pediatric cardiac anesthesia. Curr Opin Anaesthesiol. 2019;32(3):334–42.
27. Jorgensen HS. Studies on the neuroendocrine role of serotonin. Dan Med Bull. 2007;54(4):266–88.
28. Kawano T, Takahashi T, Kaminaga S, Kadono T, Yamanaka D, Iwata H, Eguchi S, Yokoyama M. A comparison of midazolam and dexmedetomidine for the recovery of serotonin syndrome in rats. J Anesth. 2015;29(4):631–4.
29. Rushton WF, Charlton NP. Dexmedetomidine in the treatment of serotonin syndrome. Ann Pharmacother. 2014;48(12):1651–4.
30. Chi X, Liao M, Chen X, Zhao Y, Yang L, Luo A, Yang H. Dexmedetomidine attenuates myocardial injury in off-pump coronary artery bypass graft surgery. J Cardiothorac Vasc Anesth. 2016;30(1):44–50.
31. Kim MH, Lee KY, Bae SJ, Jo M, Cho JS. Intraoperative dexmedetomidine attenuates stress responses in patients undergoing major spine surgery. Minerva Anestesiol. 2019;85(5):468–77.
32. Yang CL, Tsai PS, Huang CJ. Effects of dexmedetomidine on regulating pulmonary inflammation in a rat model of ventilator-induced lung injury. Acta Anaesthesiol Taiwanica. 2008;46(4):151–9.
33. Zhang W, Zhang JQ, Meng FM, Xue FS. Dexmedetomidine protects against lung ischemia-reperfusion injury by the PI3K/Akt/HIF-1alpha signaling pathway. J Anesth. 2016;30(5):826–33.

Permissions

All chapters in this book were first published by BioMed Central; hereby published with permission under the Creative Commons Attribution License or equivalent. Every chapter published in this book has been scrutinized by our experts. Their significance has been extensively debated. The topics covered herein carry significant findings which will fuel the growth of the discipline. They may even be implemented as practical applications or may be referred to as a beginning point for another development.

The contributors of this book come from diverse backgrounds, making this book a truly international effort. This book will bring forth new frontiers with its revolutionizing research information and detailed analysis of the nascent developments around the world.

We would like to thank all the contributing authors for lending their expertise to make the book truly unique. They have played a crucial role in the development of this book. Without their invaluable contributions this book wouldn't have been possible. They have made vital efforts to compile up to date information on the varied aspects of this subject to make this book a valuable addition to the collection of many professionals and students.

This book was conceptualized with the vision of imparting up-to-date information and advanced data in this field. To ensure the same, a matchless editorial board was set up. Every individual on the board went through rigorous rounds of assessment to prove their worth. After which they invested a large part of their time researching and compiling the most relevant data for our readers.

The editorial board has been involved in producing this book since its inception. They have spent rigorous hours researching and exploring the diverse topics which have resulted in the successful publishing of this book. They have passed on their knowledge of decades through this book. To expedite this challenging task, the publisher supported the team at every step. A small team of assistant editors was also appointed to further simplify the editing procedure and attain best results for the readers.

Apart from the editorial board, the designing team has also invested a significant amount of their time in understanding the subject and creating the most relevant covers. They scrutinized every image to scout for the most suitable representation of the subject and create an appropriate cover for the book.

The publishing team has been an ardent support to the editorial, designing and production team. Their endless efforts to recruit the best for this project, has resulted in the accomplishment of this book. They are a veteran in the field of academics and their pool of knowledge is as vast as their experience in printing. Their expertise and guidance has proved useful at every step. Their uncompromising quality standards have made this book an exceptional effort. Their encouragement from time to time has been an inspiration for everyone.

The publisher and the editorial board hope that this book will prove to be a valuable piece of knowledge for researchers, students, practitioners and scholars across the globe.

List of Contributors

Pierre-Antoine Allain, Michele Carella, El-Mahdi Hafiani and Yacine Ynineb
Service d'Anesthésie-Réanimation et Médecine Péri-opératoire, AP-HP Hôpital Tenon, 4 rue de la Chine, 75020 Paris, France

Julien Burey, Francis Bonnet, Marc Garnier and Christophe Quesnel
Service d'Anesthésie-Réanimation et Médecine Péri-opératoire, AP-HP Hôpital Tenon, 4 rue de la Chine, 75020 Paris, France
Faculté de médecine Sorbonne Université (Paris VI), Paris, France

Apostolos C. Agrafiotis
Service de chirurgie thoracique, AP-HP Hôpital Tenon, 4 rue de la Chine, 75020 Paris, France

Jalal Assouad
Service de chirurgie thoracique, AP-HP Hôpital Tenon, 4 rue de la Chine, 75020 Paris, France
Faculté de médecine Sorbonne Université (Paris VI), Paris, France

Dita Aditianingsih, Pryambodho, Naufal Anasy and Aida Rosita Tantri
Department of Anesthesiology and Intensive Care, Cipto Mangunkusumo General Hospital, Universitas Indonesia, 6th Salemba Raya, DKI Jakarta 10430, Indonesia

Chaidir Arif Mochtar
Department of Urology, Cipto Mangunkusumo General Hospital, Universitas Indonesia, DKI Jakarta, Indonesia

Ferda Yaman
Department of Anesthesiology and Reanimation, Faculty of Medicine, University of Eskişehir Osmangazi, 26040 Eskişehir, Turkey

Devrim Tuglu
Department of Urology, Faculty of Medicine, University of Kırıkkale, Kırıkkale, Turkey

Luning Chen, Jingjing Ji, Yali Tian, Qing Sun and Bingbing Li
Department of Anesthesiology, Drum Tower Hospital Affiliated Nanjing University Medical School, Road 321#, Nanjing, Zhongshan 210008, China

Xuefeng Qiu and Xiaogong Li
Department of Surgery, Urology Surgery, Drum Tower Hospital Affiliated Nanjing University Medical School, Road 321#, Nanjing, Zhongshan 210008, China

Jung-Woo Shim, Yun Jeong Cho, Sang Hyun Hong, and Min Suk Chae
Department of Anesthesiology and Pain medicine, Seoul St. Mary's Hospital, College of Medicine, The Catholic University of Korea, 222, Banpo-daero, Seocho-gu, Seoul 06591, Republic of Korea

Minhee Kim
Department of Anesthesiology and Pain medicine, Bucheon St. Mary's Hospital, College of Medicine, The Catholic University of Korea, Seoul, Republic of Korea

Hyong Woo Moon and Sung Hoo Hong
Department of Urology, Seoul St. Mary's Hospital, College of Medicine, The Catholic University of Korea, Seoul, Republic of Korea

Huai Jin Li and Zhi Yu Geng
Department of Anesthesiology, Peking University First Hospital, Beijing, China

Shan Liu
Department of Anesthesiology, Beijing Shangdi Hospital, Beijing, China

Xue Ying Li
Department of Biostatics, Peking University First Hospital, Beijing, China

Chaosheng Qin, Jijun Xiong, Xiaogang Wang, Qinghua Dong and Jingchen Liu
Department of Anesthesiology, The First Affiliated Hospital of Guangxi Medical University, Nanning, Guangxi 530021, People's Republic of China

Yuanming Liu
Department of Ultrasound, Affiliated Hospital of Guilin Medical University, Guilin, Guangxi 541001, People's Republic of China

Tingshi Su
Department of radiotherapy, Affiliated Tumor Hospital of Guangxi Medical University, Nanning, Guangxi 530021, People's Republic of China

Peng-fei Gao, Shun Wang, Yun-feng Zhang, Guo-qiang Wang, Qi Xu and Xiao Guo
Department of Anesthesiology, North Sichuan Medical College, Nanchong 637000, Sichuan, China

Jing-yan Lin
Department of Anesthesiology, North Sichuan Medical College, Nanchong 637000, Sichuan, China
Department of Anesthesiology, Affiliated Hospital of North Sichuan Medical College, Nanchong 637000, Sichuan, China

Hamdy A. Hendawy
Faculty of Medicine, Suez Canal University, Ismailia, Egypt

Mohamed E. Abuelnaga
Department of Anesthesia, Intensive Care and Pain Management, Faculty of Medicine, Suez Canal University, Ard Elgameiat, Ismailia City, Egypt

Josephine Zachodnik, Jens Laigaard and Laura S. Kruuse
Department of Anesthesiology, Zealand University Hospital, Lykkebækvej 1, 4600 Koege, Denmark

Magnus Sandberg and Eva I. Persson
Department of Health Sciences, Faculty of Medicine, Lund University, Lund, Sweden

Anja Geisler
Department of Anesthesiology, Zealand University Hospital, Lykkebækvej 1, 4600 Koege, Denmark
Department of Health Sciences, Faculty of Medicine, Lund University, Lund, Sweden

Charlotte V. Sørensen
Department of Orthopaedics, Zealand University Hospital, Koege, Denmark

Ole Mathiesen
Department of Anesthesiology, Zealand University Hospital, Lykkebækvej 1, 4600 Koege, Denmark
Department of Clinical Medicine, Faculty of Health Sciences, Copenhagen University, Copenhagen, Denmark

Zi-Ye Pan, Zhong-Hua Hu, Fan Zhang, Wen-Xiu Xie, Yong-Zhong Tang and Qin Liao
Department of Anesthesiology, The Third Xiangya Hospital of Central South University, Changsha 410013, Hunan, China

Rehena Sultana
Centre for Quantitative Medicine, Duke-NUS Medical School, 8 College Road, Singapore, Singapore

Yi An, Lei Zhao, Tianlong Wang, Wei Xiao, Ping Wang, Lixia Li, Zhongjia Li and Xiaoxu Chen
Department of Anesthesiology, Xuanwu Hospital, Capital Medical University, 45 Changchun Street, Xicheng District, Beijing 100053, China
National Clinical Research Center for Geriatric Disorders, Beijing, China

Jiapeng Huang
Department of Anesthesiology, Jewish Hospital and Department of Anesthesiology & Perioperative Medicine, University of Louisville, Louisville, KY, USA

Chin Wen Tan
Department of Women's Anaesthesia, KK Women's and Children's Hospital, 100 Bukit Timah Road, Singapore, Singapore

Daryl Jian'an Tan
Anaesthesiology and Perioperative Sciences Academic Clinical Program, Duke-NUS Medical School, 8 College Road, Singapore, Singapore

Ban Leong Sng and Alex Tiong Heng Sia
Department of Women's Anaesthesia, KK Women's and Children's Hospital, 100 Bukit Timah Road, Singapore, Singapore
Anaesthesiology and Perioperative Sciences Academic Clinical Program, Duke-NUS Medical School, 8 College Road, Singapore, Singapore

Nian-Lin Reena Han
Division of Clinical Support Services, KK Women's and Children's Hospital, Singapore, Singapore

Li Jia, Meng Xie, Jingyu Guo, Tong Tong and Yuying Xing
Department of Anesthesiology, Fourth Hospital of Hebei Medical University, No. 12, Jiankang Road, Shijiazhuang 050000, Hebei, China

Jing Zhang
Department of Anesthesiology, Fourth Hospital of Hebei Medical University, No. 12, Jiankang Road, Shijiazhuang 050000, Hebei, China
Department of Anesthesiology, Peking University Third Hospital, No. 49, North Garden Rd, Haidian District, Beijing 100191, China

Li-Qin Li
Department of Anesthesiology, Guizhou Provincial People's Hospital, Guiyang, Guizhou, People's Republic of China

Mei-Dan Fang, Hong-Liu Lu, Li-Xue Wang, Hong-Yu Xu and Hou-Zhong Zhang
Department of Anesthesiology, Jilin University Second Hospital, No. 218 Ziqiang street, Changchun, Jilin 130021, People's Republic of China

Cong Wang
Department of Anesthesiology, First Affiliated Hospital to Changchun University of Chinese Medicine, Changchun, Jilin, People's Republic of China

Stanley S. Wong, Wing S. Chan and Chi W. Cheung
Laboratory and Clinical Research Institute for Pain, Department of Anaesthesiology, Li Ka Shing Faculty of Medicine, The University of Hong Kong, Queen Mary Hospital, Room 424, Block K, 102, Pokfulam Road, Hong Kong SAR, China

Christian Fang and Frankie Leung
Department of Orthopaedics and Traumatology, Li Ka Shing Faculty of Medicine, The University of Hong Kong, Hong Kong SAR, China

Chi W. Chan
Department of Anaesthesiology, Queen Mary Hospital, Hong Kong SAR, China

Tak W. Lau
Department of Orthopaedics and Traumatology, Queen Mary Hospital, Hong Kong SAR, China

Weiling Liu, Francis Chee Kuan Tan and Hong Jye Neo
Department of Anaesthesia, National University Hospital, National University Health System, 5 Lower Kent Ridge Road, Singapore 119074, Singapore

Chunmei Li
Department of Anaesthesia, Yong Loo Lin School of Medicine, National University of Singapore, 5 Lower Kent Ridge Road, Singapore 119074, Singapore

Tat Leang Lee
Department of Anaesthesia, National University Hospital, National University Health System, 5 Lower Kent Ridge Road, Singapore 119074, Singapore
Department of Anaesthesia, Yong Loo Lin School of Medicine, National University of Singapore, 5 Lower Kent Ridge Road, Singapore 119074, Singapore

Yiong Huak Chan
Biostatistics Unit, Yong Loo Lin School of Medicine, National University of Singapore, Singapore, Singapore

Chian-Ming Low
Department of Anaesthesia, Yong Loo Lin School of Medicine, National University of Singapore, 5 Lower Kent Ridge Road, Singapore 119074, Singapore
Department of Pharmacology, Yong Loo Lin School of Medicine, National University of Singapore, 16 Medical Drive, Singapore 117600, Singapore

Kimberly Gonsette, Willy Terram, Isabelle Huybrechts, Luc Barvais and Edgard Engelman
Department of Anesthesia and Perioperative Care, CUB Erasme University Hospital, Université Libre de Bruxelles, 808, Route de Lennik, 1070 Brussels, Belgium

Sarah Saxena
Department of Anesthesia and Perioperative Care, CUB Erasme University Hospital, Université Libre de Bruxelles, 808, Route de Lennik, 1070 Brussels, Belgium
Department of Anesthesia and Perioperative Care, Zuckerberg San Francisco General Hospital & Trauma Center, University of California, San Francisco, USA

Daniel A. Nahrwold
Department of Anesthesia and Perioperative Care, Zuckerberg San Francisco General Hospital & Trauma Center, University of California, San Francisco, USA
Department of Anesthesiology, H. Lee Moffitt Cancer Center & Research Institute, University of South Florida, Tampa, USA

Matteo Cappello
Department of Cardiothoracic Surgery, CUB Erasme University Hospital, Université Libre de Bruxelles, Brussels, Belgium

Ivana Vuka and Tihana Marciuš
Laboratory for Pain Research, University of Split School of Medicine, Šoltanska 2, 21000 Split, Croatia

Svjetlana Došenović
Department of Anesthesiology, Reanimatology and Intensive Care, University Hospital Split, Spinčićeva 1, 21000 Split, Croatia

Lejla Ferhatović Hamzić
Center for Translational and Clinical Research, Department of Proteomics, University of Zagreb School of Medicine, Šalata 3, 10000 Zagreb, Croatia

Katarina Vučić
Department for Safety and Efficacy Assessment of Medicinal Products, Agency for Medicinal Products and Medical Devices, Ksaverska cesta 4, 10000 Zagreb, Croatia

Damir Sapunar
Laboratory for Pain Research, University of Split School of Medicine, Šoltanska 2, 21000 Split, Croatia
Center for Evidence-Based Medicine and Health Care, Catholic University of Croatia, Ilica 242, 10000 Zagreb, Croatia

Livia Puljak
Center for Evidence-Based Medicine and Health Care, Catholic University of Croatia, Ilica 242, 10000 Zagreb, Croatia

Zhengfeng Gu, Lian Xin, Haoxing Wang, Chunxiao Hu, Zhiping Wang, Shunmei Lu, Jingjing Xu and Yiling Qian
Department of Anesthesiology, Wuxi People's Hospital Affiliated to Nanjing Medical University, 299 Qingyang Road, Wuxi 214023, Jiangsu, China

Jun Wang
Department of Anesthesiology, Wuxi People's Hospital Affiliated to Nanjing Medical University, 299 Qingyang Road, Wuxi 214023, Jiangsu, China
Department of Anesthesiology, Peking University Third Hospital, No. 49, North Garden Rd, Haidian District, Beijing 100191, China

Jefferson Tang, Chong Oon Tan, Raymond Hu, Brett Pearce and Luka Cosic
Department of Anaesthesia, Austin Health, Heidelberg, Victoria, Australia

Leonid Churilov
Melbourne Medical School, University of Melbourne, Heidelberg, Victoria, Australia

Laurence Weinberg
Department of Anaesthesia, Austin Health, Heidelberg, Victoria, Australia
Department of Surgery, University of Melbourne, Austin Health, Heidelberg, Victoria, Australia

Christopher Christophi
Department of Surgery, University of Melbourne, Austin Health, Heidelberg, Victoria, Australia

Xiaona Lin, Yang Zhou, Hongcai Zheng, Kaixi Liu, Xiangyang Guo, Zhengqian Li and Bin Han
Department of Anesthesiology, Peking University Third Hospital, No. 49, North Garden Rd, Haidian District, Beijing 100191, China

Xiaoxiao Wang
Research Center of Clinical Epidemiology, Peking University Third Hospital, Beijing 100191, China

Junwei Zheng, Jie Wang, Bin Li, Tao Ma and Kaimei Lu
Department of Anesthesiology, Ningxia Medical University, Yinchuan 750004, China

Yang Gu
Department of Anesthesiology, Ningxia Medical University, Yinchuan 750004, China
Department of Anesthesiology, People's Hospital of Ningxia Hui Autonomous Region, Yinchuan 750002, China

Fan Yang, Yonghai Zhang, Xiang Cui and Hanxiang Ma
Department of Anesthesiology, General Hospital of Ningxia Medical University, Yinchuan 750004, China

Xue Li, Zhen-Zhen Xu, Ting-Ting Jiang, Zeng-Mao Li and Dong-Xin Wang
Department of Anesthesiology, Peking University First Hospital, No. 7 Xishiku Street, Xicheng District, Beijing 100034, China

Xue-Ying Li
Department of Biostatics, Peking University First Hospital, No. 7 Xishiku Street, Xicheng District, Beijing 100034, China

Jingxiong Zhang, Yuting He, Shi Wang, Zhengjie Chen, Yu Zhang, Yuan Gao, Quanguang Wang and Riyong Zhou
Department of Anesthesiology, the First Affiliated Hospital of Wenzhou Medical University, Zhejiang, China

Yun Xia
Department of Anesthesiology, Ohio State University Wexner Medical Center, Columbus, OH, USA

Thomas J. Papadimos
Department of Anesthesiology, the First Affiliated Hospital of Wenzhou Medical University, Zhejiang, China
Department of Anesthesiology, Ohio State University Wexner Medical Center, Columbus, OH, USA

Hanhua Wu, Jiamei Pan, Ming Han, Huijun Cai and Hong Zhang
Department of Anesthesiology, Affiliated Hospital of Zunyi Medical University, No. 149 Dalian Road, Huichuan District, Zunyi 563003, Guizhou Province, China

Jinqing Tang
Department of Anesthesiology, Third Affiliated Hospital of Zunyi Medical University, Zunyi 563003, Guizhou Province, China

Index

A

Abdominal Hysterectomy, 53, 72-73, 79, 93, 104, 107

Abdominal Surgery, 10-11, 17, 19, 36, 42, 55-56, 60, 62-63, 79, 88, 91, 93, 100, 107, 125, 150, 188, 202, 210-211, 215, 217

Abnormal Sensation, 129, 133

Analgesia, 1-12, 14-21, 23, 25-26, 28-30, 33-35, 37-39, 41-42, 44-50, 53-56, 58, 62-63, 65, 68, 70-76, 78-79, 88-95, 97, 99-105, 125-126, 134-136, 145, 147-148, 173, 176, 178-181, 183-191, 193, 201-203, 206-207, 209-211, 215, 217, 219

Anti-inflammatory Drug, 7

B

Bispectral Index, 11, 39, 50, 65, 70, 89, 99, 109, 113, 145, 176, 194-195, 199-200, 209, 218, 225

Blood Pressure, 2, 11-12, 21, 26, 29-30, 42, 46, 50, 65, 69-70, 73, 76, 89, 95, 104, 109, 113, 127, 145, 196, 211, 219

Bupivacaine, 10, 12-14, 17-20, 25-26, 37-39, 42, 44-47, 58, 73-74, 81, 99, 107, 115-119, 121, 123, 125, 155, 158, 180-181, 184, 190, 192, 217

C

Cardiopulmonary Bypass, 218-221, 225

Chronic Pain, 19, 46, 65, 79, 88, 92-93, 95, 99, 127, 137-138, 142-143, 152, 164, 168-171, 188, 191

Clinical Trial, 19, 26, 37, 49, 54, 63, 72-73, 114, 135-136, 151, 153-154, 170-171, 173, 176, 209, 211, 217, 219, 225

Colonoscopy, 108-114, 173, 175-176

Colorectal Surgery, 58, 63, 88-89, 91-93, 136

Coronary Artery, 206, 219, 225-226

Coughing, 3, 5, 25, 37-38, 40-41, 43, 203, 205, 208, 219

Cytokine, 138-141, 143

D

Dexmedetomidine, 25, 27, 48-49, 52-54, 69-71, 108-114, 123, 125, 176-177, 194-195, 199-200, 202, 204, 206, 218, 225-226

Dorsal Root Ganglion, 151-152, 160-162, 165, 170-171

Doxapram, 172-177

E

Emergence Agitation, 50, 54, 128-129, 133

Epidural Analgesia, 4, 9-12, 14-20, 46, 55-56, 58, 62-63, 89, 93, 125, 179, 181, 188, 217

Epidural Anesthesia, 6, 26, 36, 47, 90, 115, 117, 119, 125, 187-188, 190

Erector Spinae Plane, 46, 210, 212-213, 215-217

G

Gastrointestinal Endoscopy, 114, 172-176

General Anesthesia, 11-12, 17, 29-30, 33, 39, 50, 58, 71, 78, 88-90, 114, 119, 126-127, 133, 135-136, 174-175, 190, 194-195, 199, 220

H

Hospital Costs, 178, 180, 183-184, 186

Hypertension, 5, 7, 29, 31, 38, 41-42, 44, 53, 68, 76, 97, 140, 173, 175, 206, 219

Hypotension, 4, 10, 17, 21, 26, 40, 42, 44, 54, 56, 59, 62, 64, 66, 68-70, 97, 108-111, 113, 115-116, 121, 174, 176, 179, 195, 198

Hysteroscopy, 64-65, 68-71

I

Infraclavicular Nerve Block, 126-127, 130, 133-136

Infusion Pump, 12, 101-105, 107, 118, 146

Intrathecal Morphine, 37-39, 44-47, 178-179, 181-188

L

Laparoscopic Nephrectomy, 10-13, 15, 18-19, 36, 100, 209

Laparoscopic Surgery, 18, 36, 42, 45, 48-49, 52, 54, 59-62, 201

Laparoscopy, 38, 42, 49, 54, 57, 62, 99

Laryngeal Mask Airway, 50, 127, 135

Linear Regression, 41, 85, 137, 139, 180

Liver Resection, 36, 44, 47, 178-179, 181, 184, 186-188

M

Magnesium Sulfate, 64, 115-125

Magnesium Sulphate, 64-65, 68, 70-71, 118, 123, 125

Meta-analysis, 17, 19, 26-27, 46, 54-57, 60-63, 70-71, 79, 93, 100, 114, 116-117, 120-123, 125, 136, 150, 153, 169, 185, 188, 209, 225

N

Nerve Block, 8, 26, 29, 36, 47, 126-128, 130, 133-136, 164, 189-190, 192-193, 202-203, 210, 216-217

Neuromuscular Block, 12, 19, 50, 70

Non-neuropathic Pain, 151-152, 169-170

O

Opioid, 2-3, 6, 11-13, 17-23, 31, 36, 39-40, 42, 44-47, 49, 52-54, 56, 58, 61, 63-65, 68-71, 73, 76, 78-79, 82, 84-85, 89, 91-93, 95, 98-104, 106-107, 114, 127, 134, 144-146, 149-150, 174, 176-181, 183-188, 195, 198, 201-207, 209, 226

Opioids, 3, 25, 28, 37-38, 40-41, 52, 62, 64-65, 68, 70-71, 74, 76, 81-82, 88, 91, 95, 97-98, 100, 102, 106-107, 111, 115, 127-128, 147, 181, 184, 186, 224

Osteoarthritis, 46, 137-138, 141, 143, 160, 163, 170, 188-191, 193

Oxycodone, 56, 81, 85, 94-100

Oxygen Desaturation, 68, 101-102, 104-107

P

Pain Intensity, 3, 6, 18, 30-31, 36, 50, 52, 54, 80, 82, 85-87, 89, 91, 114, 136, 151-152, 155-156, 158-160, 201-202, 205, 209

Pain Management, 1, 8, 10, 12, 19, 26, 47, 55, 62, 68, 72, 78-79, 86-87, 89, 99, 104, 107, 116, 122-123, 135-136, 152, 170, 189-190, 192-193, 209

Pain Responder, 82, 84-85

Paravertebral Block, 1-6, 8, 20-21, 25-27, 29, 36, 211, 216-217

Patient-controlled Analgesia, 6, 8, 10-11, 26, 37, 42, 44, 46, 48-50, 54, 63, 72-73, 102, 107, 188-190, 193, 202

Percutaneous Nephrolithotomy, 20, 25-29, 35-36

Pneumothorax, 1-8, 21, 23, 26, 158, 166

Postoperative Analgesia, 2, 6, 8, 10-12, 19, 28-29, 35, 44, 46, 49, 54, 63, 68, 72-73, 79, 93, 100, 115-116, 118-119, 121, 123, 125-126, 134-135, 178-180, 186, 188, 190-191, 193, 209, 211, 215, 217

Postoperative Nausea, 2-3, 5, 8, 10-11, 17, 19, 28, 31, 34-35, 44, 46, 48-49, 52, 54, 64-65, 68, 70, 73, 95, 99, 201, 203, 208-209

Postoperative Pain, 1-3, 6-8, 10-12, 15, 18-20, 26, 28-31, 33-34, 36, 41, 45-47, 52, 54-55, 62-66, 68, 70-73, 78-81, 85-89, 92-95, 98-101, 114-116, 123, 125-127, 131, 133-136, 145, 150, 178-179, 184, 188-193, 202, 217

Postoperative Rehabilitation, 2, 4

Preemptive Analgesia, 94-95, 97, 100

Preoperative Education, 189, 191-193

Propofol, 2, 11, 21, 30, 39, 50-52, 64-68, 70-71, 86, 89, 95-96, 109, 111, 113-114, 127-128, 134, 136, 145, 147, 172-177, 194-196, 198-200, 202, 221, 225

Pruritus, 11, 38, 40-42, 44-47, 68, 105-106, 115, 121, 125, 128, 133

Pulsed Radiofrequency, 151-152, 160-162, 165, 170-171

Q

Quadratus Lumborum Block, 10, 12, 14-15, 17-19, 28-29, 35-36, 209

R

Rectus Sheath, 19, 37-39, 44-46

Regional Anesthesia, 46, 126-128, 133, 135-136

Remifentanil, 6, 38, 40-42, 44, 50-52, 54, 71, 89, 91, 95-98, 100, 108-114, 144-150, 176-177, 199-200, 202, 207, 225

Renal Surgery, 201-203, 209

Respiratory Depression, 11, 28, 31, 33-34, 38, 41, 53, 66, 68, 96-97, 101-102, 106-107, 109, 148, 172, 175-177, 184-186

S

Sedation, 11, 26, 30, 36, 49-51, 53-54, 65, 71, 74, 76, 94-96, 102, 104-106, 108-109, 112-114, 123, 144-146, 148-150, 172-174, 176, 180, 183-187, 198-200, 219

Sensory Block Area, 63, 210, 212-213

Serratus Plane Block, 1-6, 8-9

Standard Deviation, 14, 17, 21, 31-32, 34, 50, 56, 63, 67-68, 75, 82, 96, 99, 104, 107, 110, 116-117, 125, 128, 131, 140, 143, 146, 174-175, 204, 206, 220

Sufentanil, 2, 7, 28, 30-33, 54, 89, 91, 94-100, 176, 199-200, 202-204, 207, 220

Sufentanil Consumption, 28, 32, 91, 100

Surgical Complications, 46, 128, 180, 188

Surgical Procedure, 1-2, 4-6, 29-31, 81, 86, 88, 180

Sympathetic Nerve, 113, 219, 224

T

Total Hip Arthroplasty, 36, 79-81, 86

Total Knee Arthroplasty, 46-47, 78-79, 107, 166, 171, 189-190, 193

V

Visceral Analgesia, 17, 42

Visceral Pain, 17, 45, 62, 70, 94-100, 216

Vomiting, 2-3, 5, 8, 10-11, 17, 19, 21, 23, 31, 34, 40, 44-46, 48-54, 64-65, 68, 70, 73-78, 95-97, 99, 102, 104-106, 108, 110-111, 113, 115-116, 121-122, 126, 128-129, 133-135, 146, 174-175, 181, 186-187, 201, 203, 208-209, 213

www.ingramcontent.com/pod-product-compliance
Lightning Source LLC
LaVergne TN
LVHW060535210926
848485LV00005B/1203